VETERINARY DENTAL TECHNIQUES

for the Small Animal Practitioner

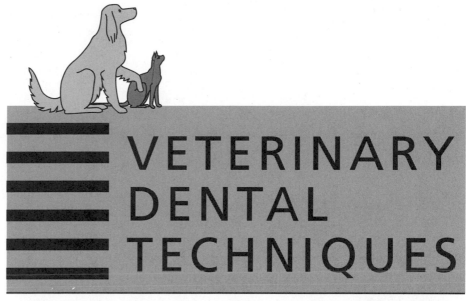

VETERINARY DENTAL TECHNIQUES

for the Small Animal Practitioner

SECOND EDITION

Steven E. Holmstrom, DVM
Diplomate, American Veterinary Dental College
San Carlos, California

Patricia Frost, DVM
Diplomate, American Veterinary Dental College
Vancouver, Washington

Edward R. Eisner, DVM
Diplomate, American Veterinary Dental College
Denver, Colorado

Illustrations by Leo Hagstrom

W.B. SAUNDERS COMPANY
A Division of Harcourt Brace & Company
Philadelphia   London   Toronto   Montreal   Sydney   Tokyo

W.B. SAUNDERS COMPANY
A Division of Harcourt Brace & Company

The Curtis Center
Independence Square West
Philadelphia, Pennsylvania 19106

Library of Congress Cataloging-in-Publication Data

Holmstrom, Steven E.

Veterinary dental techniques: for the small animal practitioner / Steven E. Holmstrom,
Patricia Frost, Edward R. Eisner; illustrations by Leo Hagstrom.—2nd ed.

p.   cm.

Includes bibliographical references and index.

ISBN 0–7216–5839–3

1. Veterinary dentistry.   2. Dogs—Diseases—Treatment.   3. Cats—
    Diseases—Treatment.   I. Frost, Patricia.   II. Eisner, Edward R.   III. Title.

SF992.M68H68   1998   636.7′08976—dc21   98–2782

VETERINARY DENTAL TECHNIQUES
FOR THE SMALL ANIMAL PRACTITIONER   ISBN 0–7216–5839–3

Printed in the United States of America.

Last digit is the print number: 9   8   7   6   5   4   3   2   1

PREFACE TO THE SECOND EDITION

We have written the second edition of *Veterinary Dental Techniques for the Small Animal Practitioner* in the same easy-to-read, easy-to-use chairside format as that of the first edition. We have attempted to create an informative, updated, practical guide to dental materials and techniques in a wide spectrum of dental procedures that includes examination and charting, routine and advanced periodontal care, endodontic treatment, restorative dentistry, orthodontics, orthopedics, dental anesthesia, and ergonomics. By so doing we aim to create an ideal book for beginning veterinary students, technicians, seasoned general practitioners, and veterinarians who are expanding their dental departments and knowledge.

Anesthesia and pain control are current "hot topics" in veterinary medicine. A new chapter has been added with practical suggestions. Another area for concern in human and veterinary dentistry is ergonomics, the study of adapting the workplace to the worker. This issue has evolved from the recognition that workers may become injured due to biological, chemical, physical, and psychosocial hazards. Employers and employees together need to create and maintain a safe workplace environment. Chapter 12 provides helpful suggestions about posture, facility adaptation, and protective exercises for the clinician's and technician's back, neck, and hands.

With the advent of the internet, information may be exchanged rapidly. The reader is invited to write the authors with any suggested techniques for future editions. The screen names are: Toothvet@aol.com (Holmstrom), PatVancVDT@aol.com (Frost), Dog2thdoc@aol.com (Eisner).

STEVEN E. HOLMSTROM, DVM, Dipl AVDC
PATRICIA FROST, DVM, Dipl AVDC
EDWARD R. EISNER, DVM, Dipl AVDC

PREFACE TO THE FIRST EDITION

Our hope in writing this text is to give veterinarians, animal health technicians, and students an understanding of dental equipment, instruments, materials, and techniques. Our goal and that of individuals practicing veterinary dentistry should be to obtain predictable results by following established protocol. This text is intended to supplement other texts, both veterinary and human dental, that discuss such topics as anatomy, pathogenesis, and theory.

The personal economic benefits that may be derived from adding dentistry to the veterinary practice must be countered with the realization that our obligation to our clients and patients goes far beyond simple disease prevention, relief of pain, treatment of disease, and performing tasks. Our duty is to perform a service that will respect the patient's need. Treatment plans also must be presented to the client with suitable alternative treatments, depending on the patient's needs and the client's desires and (unfortunately) ability to pay for these services. Our commitment is based on trust, and this trust must be upheld when we are performing all phases of our veterinary practice, including dentistry.

We hope that through the use of this text, all components of the veterinary triangle of patient, client, and veterinarian will benefit.

STEVEN E. HOLMSTROM, DVM, Dipl AVDC
PATRICIA FROST, DVM, Dipl AVDC
RONALD L. GAMMON, DVM, MS, Dipl AVDC

ACKNOWLEDGMENTS

We wish to thank Dr. Ronald Gammon for his contributions to the first edition of *Veterinary Dental Techniques for the Small Animal Practitioner,* which have laid the foundations for subsequent editions. We also thank all of the members of the American Veterinary Dental College, the Academy of Veterinary Dentistry, and the American Veterinary Dental Society for the creation of many of the techniques that are incorporated in this book. As well, we thank Carol Weldin, RDH; Stephen John, DDS; and Barry Staley, DDS, for their review of the periodontic chapters; Deborah McFall, RDH, for her review of the ergonomics chapter, and Laurie Holmstrom, RDH, for her review of the manuscript. Special thanks go to our illustrator, Leo Hagstrom, for his talent and for his patience during revisions of the art for both editions.

We are grateful to the following dentists who have contributed to our dental knowledge: Toby A. Burgess, DDS; Peter Emily, DDS; Keith Grove, VMD, DDS; Stephen John, DDS; Charles L. Neubauer, DDS; Robert Olson, DDS; Morgan Powell, DDS; Nick Sabbia, DDS; Judith Timchula, DDS; and Walter E. Tweedie, DDS.

Finally, we also thank the American Dental Association and the California Dental Association for their generosity in admitting interested veterinarians to their annual meetings and symposia. Without the sharing of knowledge, veterinary dentistry would not have progressed as rapidly.

CONTENTS

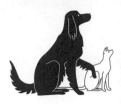

Chapter 1

DENTAL RECORDS

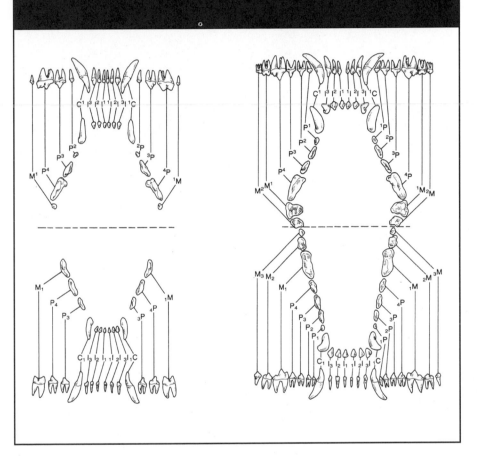

General Comments

- Written records are necessary to identify the patient; to record the patient's status before, during, and after treatment procedures; to document client acceptance or rejection of the treatment plan; to record therapy sequence, prognosis, results, and sequelae; to measure progress at successive appointments; to document consultations and referrals; and to provide ease of transfer to another practitioner.[1]
- The reader has the authors' permission to use the dental charts in this text in the course of practice.

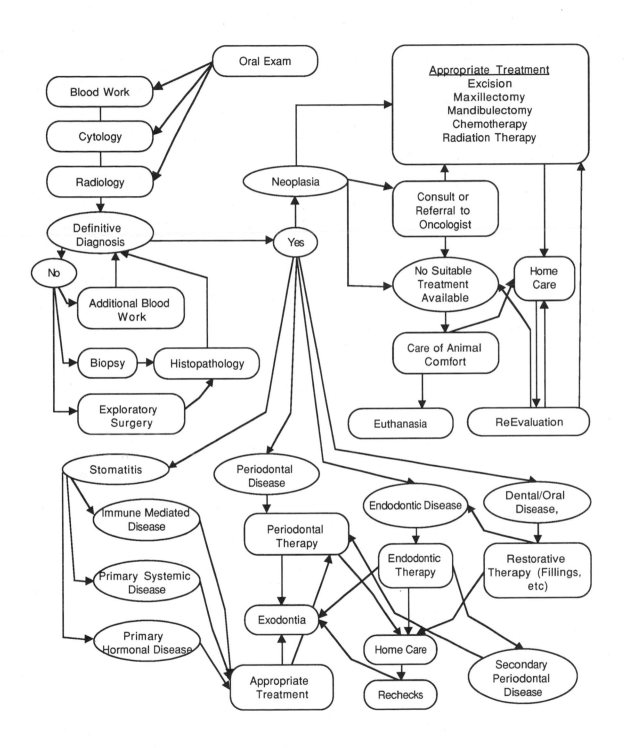

TOOTH IDENTIFICATION SYSTEMS

General Comments

- A number of tooth identification systems have been used for dental records.
- In some systems a number is given to each tooth, whereas other systems use numbers and symbols to designate a tooth. The systems that use numbers alone are more readily adaptable for use with computers.
- This text uses the terms "type" to refer to primary (deciduous) or secondary (permanent) dentition and "function" to refer to the four common functional groups: incisor, canine, premolar, and molar.

MODIFIED TRIADAN SYSTEM

General Comments

- Each tooth is given a three-digit number.
- The first number represents the quadrant, with the upper right quadrant being 1. Look at the chart, set up to reflect the clinician and the patient facing each other, which goes clockwise from the upper right to the lower right quadrant.
- For permanent teeth, the maxillary (upper) right quadrant is 1, the maxillary left quadrant is 2, the mandibular (lower) left quadrant is 3, and the mandibular right quadrant is 4. Quadrants for primary teeth are represented by 5, 6, 7, and 8, beginning again with the upper right quadrant as 5 and ending with the lower right as 8. The individual teeth are represented by two digits, with 01 being the first tooth from the midline and continuing distally along the arch to the last tooth. For dogs, the last number is normally 10 for the upper arches and 11 for the lower arch. The Rule of Four and Nine is used to simplify the annotations among the various species. Tooth 4 is always the canine tooth, and tooth 9 is always the first molar. For example, 504 represents the primary maxillary right canine tooth, and 309 represents the secondary mandibular left first molar. In species such as the cat, where the maxillary first premolar is missing, the teeth on the maxillary right side are 101, 102, 103, 104 (105 is missing), 106, 107, 108, and 109.

Advantages

- Is adaptable for computer use if computer is nonalphanumeric.
- Each tooth has an individual number.
- Easy to use in dealing with a single species or when records with anatomic charts printed on them are used.
- If the Rule of Four and Nine is used, may chart a variety of species.

Disadvantages

- Difficult to learn and remember if not used frequently.
- Tooth function is not identified by this system

DENTAL SHORTHAND/ANATOMIC IDENTIFICATION SYSTEM

General Comments

- Each tooth is given a letter corresponding to tooth function and type.
- Uppercase letters are used for secondary (permanent) teeth, and lowercase letters are used for primary (deciduous) teeth.
  I = incisor   i = primary incisor
  C = canine   c = primary canine
  P = premolar   p = primary premolar
  M = molar

- Each quadrant of the mouth corresponds to a corner around the letter.
- Maxillary teeth are indicated by superscript numbers, and mandibular teeth are indicated by subscript numbers.
- Teeth on the patient's right are indicated to the right side of the letter, and teeth on the patient's left are indicated to the left side of the letter.
- The teeth are numbered consecutively, for each functional group of teeth, starting from the midline. This number is placed in the appropriate corner around the letter. For example:

  Superscript and subscript numerals for the teeth on the animal's right side are placed on the right side of the letter designating the functional group.

  The permanent upper right central incisor is represented by the number 1 placed as a superscript on the right side of the letter I as: I^1.

Second and third secondary lower left premolars are represented by the numbers 2 and 3 placed as a subscript on the left side of the letter P as: $_{3,2}P$.

The primary upper left canine is represented by the number 1 placed as a superscript on the left side of the letter c = ^1c.

Advantages

- Easy to learn because it is more self-explanatory.
- Identifies tooth function and type.
- The same tooth number is used for the same corresponding tooth in different species.
- Several teeth can be listed with one letter: $P^{1,2,3,4}$
- May be used with alphanumeric systems by placing "U" or "L" or "+" or "−" before or after the tooth number.

The permanent upper right central incisor = IU1 or I + 1, URI1.
Second permanent lower left premolar = L2P or −P, LLP2.
Primary upper left canine = U1c or +1c.

- The letters L or R may also use used: UR 1C

Disadvantages

- May not be used with all computer systems without the above modifications.
- May be confusing to an uninformed reader as to whether reference is to patient's or observer's right or left.
- Is easier to use in written than oral form.

PALMER NOTATION SYSTEM

General Comments

- Each tooth is given a letter corresponding to its function.
- Capital letters are used for permanent teeth, and lowercase letters are used for primary teeth.
- The teeth are numbered consecutively within their functional group, and a symbol is used to denote the quadrant. Note that right and left are as viewed and do not indicate the patient's right and left.

P $\lfloor$2 = upper left second permanent premolar.
P $\lceil$1 = lower left first permanent premolar.
C1$\rceil$ = lower right first permanent canine.

Advantages

- Identifies tooth function and type.
- Easy identification of quadrant.

Disadvantages

- Not easily used with a computer.
- Difficult to use to describe tooth verbally.

NUMERICAL ORDER (UNIVERSAL TOOTH NUMBERING SYSTEM)

General Comments

- Each permanent tooth is given a number 1 to 30 in the cat, 1 to 42 in the dog. Primary teeth are lettered (a to z in the cat; a to z, A to Z in the dog).
- The teeth are numbered starting in the upper left quadrant with the last tooth and continuing with consecutive numbers around the arch to the opposite last upper right tooth. The lower arch is numbered starting from the last lower left tooth continuing around the arch to the last lower right tooth.

Advantages

- Enables easy communication if both parties know the numbers and the system.
- Easily used with computers.

Disadvantages

- The same tooth from species to species will have a different number because of the differences in dental formulas.
- Difficult to memorize all the numbers, especially if the system is used infrequently or if numerous species are treated.
- Does not identify tooth function.

HADERUP SYSTEM

General Comments

- This system numbers each tooth in a quadrant consecutively, starting at the midline.
- The upper or lower arch is indicated by a + or − next to the number, with + corresponding to the upper jaw and − to the lower jaw.
- The right or left is indicated by the side of the tooth on which the symbol is placed: +2 = left upper second incisor, 6− = right lower second premolar.

Advantages

- Readily usable with computerized records.
- Easier to use in oral communication than the anatomic system. However, all parties involved must know the system.

Disadvantages

- The practitioner must memorize the numbering for each species treated. This becomes cumbersome.
- Does not identify tooth function.

Palmer	I3⌋	I2⌋	I1⌋	I⌊1	I⌊2	I⌊3
Tridan	103	102	101	201	202	203
Anatomic	I³	I²	I¹	¹I	²I	³I
Universal	13	12	11	10	9	8
Haderup	3+	2+	1+	+1	+2	+3
Zsigmondy	3⌋	2⌋	1⌋	⌊1	⌊2	⌊3
Federali	1,3	1,2	1,1	2,1	2,2	2,3

Palmer	Tridan	Anatomic	Universal	Haderup	Zsigmondy	Federali		Federali	Zsigmondy	Haderup	Universal	Anatomic	Tridan	Palmer
C1⌋	104	C¹	14	4+	4⌋	1,4		2,4	⌊4	+4	7	¹C	204	C⌊1
P1⌋	105	P¹	15	5+	5⌋	1,5		2,5	⌊5	+5	6	¹P	205	P⌊1
P2⌋	106	P²	16	6+	6⌋	1,6		2,6	⌊6	+6	5	²P	206	P⌊2
P3⌋	107	P³	17	7+	7⌋	1,7		2,7	⌊7	+7	4	³P	207	P⌊3
P4⌋	108	P⁴	18	8+	8⌋	1,8		2,8	⌊8	+8	3	⁴P	208	P⌊4
M1⌋	109	M¹	19	9+	9⌋	1,9		2,9	⌊9	+9	2	¹M	209	M⌊1
M2⌋	110	M²	20	10+	10⌋	1,10		2,10	⌊10	+10	1	²M	210	M⌊2
M3	411	M_3	42	11−	11⌋	4,11		3,11	⌊11	−11	21	₃M	311	M⌊3
M2	410	M_2	41	10−	10⌋	4,10		3,10	⌊10	−10	22	₂M	310	M⌊2
M1	409	M_1	40	9−	9⌋	4,9		3,9	⌊9	−9	23	₁M	309	M⌊1
P4	405	P_4	39	8−	8⌋	4,8		3,8	⌊8	−8	24	₄P	308	P⌊4
P3	407	P_3	38	7−	7⌋	4,7		3,7	⌊7	−7	25	₃P	307	P⌊3
P2	406	P_2	37	6−	6⌋	4,6		3,6	⌊6	−6	26	₂P	306	P⌊2
P1	405	P_1	36	5−	5⌋	4,5		3,5	⌊5	−5	27	₁P	305	P⌊1
C1	404	C_1	35	4−	4⌋	4,4		3,4	⌊4	−4	28	₁C	304	C⌊1

Right   Left

Federali	4,3	4,2	4,1	3,1	3,2	3,3
Zsigmondy	3⌋	2⌋	1⌋	⌊1	⌊2	⌊3
Haderup	3−	2−	1−	−1	−2	−3
Universal	34	33	32	31	30	29
Anatomic	I₃	I₂	I₁	₁I	₂I	₃I
Tridan	403	402	401	301	302	303
Palmer	I3⌋	I2⌋	I1⌋	I⌊1	I⌊2	I⌊3

ZSIGMONDY SYSTEM

General Comments

- This system uses a plus sign to identify quadrants. With the head of the patient facing the observer, visualize a horizontal line between the upper and lower jaws and a vertical line separating the right from the left side.
- The intersecting lines of this sign are used to show the corresponding quadrant. These are notated as viewed (not the patient's right or left).
- The permanent teeth are numbered consecutively in each quadrant, starting from the midline. The primary teeth are lettered consecutively, starting with the letter A for the first tooth from the midline.

  $\underline{5|}$ = permanent upper right first premolar in the dog.

  $\overline{|4}$ = permanent lower left canine in the dog.

  $\underline{|B}$ = primary upper left second incisor in the cat or dog.

Advantage

- Clearly defines maxillary versus mandibular quadrant and right versus left quadrant.

Disadvantage

- Inconsistent with other systems except for, e.g., the Palmer Notation System; in this system the tooth is identified by the observer's view of the tooth rather than by where the tooth is in the patient's mouth.

FÉDÉRATION DENTAIRE INTERNATIONALE SYSTEM

General Comments

- This system identifies each quadrant by 1 to 4 for permanent teeth and 5 to 8 for primary teeth. 1/5 = upper right maxillary teeth, 2/6 = upper left maxillary teeth, 3/7 = lower left mandibular teeth, and 4/8 = lower right mandibular teeth.
- The teeth are numbered consecutively in each quadrant from the midline, with the corresponding quadrant number for the permanent or primary tooth in front of it. In the dog 1,1 = upper right maxillary permanent central incisor.
- In the cat 6,4 = upper left maxillary primary canine.

Advantages

- Easy identification of quadrant (upper maxillary or lower mandibular, left or right).
- Can be used easily with computerized records.

Disadvantages

- Difficult to learn.
- Does not identify tooth function.
- Not good for use with multiple species.

VETERINARY MEDICAL RECORDS

General Comments

- Written records must be dated, accurate, and readable, and they should be signed.
- In recording dental findings, written justification for treatment and procedures performed is necessary to provide a substantiation in a legal record. If that treatment is ever questioned, the record will reflect continuity of periodic treatment for various dental disorders.
- The medical record should contain the client's name, address, and telephone number(s) and the name, breed, age, and gender of the patient.
- Having a telephone number where the client can be contacted during a patient's dental procedure can be beneficial if additional abnormalities are found while the patient is anesthetized.

Client number _____

Pet Clinic
Initial Oral Exam

Medical Alert

Owner _____ Patient _____ Date _____
Species _____ Breed _____ Sex _____ Date of Birth _____
Chief complaint _____
Past dental history _____
General medical history _____
Diet _____
Home oral hygiene _____
Other _____

Skull type:

- ☐ Brachycephalic
- ☐ Mesocephalic
- ☐ Dolichocephalic
- ☐ _____

Oral Hygiene

☐ Plaque	N S M H
☐ Calculus	N S M H

Normal Slight Moderate Heavy

Periodontal Exam

- ☐ Inflammation   I C P M
- ☐ Gingival Edema   I C P M
- ☐ Pockets >3mm   I C P M
- ☐ Pockets >5mm   I C P M
- ☐ Recession   I C P M
- ☐ Hyperplasia   I C P M
- ☐ Mucogingival loss   I C P M
- ☐ Tooth Mobility   I C P M
- ☐ Further evaluation   I C P M

Incisor Canine Premolar Molar

Occlusion:

- ☐ Scissors
- ☐ Brachygnathic
- ☐ Prognathic
- ☐ Wry
- ☐ Level
- ☐ Crossbite
- ☐ Occlusal wear   I C P M

Tooth Abnormalities

- ☐ Ret. Primary   I C P
- ☐ Missing   I C P M
- ☐ Supernumerary   I C P M
- ☐ Caries   I C P M
- ☐ Resorptive   I C P M
- ☐ Injured   I C P M

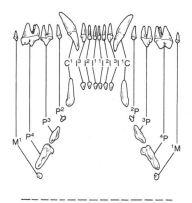
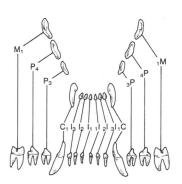

FELINE

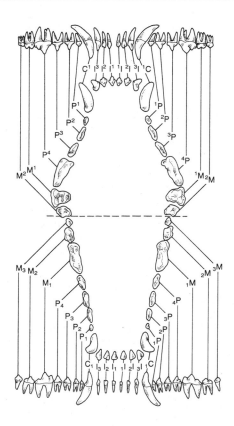

CANINE

DENTAL RECORDS

General Comments

- Dental records also have legal ramifications and can consist of fill-in or check-off formats, dental anatomic charts, or a combination of these to provide convenient recording.
- An adequate dental record provides subjective and objective information. It should contain enough information to justify the treatment performed and the materials used in that treatment, tooth by tooth. To provide an efficient record-keeping system, a chart should include a dental diagram with a key so that abbreviations and diagrams, augmented by a brief description to clarify disease(s) and treatment protocols, can be read accurately by a person not in the field. An assessment of procedure(s) performed, a therapeutic plan, and a prognosis completes the functional dental record.
- Dental anatomic charts are important because three-dimensional objects are described that are often difficult to discuss in written terms. An anatomic chart facilitates the recording of sequential treatments. If repetitive and extensive treatment is performed, additional pages with ongoing notations permit treatment progress review at a glance.
- The type of record used will vary in each practice but should include patient/client identification, chief complaint, a general health history, dental history, tooth identification system used, specific findings, treatment plan, anesthetic protocol procedures performed, follow-up care, radiographic interpretation, assessment of treatment, prognosis, documentation of discussions and consultations, missed appointments, or deviation from recommended follow-up, and documented informed consent.
- Labels with dental charts are available from a variety of sources. These peel-off labels can be charted and placed in the dental record.

INITIAL ORAL EXAMINATION

General Client/Patient Information

- This includes the names of the client and patient, date of examination, species, breed, sex, and date of birth (or age).

Chief Complaint

- Listing the chief complaint ensures that this problem is addressed even though additional dental problems may be found on examination.

Past Dental History

- This includes dates and descriptions of past dental problems, their treatment, and any complications.

General Medical History

- The general health of the patient is extremely important during dental procedures because treatment of most dental diseases requires a general anesthetic. Metabolic and endocrine abnormalities and ongoing medical treatment affect decisions concerning a safe anesthetic protocol.

Diet

- The patient's current diet and amounts fed—whether moist, dry, or table scraps—should be recorded. Other treats fed and chewing habits (fence, bones, rocks, etc.) are listed.

Home Oral Hygiene

- Home oral hygiene performed is noted. This should include names of products, frequency, and manner of care; e.g., brushing, oral rinse, food or water additive, and chewable/edible treat.

Recording Specific Findings

- The head and oral cavity are examined systematically, and initial findings and abnormalities are recorded.
- The skull type (brachycephalic, mesocephalic, dolichocephalic, or variation) is noted.
- The face and jaw should be examined for symmetry, swellings, and any abnormalities of the salivary glands and regional lymph nodes.
- The occlusion and any occlusal wear are noted.
- The amount of plaque and calculus present in general is recorded.
- Tooth abnormalities, including retained primary teeth, missing teeth, and supernumerary teeth, should be noted. Other dental findings, such as carious lesions, resorptive lesions, dental trauma, and any other abnormalities, are noted by indicating the tooth involved and their location on the tooth.
- The periodontal status is recorded by noting gingival inflammation, gingival edema, significant periodontal pocket depth, gingival recession, gingival hyperplasia, attachment loss, and tooth mobility. Necessary further diagnostic evaluation should be noted.
- Other oral disease, if present, is noted in the dental chart.
- A permanent initial record of dental findings can be kept for future reference.
- In addition to dental tissue, the oral cavity in general should be examined for lesions. These lesions may be described in a variety of different ways, described in Table 1–1.

Table 1–1 • WORDS TO DESCRIBE ORAL INFLAMMATORY DISEASE

Type Categories	Descriptive Term	Definition
Duration	Acute	Having a short course
	Chronic	Having a long, continued course
Physical appearance	Vesicular	Small, blister-like
	Bullous	Circumscribed, elevated lesion more than 5 mm diameter
	Ulcerative	Loss of epithelial covering causing a gradual disintegration of tissues
	Proliferative	Growth by reproduction of similar cells
	Suppurative, purulent	Inflammatory exudate formed within the tissues
	Fibrinous	Containing fibrous tissue, usually by degeneration
	Hemorrhagic	Containing the elements of blood
Severity	Mild	Appreciated only after careful observation
	Moderate	Readily apparent, but lacks visual and mental impact
	Severe	Immediate and forceful visual impact on viewer
Spread	Focal	Discrete and well circumscribed
	Multifocal	Well defined but numerous
	Diffuse	Substantial portion of affected region
Location of inflammation	Glossitis	Inflammation of the tongue
	Cheilitis	Inflammation of the lips
	Buccostomatitis	Inflammation of the inner cheek
	Pharyngitis	Inflammation of the pharynx
	Faucitis	Inflammation of the glossopalatine folds or angles of the mouth
	Palatitis	Inflammation of the palate
	Gingivitis	Inflammation of the gingiva
	Periodontitis	Inflammation of the periodontium

ANATOMIC CHARTING

- Pathologic findings can be recorded on the anatomic chart. The chart is updated as the patient's condition changes (see the canine dental chart). This becomes the continuing record of the patient's dental status.
- Symbols or letters to indicate a variety of abnormalities can be used on a dental anatomic chart to speed recording and allow a quick reference to all the abnormalities and treatments.
- Many symbols are in common usage in dentistry, or clinicians may develop their own.
- A key for symbols and letter abbreviations used should be available to eliminate confusion for others reading the record.
- The American Veterinary Dental College has adopted an extensive list of abbreviations (Tables 1–2, 1–3). The clinician can choose diagnoses and procedures most common in the practice and list these abbreviations and descriptions in an abbreviation key on the dental chart.
- The additional box rows (2 and 3) can be used for noting additional measurements, footnoting the record, and entering other descriptive abbreviations.

Remarks

- Miscellaneous remarks may be entered.

Diagnosis/Treatment Plan/ Treatment Completed

- A date, the tooth or teeth involved, radiographic assessment and number of films taken, and treatment plan or options are entered. A "P" is placed in the column to denote a plan, or a "T" is placed to denote a treatment. The date may be written alongside the "P" to indicate a plan that has been followed with a treatment.
- Complications and follow-up may be recorded in this area.
- Discussions and consultations may also be recorded in this section.

Pet Clinic
Canine Dental Treatment Chart

M2	M1	P4	P3	P2	P1	C1	I3	I2	I1	1I	2I	3I	1C	1P	2P	3P	4P	1M	2M
110	109	108	107	106	105	104	103	102	101	201	202	203	204	205	206	207	208	209	210

Right Side — Buccal / Occlusal / Palatal — Left Side — Buccal / Occlusal / Palatal

Lingual / Occlusal / Buccal (Right Side) — Lingual / Occlusal / Buccal (Left Side)

M3	M2	M1	P4	P3	P2	P1	C1	I3	I2	I1	1I	2I	3I	1C	1P	2P	3P	4P	1M	2M	3M
411	410	409	408	407	406	405	404	403	402	401	301	302	303	304	305	306	307	308	309	310	311

Remarks and Diagnosis: _____

_____

_____

Radiographic Evaluation and Assessment: _____

_____

_____

Treatment Summary and Plan: _____

_____

_____

Client Instructions: _____

_____

_____

Table 1–2 • LIST OF DIAGNOSTIC CODES[2]

2D	Secondary dentin
AB	Abrasion
AL	Attachment loss
APG	Apexigenesis
APX	Apexification
AT	Attrition
AXB	Anterior crossbite
BF	Broken file
BG	Buccal granuloma
BL	Bone recession (or bone loss)
BSF	Broken spiral filler
C/MOD	Cavity–mesial occlusal distal surface
C1	Occlusal or pit and fissure; molars and premolars
C1N	Class 1, nonvital tooth
C1O	Class 1 occlusion: normal with one or more teeth out of alignment or rotated
C1V	Class 1, vital tooth
C2	MOD: Mesio-occlusodistal, mesio-occlusal, occlusodistal, molars and premolars
C2O	Class 2 occlusion: brachygnathism; overshot; retrusive mandible; distal mandibular excursion
C3	M or D; incisor no ridge
C3O	Class 3 occlusion: prognathism; undershot; protrusive mandible; mesial mandibular excursion
C4	MID: mesioincisodistal, mesioincisal, incisodistal; incisor with ridge
C5	Lingual or facial
C6	Cusp
C7	Root
C8	Root apex
CA	Cavity: fracture or defect (1–8)
CAL	Calculus
CC	Curettage closed
CFL	Cleft lip
CFP	Cleft palate
CI	Calculus index
CMO	Craniomandibular osteopathy
CO	Curettage open
CON	Consultation
CU	Contact ulcer (kissing ulcer)
CWD	Crowding
DB	Dentinal bonding agent
DC	Dentigerous cyst
DR	Dilacerated root
DT/D	Deciduous tooth
ED	Enamel defect
EG	Eosinophilic granuloma
EGC	EG lip/cheilitis (lip)
EGL	EG lingual/tongue
EH	Enamel hypocalcification/hypoplasia
EP	Epulis (fibromatous)
EX	Excision
EXT	Extrusion
FB	Foreign body
FE	Furcation exposure
FE1	Furcation exposure class 1: probe can barely detect the entrance to the furcation
FE2	Furcation exposure class 2: probe can enter furcation but not reach other side
FE3	Furcation exposure class 3: probe can pass through furcation to the other side
FEN	Fenestration
FRE	Frenectomy
FRN	Frenotomy
FX	Fracture
GCF	Gingival crevicular fluid
GH	Gingival hyperplasia/hypertrophy
GI	Gingival Index (Loe and Silness)
GI0	Gingival Index Grade 0: normal gingiva
GI1	Gingival Index Grade 1: mild inflammation
GI2	Gingival Index Grade 2: moderate inflammation
GI3	Gingival Index Grade 3: severe inflammation
GLS	Glossitis
GM	Gingival margin
GP	Gutta-percha
GR	Gingival recession
HT	Hairy tongue
INT	Intrusion
KL	Kissing lesion
LFD	Lip fold dermatitis
LG	Lingual granuloma
LPS	Lymphocytic plasmacytic stomatitis
LUP	Lupus erythematosus
M0	Mobility: normal or none
M1	Mobility: slight
M2	Mobility: moderate
M3	Mobility: severe
MAL	Malocclusion (modified angle classification)
MAL1	Crossbite
MAL2	Brachygnathia
MAL3	Prognathia
MGL	Mucogingival loss
MGM	Mucogingival margin
MM	Mucous membrane
MN/FX	Mandible fracture
MX/FX	Maxillary fracture
NE	Near exposure
NV	Nonvital
◯	Circle around missing tooth on chart
OAF	Oroantral fistula
OM	Oral mass (mm)
ONF	Oronasal fistula
OST	Osteomyelitis
OW	Occlusal wear
P&F	Pit and fissure
P3	Periodontal pocket 3 mm
P4	Periodontal pocket 4 mm
P5	Periodontal pocket 5 mm
P6	Periodontal pocket 6 mm
P7	Periodontal pocket 7 mm
P8	Periodontal pocket 8 mm
P9	Periodontal pocket 9 mm
PAP	Papillomatosis
PD	Palatal defect
PD1	Periodontal disease stage 1: initial stage
PD2	Periodontal disease stage 2: early stage
PD3	Periodontal disease stage 3: established stage
PD4	Periodontal disease stage 4: advanced stage
PDI	Periodontal Disease Index
PDL	Periodontal ligament
PE	Pulp exposure
PEM	Pemphigus
PERF	Perforation
PG	Periodontal pocket gingival (pseudopocket)
PI	Plaque Index (Silness and Loe)
PI0	Plaque Index Grade 0: no plaque
PI1	Plaque Index Grade 1: thin film of plaque at gingival margin visible when checked with explorer
PI2	Plaque Index Grade 2: Moderate amount of plaque along gingival margin; interdental space free of plaque; plaque visible
PI3	Plaque Index Grade 3: heavy plaque accumulation at gingival margin; interdental space filled with plaque
PIB	Periodontal pocket infrabony
PLQ	Plaque
PLT	Palate
PP	Periodontal pocket
PP	Periodontal pocket
PSB	Periodontal pocket suprabony
PT	Palatal trauma defect
PT/P	Permanent tooth
PXB	Posterior crossbite
RCT	Root canal therapy
RD	Retained deciduous tooth
RE	Root exposure

Table 1–2 • LIST OF DIAGNOSTIC CODES[2] *Continued*

RL	Resorptive lesion (FORL = feline odontoclastic resorption lesion)	SYM/S	Symphysis separation
ROT	Rotation	SZ	Zygomatic salivary gland
RR	Retained root	TA	Tooth avulsed
RTR	Retained root	TIP	Tipping
SAL	Salivary gland	TL	Tooth luxated
SBI	Sulcus Bleeding Index	TMJ/DL	TMJ (temporomandibular joint) dislocation
SE	Staining extrinsic (metal)	TMJ/DP	TMJ dysplasia
SER	Supereruption	TMJ/FX	TMJ fracture
SI	Staining intrinsic (blood)	TMJ/L	TMJ luxation
SL	Sublingual	TRANS	Translation or bodily movement
SLG	Sublingual granuloma	VBL/NV	Vital/nonvital bleaching
SM	Mandibular SG (surgery, mandibulectomy)	VT	Vital tooth
SMo	Molar SG (molar salivary gland)	VWD	von Willebrand disease
SN	Supernumerary	W1	Periodontal bony pocket 1 wall
SP	Parotid salivary gland	W2	Periodontal bony pocket 2 wall
SS	Sublingual salivary gland	W3	Periodontal bony pocket 3 wall
STM	Stomatitis	W4/CUP	Periodontal bony pocket 4 wall cup lesion
SUL	Sulcus	WRY	Wry mouth
SYM	Symphysis	XRFM	X-ray full mouth
		ZOE	Zinc oxide eugenol

[2]As adapted from the American Veterinary Dental College Tracking Committee recommendations.

Table 1–3 • LIST OF TREATMENT CODES[2]

ACY	Acrylic	OAA	Orthodontic appliance: adjust
AP	Alveoloplasty	OAI	Orthodontic appliance: install
AS	Apical sealer/cement	OAR	Orthodontic appliance: remove
BE	Biopsy excisional	OC	Orthodontic consultation (genetic counseling)
BFR	Buccal fold removal		
BG	Bone graft	OI	Osseous implant
BI	Biopsy incisional	OL	Onlay
BKT	Bracket	ONF/R	Oronasal fistula repair or restore
BP	Bridge pontic	OP	Odontoplasty
BR	Bridge	OR	Orthodontic recheck
BRC	Bridge cantilever	OSW	Osseous wiring
BRM	Bridge Maryland	P&FS	Pit and fissure sealer
CAM	Crown amputation reduction	PC	Pulp capping
CBU	Core build-up	PCD	Direct pulp capping
CFP/R	Cleft palate repair	PCI	Indirect pulp capping
CFW	Circumferential wiring	PFM	Crown porcelain fused to metal
CM	Crown metal (CMG = gold; CMB = base metal; etc.)	PRO	Prophylaxis complete
		PS	Periodontal surgery
CON	Consultation	R	Restoration
CR	Crown	R/A	Restoration amalgam
CS	Culture/sensitivity	R/C	Restoration composite
CT	Citric acid treatment	R/I	Restoration glass ionomer
CUL	Culture	RCS	Surgical root canal
EC	Elastic chain (power chain)	RCT	Root canal therapy
EX	Excision	RGF	Retrograde filling (RGF/A = amalgam, etc.)
FAR	Flap apically repositioning	RP	Root planing
FCR	Flap coronally repositioning	RPC	Closed root planing
FG	Fluoride gel	RPO	Open root planing
FGG	Flap free gingival graft	RRX	Root resection (hemisection)
FLS	Flap lateral sliding	SC	Subgingival curettage
FR-P/P	Fracture repair pin/plate/splint/screw (SC)/wire(W)	SM	Surgery: Mandibulectomy
		SO	Surgical orthopaedics
FRB	Flap reverse bevel	SP	Surgery: palate
FV	Fluoride varnish	SPF	Scale polish fluoride
GP	Gingivoplasty	SPL	Splint
GTR	Guided tissue regeneration	SX	Surgery: maxillectomy
GV	Gingivectomy	T	Bracket marked on chart
HS	Hemisection	TP	Treatment planning
IDW	Interdental wiring	TRX	Tooth resection (hemisection)
IL	Inlay	VER	Veneer
IM	Impressions/models (orthodontic or restorative)	VP	Vital pulpotomy
IMP	Implant	WIR	Wire
IO	Interceptive orthodontics	X	Simple extraction
IOD	Interceptive orthodontics deciduous tooth	XR	X-ray
IOP	Interceptive orthodontics permanent tooth	XS	Extraction with sectioning of tooth
OA	Orthodontic appliance	XSS	Surgical extraction

[2]As adapted from the American Veterinary Dental College Tracking Committee recommendations.

PERIODONTAL CHARTING

- Periodontal charting is a more specialized record of the periodontal status of each tooth (see the feline dental chart). It can include evaluation of the various indices to quantitate gingival health, such as gingival bleeding and edema (gingival index); amount of plaque and calculus (plaque index or calculus index); probing depths; mobility; and attachment levels. These measurements are important in quantitating the degree of periodontitis present generally as well as the involvement of individual teeth, and they allow for greater assessment of treatment and home-care procedures needed. The level of the patient's periodontal disease is determined by the most-involved teeth. This level may change with successive treatment. This is a fairly subjective evaluation, and a patient may have a generalized stage and a local stage, e.g., generalized stage 2 with localized stage 4.

Periodontal Indices

- Changes in the periodontium in response to disease can be quantitated by the use of various indices. This helps to assess the severity of the pathologic process and can be used to evaluate success of treatment.
- Epidemiologic studies use indices in order to have a consistent evaluation of disease and to be able to compare data statistically.

Plaque Index (Silness and Loe[3])

Grade
0   No plaque.
1   Thin film of plaque at gingival margin visible when margin checked with explorer.
2   Moderate amount of plaque at gingival margin. Interdental space is free of plaque. Plaque is visible to the naked eye.
3   Heavy plaque accumulation at gingival margin. Interdental space filled with plaque.

Gingival Index (Loe and Silness[3])

Grade
0   Normal gingiva. No inflammation, discoloration, or bleeding.
1   Mild inflammation, slight color change, mild alteration of gingival surface, no bleeding on probing.
2   Moderate inflammation, erythema, swelling bleeding on probing or when pressure applied.
3   Severe inflammation, severe erythema and swelling, tendency toward spontaneous hemorrhage, some ulceration.

Mobility

Grade I—slight mobility: represents the first detectable sign of movement greater than normal.

Grade II—moderate mobility: movement of 1 mm.

Grade III—marked mobility: movement of more than 1 mm in any direction and/or intrusive movement.

Furcation Exposure

Class I—The periodontal probe can barely detect the entrance to the furcation.

Class II—The periodontal probe can enter the furcation but does not extend to the other side. Early radiographic changes may be seen.

Class III—The periodontal probe can pass through the furcation to the other side.

Pet Clinic
Feline Dental Treatment Chart

| | M1 | P4 | P3 | P2 | C1 | I3 | I2 | I1 | 1I | 2I | 3I | 1C | 2P | 3P | 4P | 1M |
| | 109 | 108 | 107 | 106 | 104 | 103 | 102 | 101 | 201 | 202 | 203 | 204 | 206 | 207 | 208 | 209 |

Right Side

Buccal

Occlusal

Palatal

Lingual

Occlusal

Buccal

Left Side

Buccal

Occlusal

Palatal

Lingual

Occlusal

Buccal

| | M1 | P4 | P3 | C1 | I3 | I2 | I1 | 1I | 2I | 3I | 1C | 3P | 4P | 1M |
| | 409 | 408 | 407 | 404 | 403 | 402 | 401 | 301 | 302 | 303 | 304 | 307 | 308 | 309 |

Remarks and Diagnosis: _____

_____

_____

Radiographic Evaluation and Assessment: _____

_____

_____

Treatment Summary and Plan: _____

_____

_____

Client Instructions: _____

_____

_____

_____

_____

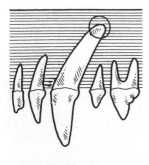

Periapical
pathology
(PA)

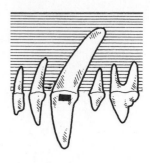

Restoration
(R)

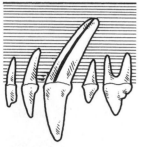

Root canal
treatment
(RCT)

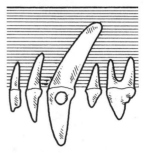

Caries
(C5–CA)

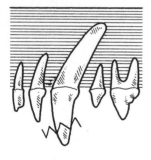

Fractured
crown
(FX–C6)

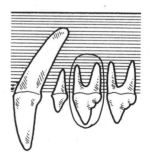

Missing
tooth

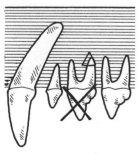

Retained
root
(RTR)

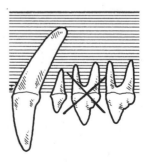

Extracted
tooth
(XS)

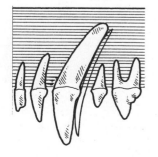

Retained
primary
tooth
(RD)

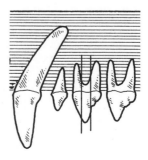

Planned
extracted
tooth

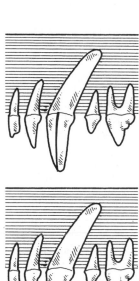

Posts

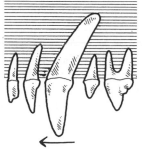

Malpositioned tooth

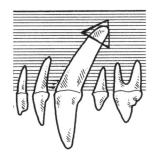

Apicoectomy
(RCS)

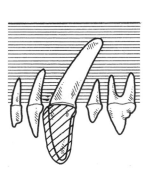

Crown
(CR)

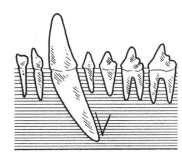

Frenula
problem

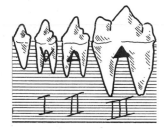

Furcation Exposure
(FE I)
(FE II)
(FE III)

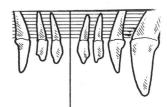

Bridge
(BR)

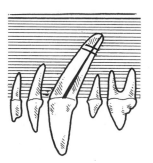

Implant
(IMP)

SAMPLE DENTAL CHART WITH DISEASE

Various standard marks can be used to record conditions of the teeth and gums. The sample chart on the facing page shows many of these marks. The numbers of the following list refer to points on the chart.

1. Periapical disease is indicated by a circle around the root tip in the buccal view.

2. Fractured crown is indicated by a jagged line over the crown in all three views, with an attempt made to show the missing area.

3. Retained root is indicated by an X over the crown in the buccal, occlusal, or palatal (lingual) view and by drawing in the root portion retained in the buccal view.

4. Retained primary tooth is indicated by drawing in the tooth on the buccal view, including the root.

5. Cavities are indicated by an irregular circle on the appropriate views in the area of the lesion (do not fill in, because that indicates a restoration).

6. Missing teeth are indicated by a circle around the tooth in all three views.

7. Planned extractions are indicated by parallel lines over all three views.

8. Malpositioned teeth are indicated by an arrow in the direction of malposition in the appropriate views.

9. A need for a frenectomy is indicated by a V-shaped figure in the buccal view at the involved area.

10. An exposed furcation (class 1) is indicated by a V.

11. An open triangle denotes a class 2 furcation.

12. A filled-in triangle denotes a class 3 furcation.

13. A hatched line over the V indicates that a frenectomy has been performed.

14. Probing depth measurements can be recorded in the first row of boxes.

15. A line is drawn on the buccal view to show the level of the gingival margin. Combining the charted gingival margin line with the charted probing depth allows the practitioner to determine the level of gingival attachment. See the Periodontal Charting section in this chapter for more specific information.

16. Root canal treatment is indicated by a solid line in the root canal (not in the pulp chamber) in the buccal view.

17. A restoration is indicated by filling in the area of restoration on appropriate views.

18. Extracted teeth or roots are indicated by an X over the tooth/root extracted in all three views.

19. Posts are indicated by a line in the pulp chamber (not in the root canal, which would indicate root canal therapy).

20. Apicoectomy is indicated by an open triangle around the apex.

21. A crown/cap is indicated by a circle around the coronal views. If porcelain, it is left clear; if metal, it is filled in with hatch lines.

22. A bridge is indicated by parallel lines connecting the involved crowns in the occlusal view.

23. An implant is indicated by a line in the root area, with perpendicular lines on the buccal view.

24. Pulp capping is indicated by a straight line across the crown and a solid rectangle in the coronal pulp chamber below the line.

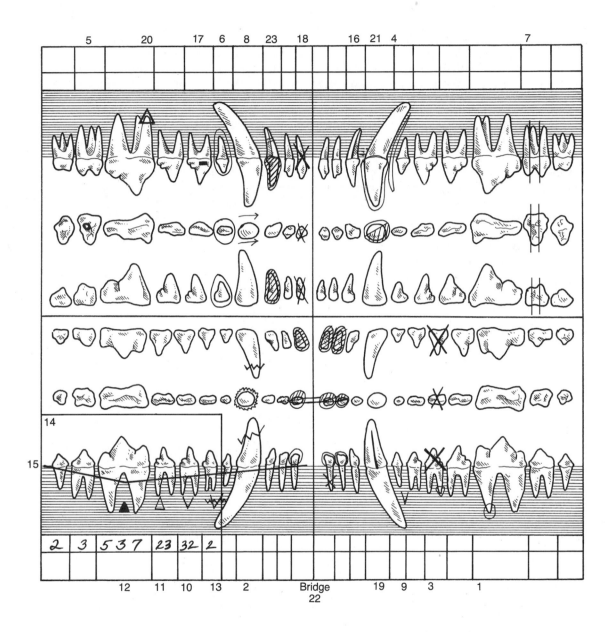

INTRAORAL PHOTOGRAPHY

General Comments

- Oral photography is an important tool in veterinary dentistry. For years it has been used in the educational process. In the office, the veterinarian can document written and oral case studies and reports, peer review, and self-evaluation; record progress on cases; train staff in understanding the disease process, equipment care, and procedures; consult with colleagues across the country; and educate clients as well as the general public. It is important that these photographs be of good quality so that the viewer can appreciate the subject matter. General-use cameras do not allow the photographer to get close-ups that focus on oral subject matter.
- There are many types of cameras for oral photography. The camera must be suited to each individual photographer. For those with little camera knowledge or little willingness to learn, a "point and shoot" camera may be the best choice. Experienced photographers may already have the equipment; with a few equipment modifications, they can get excellent results.

RANGE FINDER CAMERAS

General Comments

- Both Kodak and Polaroid have close-up kits that use the fixed focus technique.
- These cameras have lenses that attach to the camera with a frame in front that serves as an aiming mechanism for the area of the photograph and the distance.

Advantages

- Can be used by anyone.
- Are uncomplicated and range in price from $250 to $400.

Disadvantages

- Polaroid camera produces prints only, which are available instantly; Kodak camera can produce prints and slides.

- May be difficult to position camera in patient's mouth.

SINGLE REFLEX CAMERAS

General Comments

- "Single lens reflex" indicates a viewing system in which mirrors are used inside the camera that allow the photographer to view the image through the lens prior to exposure of the film.
- As the camera shutter is opened, a mirror inside the camera swings out of the way, exposing the film.
- The "state of the art" camera is the Single Lens Reflex, Through-the-Lens 35 mm camera (SLR-TTL).
- The camera is able to sense the light and deliver the correct amount of flash, time exposure, and size of the aperture (f-stop).
- These cameras can be equipped with motor drive, automatic ASA (film speed) setting, data backs, and automatic film loading.
- Usually, these cameras provide excellent pictures; however, sometimes the camera can make a mistake and produce a less-than-desirable picture.
- These auto-exposure systems generally start around $600.

LENSES

- A lens of either approximately 50 mm or 100 mm will work well for close-up oral photography.
- The lens should have macro-capabilities; that is, it should have the ability to focus down to 1:1 life-size images (if the subject is 10 mm, the image on the film is 10 mm).
- As the magnification increases, the image size on the film decreases (the 10 mm subject would be 5 mm on the film at 1:2 magnification or 1 mm at 1:10).

50 mm Lens

Advantage
- Less bulk

Disadvantage
- Greater distortion.

100 mm Lens

Advantage

- A longer working length, and the photographs can be taken at a greater distance from the mouth.

Disadvantage

- Are more expensive than equivalent 50 mm macro-lens and longer and bulkier to use.

LIGHTING SYSTEMS

- There are two types of close-up lighting systems: ring light and point light.

  With ring light, the flash strobe circles the lens.
  With ring light, there are no shadows, unless switches are purposely turned off or on, and it is best used for lighting the total subject.
  Because ring light can eliminate shadows, it also can eliminate contrast that is gained by the shadows.
  For that reason, small point lights are available.

- Point light is best for work that is cosmetic in nature or where contrast and detail are desirable.
- There are systems that use both point light and ring light.
- In addition, many systems come with modeling lights to aid in focusing.

FILM

- There are two types of film: print film and slide film.

Print Film

Advantages

- Does not need a special viewer to look at it.
- Greater latitude of exposure.

Disadvantages

- Less detail.
- Without converting to slides, cannot be shown to a large audience.

Slide Film

Advantages

- Greater detail.
- Can be shown to large audience.

Disadvantages

- Must be converted to prints or seen with a special viewer (photographic loop or projector).

Film Speed

- Film speed is rated in ASA: the higher the ASA number, the faster the film.
- Fast film requires less exposure.
- Faster film has increased grain that decreases the detail as compared with slower ASA film.

Processing Date

- Due to color changes that occur in time, check the dating on the box of film and beware of buying "outdated" or "short-dated" film, regardless of the price "bargain."

MIRRORS

- Areas difficult to photograph may be visualized with dental mirrors.
- These mirrors are finely polished and yield excellent results.
- Care must be taken to retain their clean, smooth finish.
- To prevent moisture condensation, a mirror can be warmed slightly with a surgical lamp, warm water, or hair dryer before inserting into the patient's mouth.

TAKING PHOTOGRAPHS

- Ensure the subject is in the unobscured field of view.
- Pay strict attention to distracting factors, such as improper instrument technique, blood, dirty fingernails, matted hair, etc.
- If the patient's lips or tongue must be held back, it is best to do this mechanically or use gloves.

- When working with slides, crop the slide to focus on the center object by using Mylar masking tape.
- With prints, distractions can be cropped out.
- To take a photograph, check the strobe to ensure it is operational.
- If the strobe is fitted with ring and point, the appropriate selection is made.
- Choose the magnification and setting on the lens.
- Set the shutter speed and f-stop.
- To take a photograph, move the camera back and forth until the image is in focus. Once the image is focused, gently press the shutter.

Additional Tips

- Setting the magnification rather than adjusting the focus makes the photographs standardized and allows comparison of cases and standardization of photographic technique.
- A log should be kept in a notebook (pieces of paper tend to get lost in most offices) recording the date, patient/condition, f-stop setting, magnification (distance from subject), type of strobe (ring or point), and any other information.

The Future of Intraoral Photography

- At the current time, digital cameras are becoming more reliable.
- Some digital cameras are combination still-and-video systems.
- Some digital cameras have their own image storage systems; images may be stored on a computer.
- As computers and software become more sophisticated, veterinary practices will be incorporating photographic records into patient records on a computer.

DENTAL TERMINOLOGY

• A knowledge of dental terminology is important for understanding a technique; discussing a case with another veterinarian, dentist, or student; and reporting a finding or procedure in a record. A list of common dental and anatomic terms follows.[4, 5, 6]

GLOSSARY

Anatomic Terms

Alveolar bone. Cancellous bone directly surrounding the tooth roots.

Alveolar crest. The most coronal ridge of bone between two adjacent teeth or between the roots of a tooth.

Alveolar mucosa. Less densely keratinized gingival tissue covering the bone.

Alveolus. The cavity or socket in either jawbone that surrounds and supports the root of the tooth.

Anterior teeth. The canine and incisor teeth.

Apex. The terminal portion of the root.

Apical delta. The diverging branches of the root canal at the apical end of the tooth root.

Apical foramen. The opening(s) in the apex of the root through which nerves and vessels pass into the root canal.

Arch, dental. The dentition and alveolar ridge of either the maxilla or the mandible; sometimes called either the upper or lower arch.

Attached gingiva. The gingiva that extends apically from the free gingival groove to the mucogingival junction.

Attachment apparatus. The periodontal ligament, cementum, and alveolar bone that hold the tooth in place.

Canine tooth. Large, single-rooted tooth designed for puncturing, tearing, and grasping.

Carnassial tooth. Shearing tooth. Upper P4 and lower M1 in the dog and cat.

Cementoenamel junction. The junction at the neck of the tooth where the enamel and the cementum meet.

Cementum. A specialized calcified connective tissue covering the root surface and serving as attachment for the periodontal ligament from the bone to the tooth.

Cingulum. The ledge on the cervical third of the palatal surface of the crowns of the incisor teeth.

Col. The interdental connection between the junctional epithelia of any two adjacent teeth.

Crown. The portion of the tooth covered with enamel.

Cusp. The tip or pointed prominence on the occlusal surface of the crown.

Deciduous teeth. Teeth of primary dentition ("baby teeth") that will be replaced by secondary (adult) teeth.

Dental arch. Formed by the curve of the crowns of the teeth in their normal position or by the residual ridge if the teeth are missing.

Dental quadrant. An upper or lower dental arch on one side of the patient.

Dentin. The main component of the tooth, consisting of multiple tubules that radiate from the pulp to the tooth's outer surface. The tubules contain sensory nerve fibers that register various degrees of pain. Harder than bone, dentin is covered by enamel on the crown and by cementum on the root.

Dentition. Natural teeth as a unit in the dental arches.

Diastema. The space between two adjacent teeth that are not in contact with each other in an arch.

Embrasure. The space between teeth occlusal to areas of contact of teeth.

Enamel. The hard, shiny outer layer of the crown, composed of hexagonal rods of hydroxyapatite crystalline components organized with their long axis approximately at right angles to the surface.

Epithelial attachment. The epithelium attaching the gingiva to the tooth.

Fauces. The arch between the pharyngeal and oral cavities, formed by the tongue, tonsillar pillars, and soft palate.

Free gingiva. Portion of the gingiva not directly attached to the tooth that forms the gingival wall of the sulcus.

Free gingival groove. On the surface of the gingiva, a slight concavity or line separating free from attached gingiva.

Free gingival margin. The unattached edge of the gingiva that lies against the tooth surface.

Furcation. The space between tooth roots where the roots join the crown.

Gingiva. The soft tissue surrounding the teeth.

Gingival sulcus. The normal space created between the free gingiva and the tooth.

Gnathic. Referring to the jaw.

Halitosis. Foul, offensive, or unpleasant breath.

Incisal edge. The cutting edge of the incisors.

Incisive papilla. The small protuberance palatal to the maxillary incisors. The nasopalatine ducts exit on each side of the incisive papilla.

Incisor. Small anterior tooth with a single root.

Infrabony pocket. A periodontal pocket whose base is apical to the crest of the alveolar bone.

Interdental. The area between the proximal surfaces of adjacent teeth in the same arch.

Interproximal. The area between adjacent surfaces of adjoining teeth.

Interradicular. The area between roots of multirooted teeth.

Juga. The prominent bulge of bone formed by roots in the alveolar process on the mandible, the premaxilla, and the maxilla.

Lamina dura. A radiographic term referring to the dense cortical bone forming the wall of the alveolus. The lamina dura appears on a radiograph as a bony white line next to the dark line of the periodontal ligament.

Lateral or accessory canal. The small canal branching from the root canal to the outer surface of the root, usually occurring in the apical third of the root.

Mental foramen. Openings in the lateral wall of the mandible through which nerves and vessels pass to supply the tissues of the lip.

Molar. The large, multicusp tooth designed primarily for grinding.

Mucogingival junction. The line of demarcation where the attached gingiva and alveolar mucosa meet.

Neck (cervical line). The junction between the crown and root.

Odontoblast. The outer cells of the pulp that produce dentin throughout the life of the tooth.

Palate. The bone and soft tissue that separate the oral and nasal cavities.

Periodontal ligament. A network of collagenous fibers suspending the tooth in its alveolus attaching it to its supporting bone.

Periodontium. The supporting tissues of the teeth including the periodontal ligament, gingiva, cementum, and alveolar supporting bone.

Pockets, periodontal. An area of diseased gingival attachment, characterized by its loss of attachment and eventual damage to the tooth's supporting bone.

Posterior teeth. The premolar and molar teeth.

Premolar. The teeth distal to the canine and mesial to the molars that have one to three roots in the dog and cat.

Primary (deciduous) teeth. The first teeth to erupt; they are replaced by secondary (adult) teeth.

Proximal surface. The surface of a tooth or cavity that is closest to the adjacent tooth.

Pulp. Soft-tissue component of the tooth consisting of blood, vascular tissue, nerve tissue, loose connective tissue, and cellular elements such as odontoblasts that form dentin.

Pulp chamber. The portion of the crown containing the pulp.

Root. The portion of the tooth apical to the crown and normally covered by cementum.

Root canal. Portion of the root containing the pulp.

Ruga palatina. The irregular ridges in the mucous membrane covering the anterior part of the hard palate.

Sulcus. A groove. In veterinary dentistry it usually refers to the gingival sulcus present, in healthy patients with healthy gingiva, between the free gingiva and the surface of the tooth and extending around the tooth's circumference.

Suprabony pocket. A periodontal pocket, the base of which is above the level of the crestal alveolar bone.

Vestibule of oral cavity. The part of the oral cavity between the cheeks or lips and alveolar ridge.

Dental Positioning/Surfaces

Apical. Toward the apex.

Buccal. The surface of the tooth nearest the cheek (posterior teeth).

Coronal. Toward the crown.

Distal. Away from the midline of an imaginary line following the curve of the dental arches.

Facial. The surface of the tooth nearest the face. This term is awkward to apply to most veterinary patients because there is little delineation of face and cheek. Buccal and labial are more accurate.

Incisal. The biting surface of anterior teeth.
Interproximal. Between closest surfaces of adjoining teeth.

Labial. The surface of the tooth nearest the lips (anterior teeth).
Line angle. Imaginary line formed by the junction of two adjacent vertical surfaces/walls of a tooth.
Lingual. The surface of the tooth nearest the tongue.

Mandible. The bone that forms the lower jaw.
Maxilla. The bone that forms most of the upper jaw and contains the sockets of all the upper teeth except the incisors.
Mesial. Toward the midline along the curve of the dental arch.

Occlusal. The chewing surfaces of the caudal teeth.

Palatal. The surface of the tooth toward the palate.

Sublingual. The structures and surfaces beneath the tongue.

Dental Disciplines

Endodontics. The diagnosis and treatment of diseases that affect the tooth pulp and apical periodontal tissues.

Exodontics. The branch of dentistry that deals with extraction of teeth.

Oral surgery. Pertaining to surgery of the oral cavity.
Orthodontics. The branch of dentistry that deals with the guidance and correction of malocclusion of the juvenile teeth and adult tooth positioning.

Periodontics. The branch of dentistry that deals with the study and treatment of diseases of the tooth-supporting tissues.
Prosthodontics. The branch of dentistry that deals with the construction of appliances designed to replace missing teeth and/or other adjacent structures.

Restorative/operative dentistry. The branch of dentistry that deals with restoring the form and function of teeth.

Oral Diseases/Conditions

Abrasion. The wearing away of tooth structure because of contact with structures other than teeth.
Anodontia. The absence of teeth.
Anterior crossbite. The orthodontic condition in which the maxillary/mandibular relationship is normal and in which canine, premolar, and molar occlusion is normal, but one or more mandibular incisors are anterior to the maxillary incisors.
Attrition. The wearing away of teeth by continual tooth-against-tooth contact.
Avulsion. The loss of the tooth from its alveolus.

Brachygnathia. The lower jaw is markedly shorter than the upper jaw.

Calculus. Hard, mineralized plaque deposited on the tooth surface.
Caries. A demineralization and loss of tooth structure because of action of microorganisms on carbohydrates.
Cellulitis. A diffuse inflammation of loose connective tissue.

Dilaceration. An abnormally shaped root resulting from trauma during tooth development.

Edentulous. Without teeth.

Embedded tooth. A tooth that is usually covered in bone and that has not erupted into the oral cavity and is not likely to erupt.

Erosion. Loss of tooth structure by chemical or mechanical means not involving bacteria. The surface of the defect, unlike caries, is hard and smooth.

Facet. A flattened or worn spot on the surface of a tooth.

Faucitis. Inflammation of the glossopalatine folds or arches (fauces).

Fenestration (root). A window-like opening of bone and gingiva over the root.

Freeway space. The abnormal vertical space between the opposing mandibular and maxillary premolar cusps when the mouth is closed.

Fistula. An abnormal opening associated with underlying dental disease.

Fused teeth. The joining of two teeth in development where they have developed from different tooth buds.

Gemini tooth. The partial division of a tooth bud attempting to form two teeth.

Gingival hyperplasia. A pathologic increase in the amount of gingival tissue in a normal cellular arrangement, resulting in a thickened enlargement of tissue.

Granuloma. Chronic inflammation of loose connective tissue.

Horizontal bone loss. Loss of crestal alveolar bone along an arch, usually secondary to periodontal disease.

Impacted tooth. An unerupted or partially erupted tooth that is prevented from erupting further by any structure.

Level bite (even bite). Occlusion in which the upper and lower incisors meet incisal edge to incisal edge.

Luxation (tooth). The displacement or partial displacement of a tooth from its alveolus.

Mesiodens. A supernumerary tooth appearing in the erupted or unerupted state between the two maxillary central incisors.

Odontalgia. Pain in a tooth.

Oligodontia. Reduced number of teeth.

Open bite. The failure of the upper and lower incisors to meet or overlap each other in the vertical dimension when the mouth is closed.

Oronasal fistula. An abnormal opening between the oral and nasal cavities.

Overbite. Layman's term for the upper jaw vertically overlapping the lower jaw.

Overjet. Horizontal projection of the maxillary anterior teeth in front of the mandibular anterior teeth such that the two arches do not touch.

Pellicle. The thin film composed mostly of protein that continuously forms on the surface of teeth. It forms with or without bacteria and can be removed by abrasive action.

Periapical abscess (apical abscess or periradicular abscess). An abscess at the apical region of the root, involving the pulp and surrounding periapical tissues.

Periodontal abscess. An abscess involving the periodontium as a sequela of periodontal disease.

Plaque. A thin, sticky film covering the teeth, composed of bacteria and their byproducts, saliva, food particles, and sloughed epithelial cells.

Posterior crossbite. An abnormal occlusion in which one or more mandibular premolars or molars occlude buccal to their occlusal counterpart.

Pulpitis. Inflammation of the pulp, which may be reversible or irreversible.

Pulpitis, hypertrophic. A productive type of chronic inflammation that contains a mass of tissue protruding from a pulp exposure.

Pyorrhea. Antiquated term for discharge of pus from the periodontium.

Resorption. The loss of substance by a physiologic or pathologic process.

Reverse scissor bite. Occlusion in which all the lower incisors occlude anterior to, but are overlapping vertically and touching, the labial surfaces of the upper incisors. This is a prognathic condition.

Stomatitis. Inflammation of the soft tissues of the oral cavity.

Supernumerary tooth. An additional tooth of the same type as one already present.

Vertical bone loss. Bone loss at an angle acute to the horizontal plane along a root surface, forming an infrabony pocket.

Wry bite. A malocclusion in which the midline of the lower jaw does not oppose the midline of the upper jaw. The face and jaw are asymmetric in relation to each other.

Dental Treatment

Apical repositioning. An oral surgical procedure that repositions the gingiva and/or bone.

Apicoectomy. The retrograde surgical treatment of endodontic disease, by access to the apex, removing diseased tissue and sealing the canal.

Crown lengthening. An oral surgical procedure that entails movement of the gingiva apically and reduction of the alveolar crest. This procedure is performed as treatment of periodontal disease and in restorative crown therapy when additional crown surface area is required for cementation of an artificial crown.

Electrosurgery. The use of electrically generated energy to perform the controlled cutting of tissue.

Electrocautery. The use of electrically generated energy to perform hemostasis.

Dental (Intraoral) Devices

Abutment. The tooth or implant that is used for the support or anchorage of a fixed or removable prosthesis or appliance.

Anchorage. The supporting base for orthodontic forces that are applied to stimulate tooth movement.

Articulator. The mechanical device that represents the orientation and movement of the temporomandibular joints, the mandible and maxilla used to hold the maxillary and mandibular cast in the proper occlusal relationship.

Bite register. The impression made by closing the patient's mouth on a soft imprintable sheet of material or compound used to align casts to the occlusion of the patient.

Cast. The replication of the teeth and tissues made from an impression.

Crown or cap. The dental prosthesis covering part or all of the crown of the tooth to restore its anatomy, function, and esthetics.

Helix. A loop or coil.

Impression. The negative replication (mold) of the teeth and tissues used to make a positive reproduction (cast).

Inlay. The prosthetic device that is cemented into a recessed preparation.

Onlay. The prosthetic device that is cemented to a minimally prepared tooth surface.

Orthodontic appliance. The oral device used to apply force to malpositioned teeth to provide tooth movement or to maintain tooth position.

Prosthesis. An artificial part that replaces part of the body. In dentistry it is an appliance used either for esthetics or to maintain space when replacing a missing tooth or teeth.

Splint. An apparatus designed to prevent motion or displacement of displaced or movable teeth or bone.

Spot weld. To join together two metals by heating (but not melting) electronically and fusing (recrystallizing) in a small spot.

Dental Materials and Instruments

Amalgam. An alloy of mercury with one or more metals used for dental restorations and dies.

Anneal. To apply heat and cooling to a metal to soften it.

Baseplate wax. Thin sheets of high-quality wax used for a variety of dental and laboratory procedures.

Bracket. An orthodontic device that is cemented to a tooth that provides support for an arch wire.

Burnish. To draw (spread out) polish or to flatten a malleable metal through pressure using an instrument with rounded edges.

Button. A small metal or plastic device cemented to a tooth that serves for the attachment of an orthodontic elastic.

Cavity liner. The preparation used to seal dentinal tubules, reduce microleakage, and insulate pulp against shock from thermal changes.

Cement base. The insulating layer of cement placed in the deeper portion of a prepared cavity to insulate the pulp.

Flux. The substance used to prevent oxidation on heated metals used for welding.

Formocresol. The chemical compound used to mummify the pulp tissue.

Glass ionomer. In the pure form, a mixture of polyacrylic acid and fluoroaluminosilicate glass that, when combined, is used as a cement or restorative material. Other agents have been added that change the characteristics of the material.

Methyl methacrylate liquid and powder. An acrylic resin derived from methyl acrylic acid.

Monomer. In dentistry, a short-chain hydrocarbon (the liquid) to be mixed with the polymer (long-chain hydrocarbon) for fabrication of appliances and restorations.

Polymer. In dentistry, a long-chain hydrocarbon (the powder portion) to be mixed with the monomer (short-chain hydrocarbon) (the liquid portion) for fabrication of appliances and restorations.

Pumice. Abrasive glass agent made from volcanic rock, used for smoothing and polishing.

Resin. A broad term used to indicate organic products that are soluble in ether or acetone but not soluble in water; further named according to their activation (light, chemical), chemical components (acrylic), or physical structure (filled, nonfilled).

Solder. A fusible metal alloy used in its molten state to mechanically join two metals together. Also, the process of soldering.

Spherical amalgam. Amalgam whose particles are in the form of a ball, globe, or sphere.

Sticky wax. A hard wax that breaks off easily and is useful for wires and materials in the dental laboratory.

Varnish. A solution of one or more resins that come from natural gums, synthetic resin, or rosin.

REFERENCES

1. Cohen S, Burns RC. Pathways of the Pulp. St Louis: C.V. Mosby Co., 1984:302.
2. Wiggs RB, Lobprise HB. Veterinary Dentistry: Principles and Practice. Philadelphia: Lippincott-Raven, 1997:677–696.
3. Rateitschak KH, et al. Periodontology. Stuttgart: George Thieme Medical Publishers, 1989:35–37.
4. Zwemer TJ. Bouchers Clinical Dental Terminology. St. Louis: C.V. Mosby Co., 1982.
5. Schroeder HE. Oral Structural Biology. New York: Thieme Medical Publishers, 1991.
6. Dorland's Dentistry Speller. Philadelphia: W.B. Saunders Co., 1993.

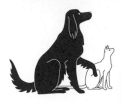

Chapter 2

DENTAL EQUIPMENT AND CARE

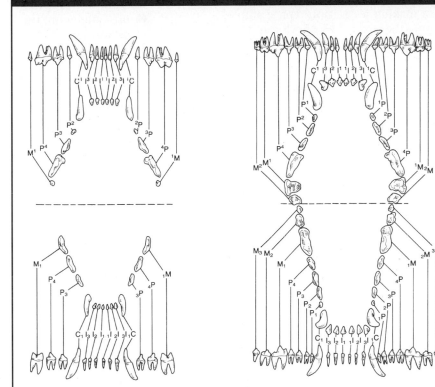

SELECTING DENTAL EQUIPMENT

A variety of equipment is available, which leads to the frequent question: "What type of dental equipment should I buy?" The question has several factors to consider, depending on the individual practice. How much and what type of dentistry will be performed? How much space is available? How much capital is available to purchase the equipment?

When purchasing dental equipment, frequency of use, type of use, space available for equipment, and the cost should be evaluated before making a decision. For example, if endodontic therapy is to be performed, purchase of an air-driven unit is recommended. Other advanced dental procedures also require specialized equipment.

After reviewing your own practice situation and goals, a choice suited to your practice should become easier to make. The purchase of dental equipment provides an excellent return on investment.[1] The dental department is one of the most cost-efficient divisions in the veterinary hospital.

POWER EQUIPMENT

When purchasing power equipment, the practitioner should consider the cost of the unit, locations available for the compressor and dental consoles, noise levels at the location, track record at the clinic for equipment maintenance, and present and future dental caseload.

Features to Consider

Foot Pedal

Advantage

- Allows hands to concentrate on working rather than switching on and off manually.

Variable Speed

Advantage

- Allows for a broader range of work with more control.

Reverse Direction

Advantages

- Can use with caution to back out of wrapped hair.
- Can use with diamond disc to cut in direction desired.

Disadvantage

- A mandrel or screw-in prophy cup may become unscrewed if turned in the direction opposite to its design.

Accessories

- Prophy angles are used to polish during prophylaxis, restorations, and other times when abrasives are used.
- Contra angles are used to change the angle of rotation of the device used on the teeth.
- Reduction contra angles are used to reduce speed at an angle.
- Acceleration contra angles are used to increase speed at which the device used on the teeth spins.
- Handpieces are used to create force and to hold contra angles, prophy angles, burs, and other instruments.

Uses

- Prophylaxis.
- Periodontics.
- Endodontics.
- Restorations.
- Exodontics.
- Orthodontics.
- Orthodontic laboratory.
- Oral surgery.

Electric-Motor-Driven Bands

Comments

- The electric motor that drives a steel, fabric, or nylon band is one of the earliest types of power equipment used in human dentistry *(A)*.
- Electric motors are still used, mostly in dental laboratories.
- They are best suited for a new practice or a practice with a small dental load or limited procedures and are available on the used dental equipment market for low cost.
- They have a speed range of 3000 to 30,000 rpm.

Advantages

- Lower cost than air-driven systems.
- Portability.
- Small size.

Disadvantages

- Slow speed.
- Breaking the band and difficulty in replacing parts.
- No water for cooling.
- Catching hair in the mechanism.
- Less convenient than electric-motor-driven or air-driven handpieces.

Maintenance

- Replacement of band.
- Lubrication according to manufacturer.

Electric-Motor-Driven Handpieces Connected to Cable

Comments

- Cable mechanisms that are hooked to electric motors come in several types.
- They are fairly inexpensive and are suited to a practice with a low volume and limited load, or they may be used as secondary units to handle additional patients when primary units are in use.
- Speed range is usually less than 3000 rpm.

Advantages

- Lower cost than compressed-air systems.
- Low maintenance.
- Portability.
- Small size.

Disadvantages

- Breaking the cable.
- No water for cooling.
- Slow speed.
- Inability to do dental procedures other than polishing.

Maintenance

- Lubrication as directed by manufacturer.

Electric Motor Handpieces

Comments

- These are handpieces with electric motors built in (B).
- A control box connects the handpiece electrically.
- Speed range 3000 to 20,000 rpm; with accelerating contra angles speed can be increased to 125,000 rpm. (These contra angles are expensive.)

Advantages

- Most cost less than air-driven units.
- Low maintenance.
- Portability.
- Small size.

Disadvantages

- Handpiece and motor break down with heavy use.

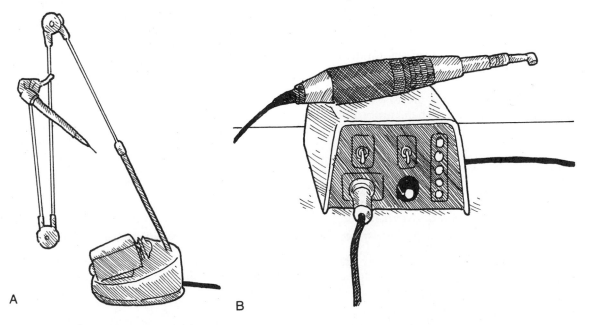

A   B

- Except for models with accessories, inability to run water through handpiece as a coolant for dental tissue.
- Slow cutting speed.
- Cumbersome to use.
- Heavier handpiece may lead to more operator fatigue.

Air-Driven Power Equipment

Comments

Air-driven systems have three components: the air power source, the "plumbing," and the handpieces. They can be powered by an air compressor or by a tank of compressed carbon dioxide or nitrogen. Compressors are rated by horsepower (hp) and the ability to deliver a flow of air. Most dental handpieces require the compressor to maintain 30 to 40 pounds per square inch (psi) at a flow of 3 cubic feet per minute. The control section is an array of air and water switches, regulators (valves), and hoses that control the flow of air and water into the hoses and, in turn, into the handpieces. The control section can be a mobile stand, cart, wall-mounted extension arm, over-the-patient unit, or small countertop unit.

Advantages

- Air acts as coolant to the handpiece.
- Water passes through the handpiece and acts as coolant/irrigant of dental tissues.
- Longer life of the compressor and handpiece.
- Ability to run at higher speeds than electric-motor-driven handpieces for rapid performance.
- Less torque than electric-motor-driven systems and therefore less heat created at the cutting surface.
- Air compressor units are easy and less expensive to maintain than carbon dioxide– or nitrogen-powered delivery systems.

Disadvantages

- Larger size than an electric delivery system.
- Noisy if not a "silent" compressor.
- More expensive than electric-motor-driven units.
- Spray mist forms aerosol.
- Accumulation of water in the oral cavity.
- Noise from a high-speed handpiece may contribute to hearing loss.

Variable Features

- These are features the practitioner should consider when purchasing these units.

Electric Foot Switches

Comment

- The electric foot switch compressor operates with an electrical circuit to turn the compressor on and off, and air is delivered directly to the handpiece without storage.

Advantage

- Require low horsepower and thus can be smaller units at tableside.

Disadvantage

- Handpiece is either on full speed or off; there is no intermediate speed.

Air Rheostat Controls

Comments

- The compressor is turned on and off by a preset pressure switch and runs only to fill the storage tank.
- Compressors of less than ¾ hp are running more than they are off. This leads to overheating and temporary shutdown.
- If the practitioner's intent is infrequent use, the smaller, chairside units work well.
- If frequent use or the use of multiple dental stations is anticipated, a larger, remote compressor with a storage tank is the best selection. At least a 1 hp compressor is recommended if either two stations or a sonic air scaler is in use.

Advantage

- Wide variability in speeds.

Disadvantage

- Greater expense than electric foot-switch units.

Remote Compressors

Comments

- Compressors can be located away from the dental operatory. This removes another item from space in the dental area and allows for multiple-station use.

Advantages

- Can be used to power multiple stations.
- Many smaller, tableside compressor control units without compressors are compact, can be moved around, can be used at different locations, and stored out of the way.
- Removes compressor noise from dental area.

Disadvantages

- Requires space with ventilation for cooling.
- Requires personnel safety considerations regarding noise level.
- Requires a location where compressor noise will not interfere with practice routine.
- Adherence to maintenance schedule is more at risk if compressor is outside the operatory.

Tableside Compressors

Comment

- Primary considerations for selection of a tableside compressor are space in the dental area, enough power and air storage for current and future use, and noise element for staff in the treatment area.

Advantages

- Can be stored in a different location when not in use.
- Can be moved easily.

Disadvantages

- Self-contained units may require additional in-line care and water filtration systems for restorative dentistry.
- Low power of some units translates into low volume of air flow and low air pressure.
- Excessive noise of some units.

Oil-Free/Oil-Containing Compressors

Comments

- Air heats up as it is compressed, and this heat is transmitted to the compressor.
- Compressors are cooled by either air or oil.
- Air-cooled oil-free compressors do not have oil to check or change.
- As a general rule, oil-free compressors are noisier and more expensive than the oil-containing variety.
- To overcome the problem of monitoring oil level with a dipstick, several oil-containing models have level view ports for observing the oil level.
- In-line filters to separate oil and water are recommended with all types of compressors.

"Whisper-Quiet" Compressors

Comments

- Traditional air compressors are fairly noisy.
- Very quiet refrigerator compressors have been converted from pumping refrigerator coolant to pumping air.
- These units are available in portable carts, portable cabinets, and countertop units.

- The single-unit compressor rates around ½ hp. If multistation use or a sonic scaler handpiece is being considered, a double-unit, 1 hp compressor should be considered.
- Because converted refrigerator compressors contain oil, the oil level must be monitored and changed according to the manufacturer's recommendation.

Advantages

- Quiet compressor.
- Available tabletop models.

Disadvantages

- Most units contain oil, and oil levels must be maintained.
- Expensive.
- If used for long periods without stopping, some models may overheat and shut down until cool; this may take 30 to 60 minutes.
- Air-driven alternatives other than by air compressor.

Carbon Dioxide

Comment

- Tanks can be rented from medical supply services and can be used, with a regulator gauge and quick disconnect couplings, to drive high-speed handpieces.

Advantages

- No maintenance.
- Saves the cost of an air compressor.
- Is not flammable.

Disadvantage

- Rental of tanks and ordering more carbon dioxide.

Nitrogen

Comment

- Same advantages and disadvantages as carbon dioxide; however, nitrogen is less expensive than carbon dioxide.

CAUTION NOTE: Oxygen from an oxygen tank should not be used to power dental handpieces because a spark could cause an explosion.

Delivery systems used in veterinary dentistry offer various combinations of accessories and handpieces. A typical top-of-the-line set-up consists of two high-speed handpieces, one low-speed handpiece with a straight attachment as well as a contra angle, and a three-way air/water syringe. Other useful accessories frequently seen as attachments on the delivery system are a suction apparatus, a sonic scaler that can be substituted for one of the high-speed handpieces, fiberoptics for the hand-pieces, and a curing unit for light-cure materials.

Three-Way Syringes

Comments

The three-way syringe (A) is used for the following:

- Flushing the oral cavity for better visualization.
- Rinsing chemicals off dental structures.
- Air-drying tooth structures during restorations and other procedures.
- Air-drying teeth to visualize calculus deposits that turn chalky when dry.[2]

Automatic Switches/Mechanical Switching

Comments

- Some units have switches that turn air on/off when handpieces are taken from or placed into their holders.
- Other units require mechanical switching by the operator.

Automatic Drain Valves

Comment

- When pressure is released from air storage tank, condensed water is released.

Advantages

- Valves require less maintenance because water is automatically drained.
- Compressor tank will last longer (decreases rust).

Disadvantages

- One more piece of equipment that may break down.
- Does not always work.

Oil-Level Indicators

Comment

- A view port is located at the same level as the oil stored inside the compressor (B).

Advantages

- Checking the oil level may be performed without the mess of a dipstick.
- The color of the oil may be inspected periodically.

Adjustable Chairside Air/Water Pressure Controls

Comment

- Some delivery systems have individual adjustable valves available for each handpiece.

Advantage

- More accommodating for the needs of different handpieces (e.g., a sonic scaler may require higher air pressure, which could be detrimental to certain prophy angles on a low-speed handpiece). Manufacturer recommendations should be consulted for each handpiece.

"Do-It-Yourself" versus "Turnkey" Units

Comments

- Components purchased at a department or hardware store can be used to assemble a dental unit.
- At least a 1 hp, and preferably a 2 hp compressor, is desirable.
- The control panels, regulators, and foot pedals can be purchased from dental suppliers.

Advantage

- There may be financial savings by constructing one's own dental unit, which could be offset by one's lack of engineering and mechanical knowledge.

Disadvantages

- This approach requires experimentation and time to create a functional unit (in most cases, if the time spent in researching and assembling a dental station were spent in clinical practice, the practitioner would earn enough income to purchase a fully assembled, turnkey unit).
- Turnkey units have been tested, and they are warranteed and serviceable.
- The practitioner will find, in most cases, the return on investment in a dental compressor will justify the purchase of a turnkey unit.

Compressor Maintenance

- All compressors with air storage tanks require periodic drainage of condensation from the tank (C).
- The last-stage regulator should be set between 30 and 40 psi (D).
- The pressure in the tank may be 80 to 120 psi, depending on the brand.

Compressor Accessories

- Filters to filter out oil and water from the compressed air.
- Dryers to dry the air.
- Water filters to filter the water before entering the handpiece.

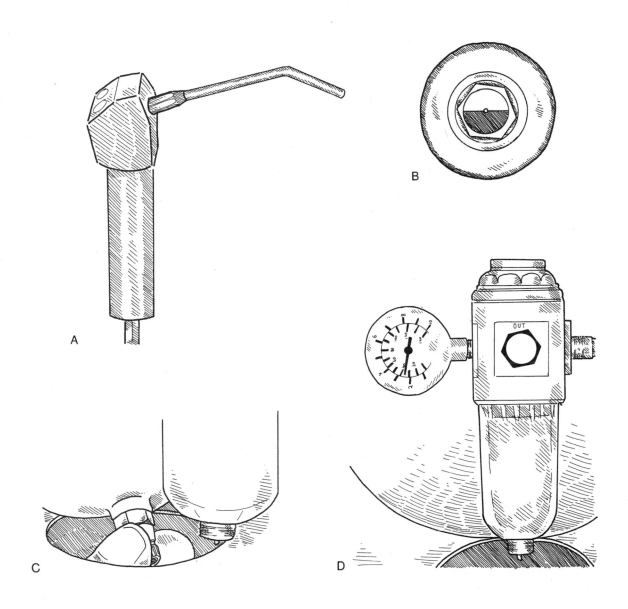

A

B

C

D

Handpieces

- Handpieces are instruments that enable the operator to work on teeth.
- Many types of handpieces are available, and they can be categorized into three basic types: low-speed, high-speed, and sonic scalers.

General Maintenance

- A handpiece should never be turned on without a bur or "blank" inserted into the chuck to prevent damage.
- Follow the manufacturer's recommendations on handpiece lubrication and air pressure.
- Lubricant should be placed in the smaller of the two large holes (A, B).

Low-Speed Handpieces

Comment

- Low-speed air-driven handpieces operate within 5000 to 20,000 rpm.

Uses

- They can be used for polishing with prophy angles.
- Contra angles can be attached to allow use of burs, endodontic files, polishing discs, and other specialized instruments requiring slower speeds and higher torques.

Advantages

- High torque; less likely to "stall out."
- Slower speed for cutting bone.

Disadvantages

- Low speed is a disadvantage when drilling into or sectioning teeth; increases working time and tissue heat.
- May shatter tooth if the bur binds while cutting the tooth.
- May create thermal injury because of the slow speed and pressure between the bur and tooth surface (drilling pressure).
- Usually do not have water as a coolant and irrigant.

Autoclave Option
Comment

- Many of the newer low-speed handpieces can be autoclaved.

Advantage

- Increases rust resistance.

Maintenance

- Lubricate according to manufacturer's instructions.
- If a heavy oil is used, spray with a light oil (WD-40) once every 2 weeks to help dissolve oil accumulations.

- Run the handpiece for 20 to 30 seconds after lubrication.
- Between patients, wipe exterior with a gauze sponge lightly soaked with alcohol.

Accessories: Prophy Angles
Comments

- Prophy angles are used to polish teeth.
- There are two types of prophy angle rubber cup attachments: snap-on and screw-on. Which to use is an individual preference, but it must match the attachment configuration of the end of the prophy angle. Some prophy angles accept either type of cup.

Circular Prophy Angles
Comments

- These prophy angles rotate 360 degrees.
- Metal models are manufactured, some to be disposed of when they break and some to be repaired.
- Plastic models are disposable and are designed for single use.

Advantages

- Circular prophy angles tend to be inexpensive.
- The inexpensive models are replaced rather than repaired.

Disadvantages

- Require disassembling and lubricating.
- May "spit" oil, contaminating the prepared dental surface.

Oscillating Prophy Angles
Comments

- The oscillating prophy angle oscillates back and forth 90 degrees.
- This style is a sealed unit.

Advantages

- This style does not require lubrication.
- Prophy paste is not thrown because the cup does not spin.
- Hair does not become trapped around the cup.

Disadvantages

- Expensive to purchase.
- Repairs, if possible, may cost more than a new prophy angle.

Maintenance of Nonsealed Prophy Angles

- The prophy angle can be disassembled and lubricated. There are usually two locations where the instrument can be opened for cleaning: the head and the cap. With most prophy angles, only one method needs to be used.

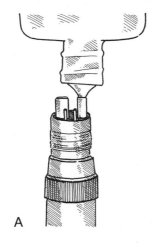

A

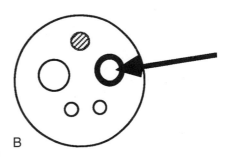

B

Removal of Head

Step 1—The head is unscrewed by turning it counterclockwise (A).

Step 2—The gears are cleaned with WD-40 or other solvent (B).

Step 3—The gears are lubricated with Prophy Lube* or other appropriate light-gear lubricant (C).

Step 4—The head is replaced by screwing it on clockwise.

Removal of Cap

Step 1—The cap is unscrewed by turning it clockwise (D).

Step 2—The gears are cleaned with WD-40 (E).

Step 3—The gears are lubricated with Prophy Lube (F).

Step 4—The cap is replaced by screwing it on counterclockwise.

---

*Young Dental Manufacturing, 13705 Shoreline Ct., Earth City, MO 63045

Accessories: Contra Angles

• Specific contra angles can increase or decrease the revolutions per minute at the working end, change angulation, or provide 90 degree rotation. Typically, a 4:1 step-up contra angle is used in low-speed electric motor handpieces and increases the speed from 20,000 to 80,000 rpm. A typical down-step contra angle is a 10:1 reduction gear and is used to reduce the speed, for example, in the employment of spiral paste fillers or in dental prosthetic procedures.

• Contra angles use right-angle (RA) or latch-type burs, which have larger-diameter shanks than high-speed burs.

• Straight low-speed handpieces use handpiece (designated HP) burs, which are longer and even greater in diameter than RA bur shanks.

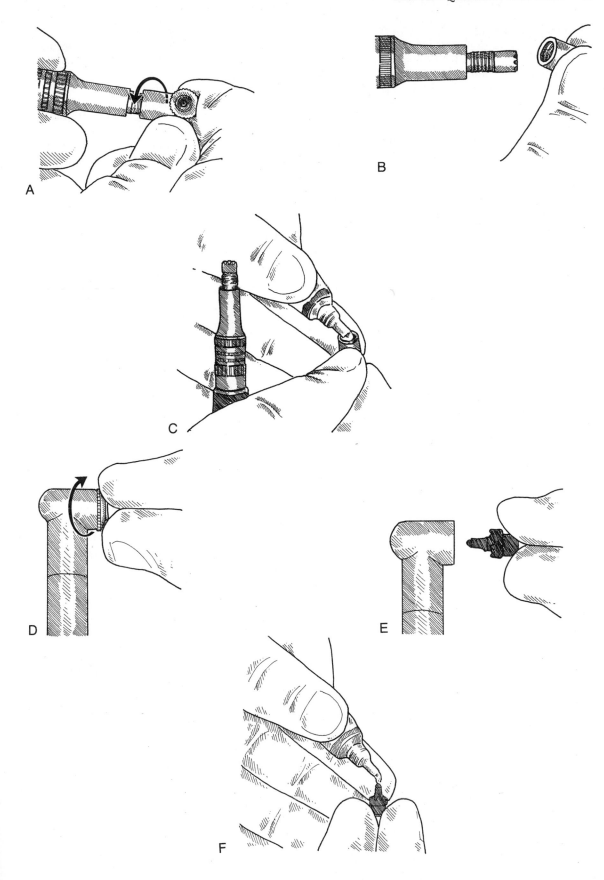

Low-Speed Burs
- Burs are held by handpieces in three ways: straight, latch, and friction grip (FG).
- The straight bur (designated HP) *(A)* fits directly into the straight low-speed handpiece.

Changing Straight Burs
Step 1—Twist the collar to open the chuck *(B)*. Proper position is usually noted by dots on the handpiece.

Step 2—Remove straight bur and replace with new bur *(C)*.

Step 3—Twist chuck latch collar to close, as noted by dots on the handpiece *(D)*.

Latch Burs
- This type of bur, also called an RA bur *(E)*, fits into a contra angle that holds the bur in place.

Changing Latch-Type Burs
Step 1—Holding the contra angle with the bur facing away from the operator, pivot the latch lever to the right *(F)*.

Step 2—Remove old bur *(G)*.

Step 3—Replace with new bur, lining up the flat portion of the bur to slide all the way in *(H)*.

Step 4—Pivot the latch back, and slide handle to the left until it clicks into place parallel to the contra angle *(I)*.

Although the FG bur can be used in appropriate low-speed handpieces, it is usually used in high-speed handpieces and is discussed in that section.

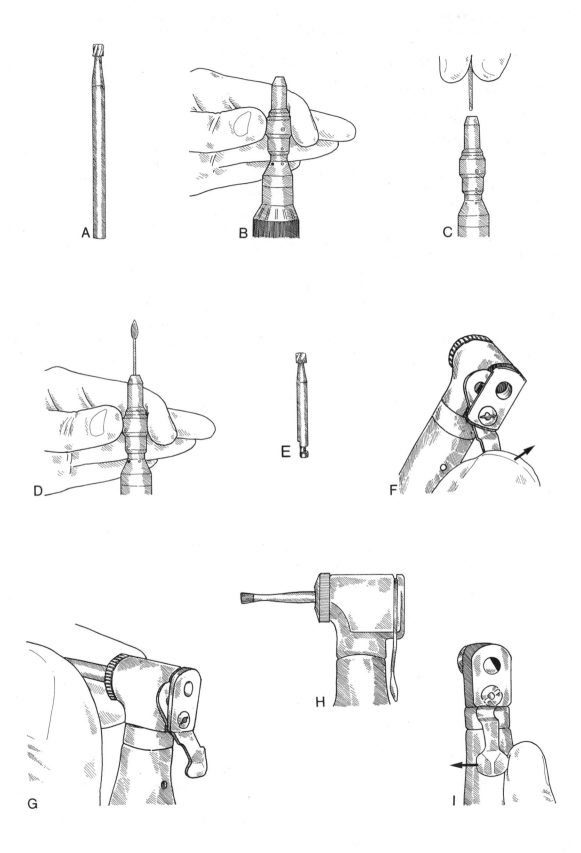

Types of Burs/Drills

- Many types of low-speed burs are similar to high-speed burs.
- Some types of burs and drills are available for low speed only.
- A bur converter is available, sold in packages of three, which allows FG burs to be used in latch contra angles *(A)*.

Gates Glidden Drills

Comments

- Have relatively long, narrow shafts with a flame-shaped boring head *(B)*.
- Have bands on the shaft to indicate size.

Uses

- Expands the opening into the endodontic system for easier instrumentation and filling of the canal during root-canal therapy.
- Tends to follow the path of a pre-existing hole.

Cautions

- If bound in the canal or bent, the drill will break, usually at the latch end of the shaft.

- Use with low-speed handpiece only.

Peeso Reamers

Comments

- Have a longer, torpedo-shaped head and shorter shaft than the Gates Glidden drill *(C)*.
- Have bands on the shank to indicate size.

Uses

- Widens the diameter of a prepared root canal in preparation for a post *(D)*.
- May cut its own path (use with caution), not necessarily following the canal *(E)*.

Mueller Bur

- The Mueller bur, like the Gates Glidden drill, has a long and narrow shaft, but the working end is that of a round cutting bur *(F)*.

Uses

- Is especially useful in performing pulpotomies on large canine teeth.
- Is usually supplied with a set of 5 burs numbered 1–5.

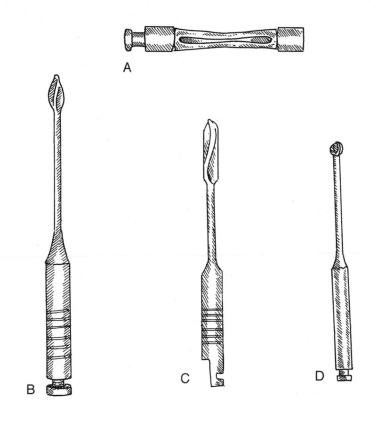

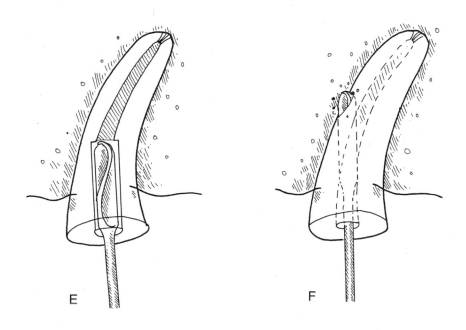

Green Stones
Comment
- Green stones are silicon carbide abrasive stones in carefully controlled grits of various shapes and sizes.

Uses
- For finishing restorations and producing a moderately rough surface.
- For bulk removal of restorative material before the final finish.

White Stones
Comment
- White stones are dense aluminum oxide abrasives of fine texture (A).

Use
- For finishing composite restorations and producing a smooth surface.

Discs
Comments
- Discs are flexible molded or cut paper, plastic, rubber, stone, porcelain, acrylic, or metal (B).
- Discs are supplied in ½ inch, ⅝ inch, ¾ inch, and ⅞ inch diameter.
- Discs may have their own shafts or may be held by a mandrel.
- Paper discs are prepared with sandpaper, cuttle, emery, or garnet finishes in extra fine, fine, medium, or coarse grits.
- Metal discs are either single-sided or double-sided, often with a diamond grit.

Use
- For finishing restorations, occlusal adjustment, and cutting tooth and material.
- Shofu polishing disc and mandrel (C).*

Wheels
Comment
- Wheels, composed of molded abrasive materials of phenolic resins or rubber with

an abrasive, come in various shapes and sizes (D).

Uses
- For laboratory procedures, finishing, and polishing.
- Shofu polishing disc (C).*

Mandrels
Comments
- Mandrels attach to the low-speed handpiece with latch, straight, or FG burs.
- Mandrels hold discs or wheels by pop-on, screw-on, or rod-type screw.
- Pop-on mandrel (E).
- Screw-on mandrel (F).
- Rod-type screw-on mandrel (G).

Use
- Hold finishing materials.

Paste Fillers
Comments
- Paste fillers are attached to the reduction gear contra angle of the low-speed handpiece (H).
- When rotated, they spin paste root-canal filling material into the canal.
- Because of their reverse spiral, they work in the forward (clockwise) rotation.
- They are manufactured in various sizes and lengths.

Advantage
- Paste fillers auger root-canal pastes or sealers apically into the canal, eliminating air bubbles.

Disadvantages
- May not fit into canal.
- Must use 10:1 reduction gear contra angles or may break spiral filler.
- Must have adequate-diameter access to prevent binding and breakage.

*Shofu Dental Corp., 4025 Bohannon Dr., Menlo Park, CA 94025

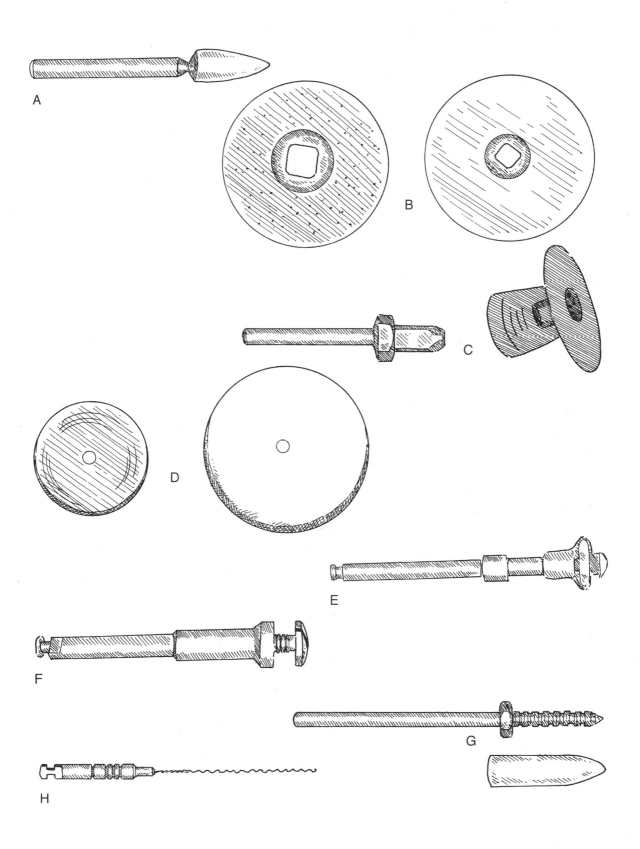

High-Speed Handpieces

Comment
- High-speed handpieces rotate in the range of 200,000 to 400,000 rpm.

Use
- Sectioning or otherwise cutting teeth, bone removal, endodontic access, cavity preparation, finishing restorations, and crown preparation.

Advantages
- High speed allows for rapid cutting of hard dental tissue.
- Water cooling protects dental tissue.
- Stalling due to low torque protects dental tissue from shattering.

Disadvantages
- Stalling may slow work.
- May create excessive heat or burning if inadequate water cooling or too much drilling pressure.
- Moisture or oil blown through the handpiece may destroy the turbine bearings.

Options
Wrenchless Handpieces
Comment
- This feature allows bur exchange without using a chuck key.

Advantage
- Speed in changing burs.

Disadvantage
- The push-button mechanism requires periodic replacement.

Fiberoptics
Comments
- Light is directed at the operating field.
- A light source provides light that is transferred by fiberoptics to the head of the handpiece.

Advantage
- Greater visualization of working area.

Disadvantages
- Bulbs can wear out.
- Models with flexible fiberoptic bundles require replacement of hoses as the fibers break during repeated use.
- Additional expense.

High-Speed Handpiece Maintenance
- Lubricant must be used on a regular basis. Follow the recommendations of the handpiece manufacturer for which spray or liquid lubricant to use. Oils are not recommended for most high-speed handpieces.
- The lubricant should be placed in the smaller of the two large holes (A).

Changing FG Burs
Overhead Chuck-Key Type
Step 1—Place chuck key over the head of the handpiece (B).

Step 2—Rotate the chuck-key knob counterclockwise (C).

Step 3—Remove old bur (D); if there is resistance, gently push in on bur to loosen the chuck grip and then pull the bur out.

Step 4—Push new bur in until completely seated (E). Caution: If the bur is not completely seated, the turbine bearings may be damaged.

Step 5—Rotate chuck-key knob clockwise just until bur is snug (F). Do not overtighten.

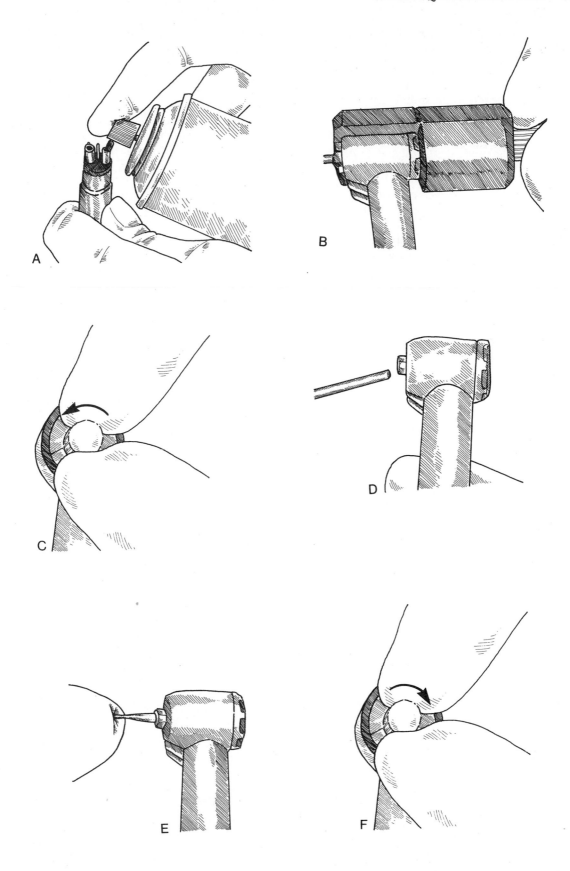

Replacement of Turbine Cartridge

Signs of defective turbine cartridge:

* Chuck does not tighten around the bur.
* Increased noise or vibration.
* Roughness felt when spinning bur by hand, with turbine in or out of handpiece.
* Handpiece stops intermittently.
* Handpiece does not work.

Cap-Style Handpiece Back

Step 1—Place "blank" bur in handpiece *(A)*. If bur that is in handpiece cannot be removed, proceed with caution to avoid cutting hands on bur.

Step 2—Place small metal ring (wrench) supplied with handpiece on cap of handpiece *(B)*.

Step 3—By rotating wrench counterclockwise, unscrew the handpiece cap and remove *(C)*.

Step 4—Press on blank or bur to remove turbine cartridge from handpiece head *(D)*.

Step 5—Place the new turbine cartridge into the handpiece head *(E)*.

Step 6—Align the new turbine cartridge with pin side up *(F)*. If the pin is not lined up with the slot, the turbine cartridge will not slide completely into the handpiece head *(G)*.

Step 7—Slide cartridge all the way into handpiece head *(H)*.

Step 8—Replace handpiece cap by twisting wrench clockwise *(I)*.

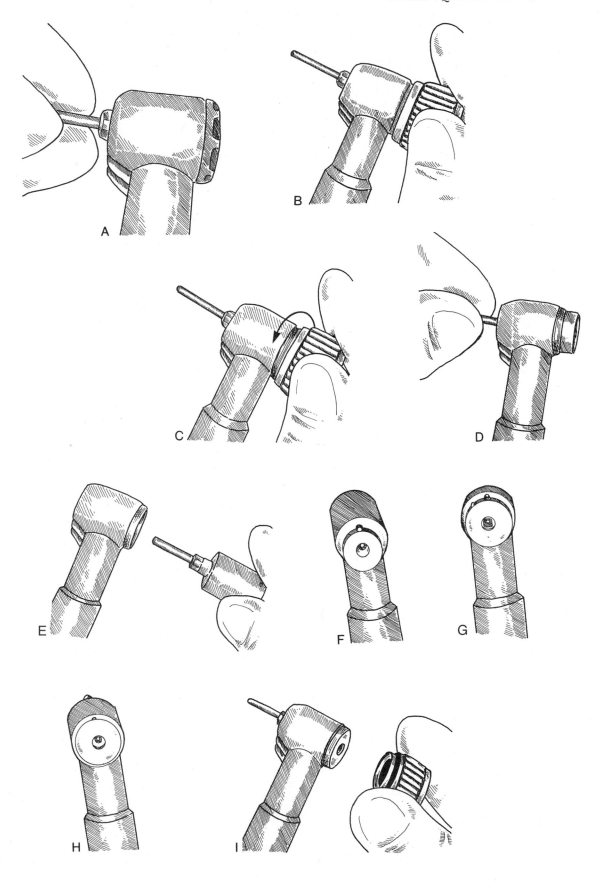

Handpiece Burs

- High-speed handpieces use FG burs.
- Only high-speed burs should be used with high-speed handpieces.
- There are three parts: shank (the portion that attaches to the handpiece); shaft (the portion from the shank to the head); and head (the working portion).
- Heads may be denoted as S (short) or L (long); if no letter, the head is standard length.
- Standard shanks are 19.0 mm long and 1.6 mm in diameter.
- Longer shanks are denoted as surgical length *(A)*. They are 25 mm long and 1.6 mm in diameter.
- The shanks of burs that fit into straight handpieces, designated in catalogs as (HP), are 44.5 mm long and 2.35 mm in diameter. Low-speed latch burs that are designated (RA) in catalogs have regular shanks that are 22 mm long by 2.35 mm in diameter and are also supplied in surgical length with shanks 26 mm long by 2.35 mm in diameter (Table 2–1).
- Flutes can be manufactured plain, without notches *(B)*; or cross-cut, with notches *(C)*.
- Most cutting burs are 6-fluted. Finishing burs have 10 or more flutes.
- "Bur type" refers to the shape of the head of the bur. Most shapes come in plain or cross-cut. Common shapes are round, cylinder (fissure), taper fissure, pear, flame, inverted cone, and wheel.
- The tips of the bur can be cutting, noncutting, square, or rounded. The noncutting tip is used to cut straight sides without cutting the floor of the cavity preparation. The cutting tip may cut into the cavity floor. The square tip creates a 90 degree angle at the interface between the floor and the wall. This may be difficult to fill with restorative material and creates a break on line angles. The round tip creates a rounded transition between the floor and wall. This interface is easier to fill and is less fragile.

Round Burs (¼, ½, 1, 2, 3, 4, 6, 8)
Uses
- The smaller burs (¼, ½) can be used to create retentive grooves in tooth structure or to mark locations for larger low-speed bur placement *(D)*. They can also be used as all-purpose cutting burs in smaller teeth, such as those in domestic cats and toy breed dogs.

Comments
- Bur tips as small as ¼ round may be easily bent or detached from the shank unnoticed by the clinician as they are installed or inadvertently bumped against a piece of equipment.
- The medium burs (1, 2) can be used for initial cavity preparation and outline.
- The larger burs are used for bulk removal of dental tissue.
- Some round burs are designed to be placed parallel to the tooth, with the shank as a limit to marking cutting depth in crown preparation.

Fissure Burs (556, 557, 558)
Comment
- The sides of the head are parallel *(E)*.

Use
- They have straight, parallel sides that create parallel cavity sides.

Tapered-Fissure Burs (plain 168, 169, 169L, 170, 170L, 171, 171L, 172, 172L, 173; cross-cut 699, 700, 701, 701L, 702, 702L, 703, 703L)
Comment
- Their head is narrower at the tip than toward the shank *(F)*.

Uses
- These are general-purpose burs that can be used for bulk removal of dental tissue, for sectioning teeth for extraction, and for endodontic access.
- When held perpendicular to a cavity preparation, they can be used to prevent an undercut.

Table 2–1 • SHANK DIMENSIONS

Bur Shank Type	Short Shank	Standard Length	Surgical Length	Shank Diameter
Friction Grip	16.0 mm	19.0 mm	36.0 mm	60.0 mm
Straight Handpiece		44.5 mm		2.35 mm
Latch Type		22.0 mm	26.0 mm	2.35 mm

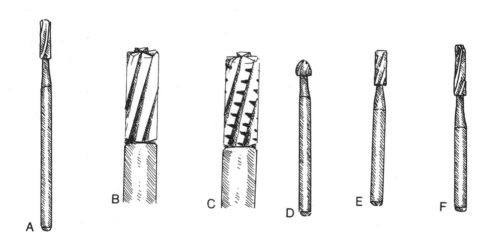

Pear-Shaped Burs (330, 331, 331L, 332)
Uses
- These are general-purpose burs that can be used for root-canal access or undercutting dentin in cavity preparation *(A)*.
- They create smoothly rounded internal line angles.

Flame Burs
- They have a pointed tip and wider body that rounds toward the shank.
- One of the commonly used Rotopro burs has the flame shape.

Inverted-Cone Burs (33½, 34, 35, 37, 38, 39)
Comment
- Their head is wider toward the tip than toward the shaft *(B)*.

Uses
- Smaller burs are used to penetrate into root canals and to create a mechanical interlock in restoration preparations in the smaller teeth.
- Larger burs are used to undercut cavity preparations to create a mechanical interlock.

Special-Use Burs
Rotopro Bur*
- Used for scaling teeth *(C)*.
- Frequency is 30,000 cycles per second at the working tip, depending on speed of air turbine and air pressure.
- See the section on Equipment for Periodontics for information.

*Ellman International, Inc., 1135 Railroad Ave., Hewlett NY 11557

Multifluted Finishing Burs
- Come in a variety of shapes.
- Have 10 to 30 flutes; the more flutes, the smoother the finish.

Diamond Burs (Many Sizes and Shapes)
- Cut by grinding and can be used for cutting *(D)* or finishing *(E)*.
- Are manufactured by electroplating diamond grit onto a one-piece bur blank by either a nickel or chromium bonding material.
- Use natural or artificial diamonds.
- Use different grits of diamonds; commonly used are extra fine, fine, medium, and coarse.

Bur Accessories
Bur-Cleaning Brush
- Bur-cleaning brushes clean the flutes of the bur but do not sharpen the flutes *(F)*.
- The brush is used by brushing the bur without running the handpiece.

Diamond-Bur Cleaning Stone
- The diamond-bur cleaning stone removes debris from the surface of the diamond bur *(G)*.
- Using the high-speed handpiece, the bur is run over a wet stone.

Bur Block
- The bur block is used to store burs *(H)*.
- Some burs are autoclavable, and some are manufactured with a hinged cover.

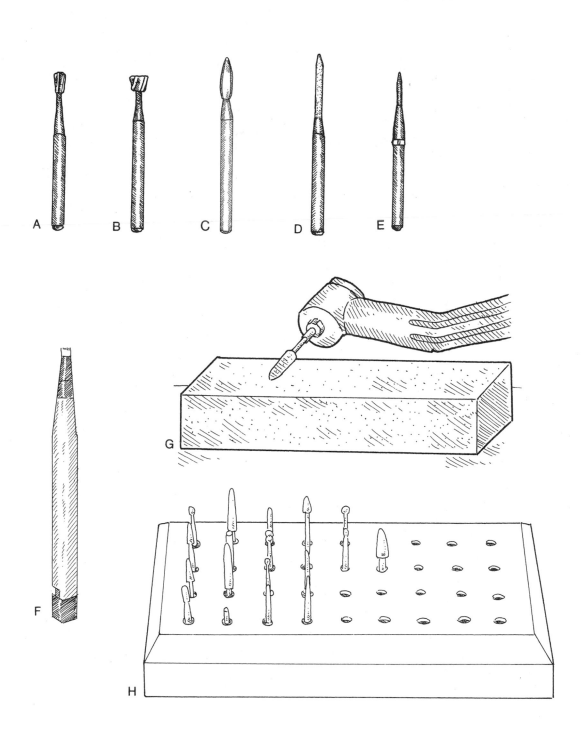

DENTAL RADIOLOGY EQUIPMENT

Veterinary Medical Units

Comment

- 50 to 500 mA veterinary medical units may be used to expose dental film.

Advantage

- No additional expense required when using standard veterinary medical machines.

Disadvantages

- The patient must be moved between the dental area and radiology area during procedures.
- The flexibility of most veterinary medical units does not allow the radiographic head to move for optimum positioning. Thus, the patient must be positioned for most radiographic views; that is more time-consuming and difficult than moving the radiographic head alone.

Dental Radiographic Units

Comments

- Used or new dental units are available.
- They are usually low-milliamperage units suited for dental film exposure.

Advantages

- Dental radiology may be carried out in the area where the dentistry is performed.
- The veterinary medical radiographic unit is available for use by the rest of the hospital while the dental procedure is performed.
- A higher-quality image is generated by parallel x-rays and a smaller focal spot than in most medical units.

Film-Processing Systems

- Film may be processed either manually or with an automatic processor.

Manual Processing

- There are three types of manual developing solutions: standard veterinary dip-tank, one-step rapid process, and two-step rapid process.

Standard Veterinary Dip-Tank Solution

Comment

- The regular developer and fixing solutions that are normally used in manual processing of veterinary radiographic film may be used to develop dental film.

Advantage

- If the hospital is already using this system, these solutions are available at no additional cost.

Disadvantages

- Loss of detail.
- Longer processing time.

One-Step Rapid Processing Solution

Comment

- A single developing solution that contains both developer and fixer to process the film in approximately 1 minute.

Advantage

- Single-step processing.

Disadvantages

- Loss of detail.
- "Greening" of processed film may occur several days after developing.

Two-Step Rapid Processing Solution

Comment

- A developing solution and a separate fixing solution designed to process film in approximately 1 minute.

Advantages

- Provide high-quality developing and rapid processing.
- If used properly, create archival-quality films that may be stored for years without loss of quality.

Automatic Processing

- There are two types of mechanical processing systems: the large-film automatic processors and the smaller dental processors.

Large-Film Processors

Comments

- Large-film automatic processors are commonly found in veterinary hospitals.
- Dental radiographic film may be taped to larger radiographic film and sent through the processor.

Advantage

- None; in most practices, manual systems are best.

Disadvantages

- Risk loss of film in the processor.
- Must use leader film to attach the smaller film.
- Possible damage to processor if improper tape is used.
- Requires more time to develop the film than manual methods.

Small-Film Processors

Comment

- Small-film processors are designed to transport dental films through the processing solutions and the dryer.

Advantages

- Greater quality control.
- No need to use leader film.

Disadvantages

- Expense.
- Requires greater time to process than manual rapid process methods.
- Location of processing is remote to the dental operatory.

Location of Processing

Dip Tanks for Darkrooms

Comment

- Tanks or containers may be used in the darkroom with rapid processing solutions to process the radiographs.

Advantages

- Inexpensive.
- Faster developing time than with traditional chemicals.

Disadvantages

- Less quality control than mechanical processors.
- Personnel must leave the dental area to go to darkroom to process the film.
- May create additional mess in the darkroom due to inadvertent spillage.

Chairside Darkrooms

Comment

- Chairside darkrooms are small, portable, lightproof boxes that have hooded hand ports for processing the film in darkness. Because this process is manual, a special see-through safety filter plastic cover allows the operator to see the film and dip tanks. The cover does not allow exposing light to affect the film.

Advantages

- Rapid (usually less than 1 minute) process.
- Avoids tying up a darkroom.

Disadvantages

- Use caution to avoid opening the lid accidentally and exposing the film during processing.
- The chemical containers are small, and the chemicals must be kept fresh.
- The amber filter will protect the film for a limited time and intensity of light.
- Must have space at tableside or in the dental area.

Maintenance

- The frequency of chemical change depends on the number of radiographs processed, the amount of exposure to air, and the age of the chemicals.
- Close lids to unused chemicals.
- Replace damaged hand porthole diaphragms.
- Clean box with mild detergent and water.
- Do not damage the porthole sleeves with jewelry.
- Chairside darkrooms need to be used in subdued-light areas. To test the location, place the chairside darkroom where you plan to use it. Open a film packet in the chairside darkroom. Lay the film on top of one of the jars and cover all but one portion of it. At 15- to 30-second intervals, uncover another portion of the film until the last portion has been exposed for the set time interval. Develop the film in the normal fashion. After fixing, examine the film for fogging. If there is no fogging, it is safe to develop film at that location under the same light-intensity conditions. If there is fogging, determine the length of time during which fogging developed and whether or not you can process films in less time at that location and light intensity. If the fogging occurred in a short time, the location or the amount of light needs to be changed.

EQUIPMENT FOR PERIODONTICS

Sonic Scalers

Comments

- Sonic scalers are used for gross calculus removal from teeth *(A)*.
- Inside most sonic scalers is a shaft that is connected to the air supply and tip.
- The vibration at the tip of the scaler is caused by air passing out of a hole in the shaft that spins a ring that encircles the shaft.
- There is little difference between the action of the ultrasonic scaler and the sonic scaler on the surface of the tooth.
- Frequency is 8000 to 18,000 cycles per second at the working tip.

Advantages

- Very little heat is created at the working tip when compared with the ultrasonic scaler.
- There is less chance of injuring the tooth with pulp hyperthermia.
- The user does not have to sharpen the instrument.
- The scaler performs a lavage function by irrigating and flushing while effecting calculus removal.

Disadvantages

- Conflicting reports regarding the relative strengths of the sonic and ultrasonic scaler. One study showed that some models of sonic scalers were as effective at calculus removal as ultrasonic scalers set at maximum power.[3] However, another study claimed that the ultrasonic scaler cleared hard deposits of calculus faster.[4]
- Some units must be cleaned and lubricated periodically.
- Sonic scalers have higher rate of breakdown than ultrasonic scalers.

Ultrasonic Scalers

Comments

- The ultrasonic scaler has long been the mainstay of cleaning teeth in veterinary dentistry.
- Several types of ultrasonic scalers are available (Table 2–2).
- Generally, the higher the frequency, the shorter the working time, and the smaller the excursion, the less trauma that is delivered to the surface of the tooth.

Uses

- Removes gross calculus from the teeth.
- Removes orthodontic bonding materials.

Advantages

- Durability.
- No need to sharpen instrument.
- Performs a lavage function by irrigating and flushing while effecting calculus removal.
- Odontoson designed for subgingival use; can easily deliver medicated solutions subgingivally.

Disadvantages

- Heat production and possible injury to tooth.
- Expense of replacement tips.
- With improper use, can damage enamel.

Tip-Only Replacement

Comment

- Some models are available in which only the tip needs to be replaced *(B)*.

Advantage

- Replacement of piezo tips is about half the cost of a whole leaf stack arrangement on a magnetostrictive unit.

Disadvantages

- Piezo tips, due to higher frequency of operation, suffer metal fatigue and require re-

Table 2–2 • TYPES OF ULTRASONIC SCALERS

Type of Scaler	Type of Action of Working Tip	Frequency (cps)	Excursion at Tip (mm)
Magnetostrictive (Cavitron-like)	Figure-of-eight	25,000 or 30,000	0.8–1.1
Piezo electric	Linear	45,000	0.2–0.4
Ferromagneto-strictive (Odontoson)*	Circular	42,000	0.01–0.2

*Odontoson-Periogiene, P.O. Box 9, Fort Collins, CO 80522

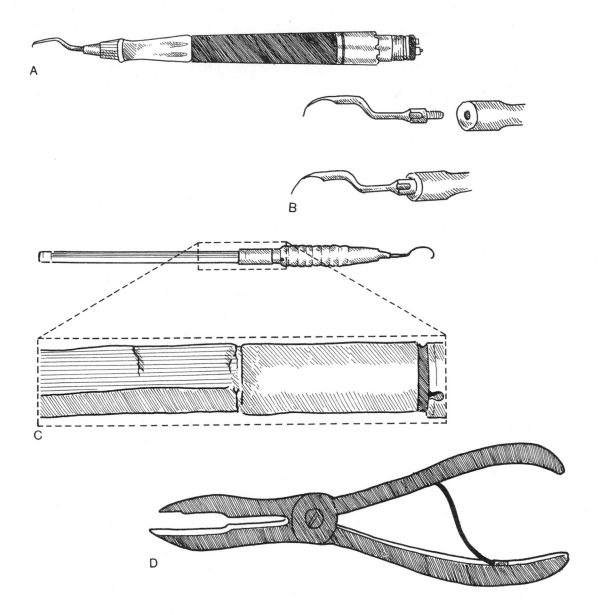

placement twice as often as the magnetostrictive stack.
- May require entire handpiece to be repaired or replaced.

Pot/Stack Magnetostrictive Model Maintenance

- The leaves should be inspected periodically
  for fracture and replaced if fractures are
  found *(C)*.
- The ferroceramic rod attached to the ferroceramic magnetostrictive tip, although
  inexpensive and easy to replace, will break
  readily if dropped.
- The longevity of any of the tip parts for all
  the units can be increased by adjusting the
  power of the unit during the procedure
  and using only the energy required for that
  particular task.

Calculus-Removal Forceps

Comment

- Calculus-removal forceps are specially designed forceps used for the removal of
  gross calculus *(D)*.

Advantage

- Quick removal of large pieces of gross calculus.

Disadvantages

- Remove only gross supragingival calculus
  (and are only one of the first steps of a
  complete and thorough prophylaxis).
- Can damage the crown, enamel, or gum
  tissue if used improperly.

Large Hand Instruments

Dental Hoe (Chisel)

Comment

- The working tip is a wide, chisel-like blade *(A)*.

Use

- Supragingival gross calculus removal.

Advantage

- Strong instrument.

Disadvantage

- For removal of large deposits only, not for removal of subgingival or small calculus and plaque.

Dental Claw

Comments

- The dental hoe and claw were once the mainstay hand instruments of veterinary dentistry.
- The claw is a large, thick, sickle-shaped universal scaler *(B)*.

Use

- To break off large pieces of supragingival gross calculus.

Advantage

- Removal of gross calculus in absence of sonic or ultrasonic scalers or calculus-removing forceps.

Disadvantages

- Slow speed.
- Some personal hand strength required.
- Potential damage to the tooth and gingival structures.

Fine Hand Instruments

- The selection of a curette or scaler is a matter of personal preference.
- If you do not like a particular instrument, do not replace it with the same one.
- Even if properly used and sharpened, these instruments need to be replaced periodically.

- When properly performed, some authorities believe hand scaling is preferable to ultrasonic scaling. It causes less damage to the tooth structure and is more efficient.[2]
- Hand scaling requires special training to avoid fatigue and repetitive-stress occupational injuries. A combination of hand scaling and mechanical scaling is desirable in veterinary medicine.
- Use of fine scalers lets the operator remove calculus and plaque from above and below the gumline.[5] It also provides for access to remote surfaces not available to mechanical means.

Options

Comments

- Curettes and scalers are made of carbon steel or stainless steel.
- Dry storage of dental instruments is an accepted procedure in human dentistry.

Carbon Steel
Advantage

- Carbon steel instruments maintain a sharper edge than stainless steel instruments, provided they are kept rust-free.

Disadvantage

- Carbon steel instruments rust and become brittle if left for extended periods in water containing cold disinfecting solutions or if steam-autoclaved without a rust inhibitor.

Stainless Steel
Advantage

- Stainless steel instruments are rust-resistant.

Disadvantage

- Stainless steel instruments become dull if left in disinfecting solutions and do not maintain as sharp an edge as carbon steel.

Replaceable Tips
Comment

- Some manufacturers make hand instruments that have a cone-socket handle and removable tips *(C)*.

Advantages

- The tips rather than the entire instrument are replaced when the tip is worn down or broken.
- The operator can select different tips for each end of the instrument and customize the instrument.

Disadvantage

- Replaceable-tip instruments are generally expensive to purchase initially.

Scalers

Comment

- The blade of a scaler is triangular and tapers to a pointed tip, with two parallel cutting edges *(D)*.

Use

- Scalers are used for supragingival scaling.

Advantages

- The angulation of a scaler is convenient for supragingival scaling.

- The pointed tip may be used to remove calculus from pits and fissures and interproximal areas *(E)*.

Disadvantages

- Because of the shape and sharp tip, the scaler should not be used below the gumline. It can distend and lacerate soft tissues.
- Scalers and curettes are designed in universal styles. These instruments can be used on all teeth. Scalers and curettes are also supplied for area-specific use. In area-specific curettes of individual styles, as the numbers of the names of the scalers increase, their use is designed for teeth progressively farther back in the mouth. This does not necessarily hold true for universal instruments.

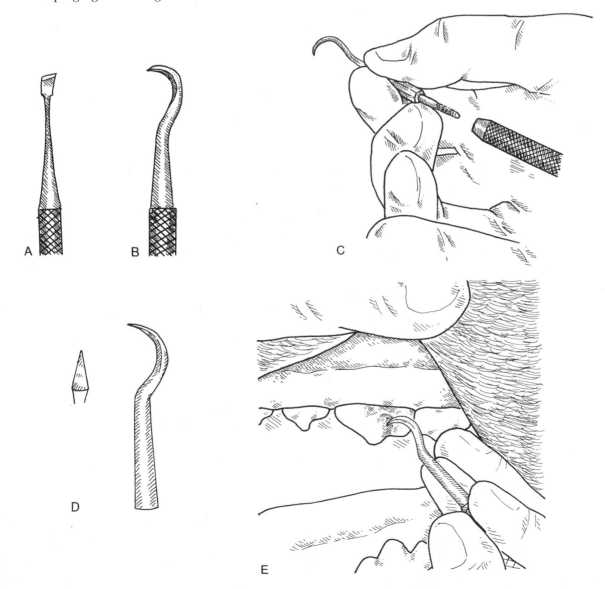

A   B   C

D   E

Types

Jacquette 2Y–3Y Scaler *(A)*
- Has medium blade, acute round angle at the blade, and no shaft; the blade is slightly longer than that of the Morse 0–00.

N135 Scaler
- Has medium shaft, thin blade with sharp curve, good for supragingival interproximal work between incisors or between maxillary fourth premolar and first molar *(B)*.

H6–H7 or N6–N7 Scaler
- Long, sickle-shaped blade of medium thickness *(C)*.

Morse 0–00 Scaler
- Has no angle; very thin, short blade; acute 90 degree angulation *(D)*.

Maintenance

- To remain functional, a scaler must be kept sharp. Sharp scalers fracture, cleave, and remove calculus; dull scalers ineffectively crush and burnish calculus.
- Ideally, hand instruments should be sharpened between each use.

Curettes

Comments

- Curettes have two sharp working edges, a flat face, and a rounded back *(E)*.
- Looking end-on, they have a half-moon shape.
- Short-shanked instruments are particularly useful in cats and small dogs. Long-shanked After Five* curettes are designed for periodontal pockets greater than 5 mm and are particularly useful on the palatal side of dog canines that have periodontal disease. Additionally, they have a shorter blade, enabling them to work well in narrow pockets.

Uses

- Removing calculus and plaque above and below the gumline.
- Subgingival curettage and root planing.

Advantage

- The rounded tip and back are less traumatic to soft tissue and adapt easily to root surfaces.

---

*After Five Curettes, Hu-Friedy Co., 3232 N. Rockwell St., Chicago, IL 60618

Disadvantages

- The rounded tip may not be able to get into all crevices.
- If used improperly, may break or cause tissue damage.

Types

Universal Curettes
- Can be used throughout the mouth; thus, they are "universal." Although the anatomy varies from humans to animals, this general concept is still valid.

Gracey Curettes
- Are area-specific; lower numbers are for incisors and canines, higher numbers are for instruments used on caudal teeth.

Columbia ¹³⁄₁₄ Curette
- Has short shank, medium-to-thin blade, and medium curve *(F)*.

Barnhart ⁵⁄₆ Curette
- Has short shank, medium blade, and small-to-medium curve *(G)*.

Columbia ¾ Curette
- Has medium shank, medium blade, and small-to-medium curve *(H)*.

Posterior Curettes
- Have a longer terminal shank for interproximal access.

4R–4L Curette
- Has a medium shank, medium blade, and medium curve, primarily for posterior teeth.

2R–2L Curette
- Has a long shaft, medium blade, and medium curve; fits shape of canine teeth, primarily anterior teeth.

Barnhart ½ Curette
- Has a long shaft, thin blade, and medium curve; good for root planing in tight fits.

Cleaning and Care of Scalers and Curettes

Step 1—The instrument should be washed with a disinfectant soap* to remove all debris.

Step 2—The instrument should be dried.

Step 3—The instrument is sharpened (see the following section, Sharpening Scalers and Curettes).

Step 4—The instrument is soaked in a disinfectant solution, autoclaved, dry-sterilized, or gas-sterilized.

---

*Nolvasan Scrub, Fort Dodge Laboratories, 800 Fifth St. NW, Fort Dodge, IA 50510

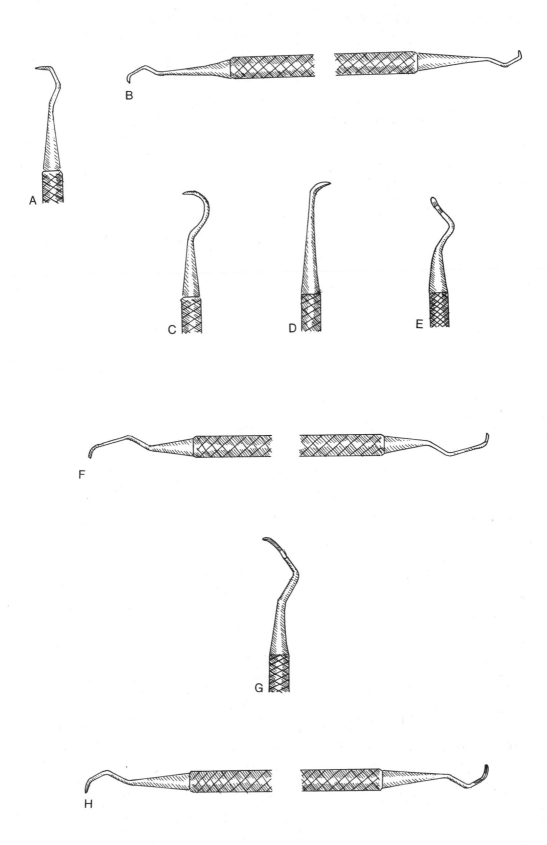

Sharpening Scalers and Curettes

Objectives

- Remove as little of the instrument as possible.
- Obtain sharp edge.
- Retain original design of the instrument.

Materials: Sharpening Stones

- Sharpening stones are used to restore the cutting edge on a dull instrument without changing the original design of that instrument.[6]
- The coarser the stone, the faster the sharpening, and the rougher the edge.
- Fine stones are used for sharpening only slightly dull instruments and for finishing sharpening to remove rough edges or flash.
- Coarse stones are used for dull instruments and for reshaping.

Arkansas Stones
Comments
- Fine stones.
- Used with oil.

Advantages
- Give a fine finish.
- Relatively little of the instrument is reduced.

Disadvantage
- May be slow if used to recontour the instrument.

Maintenance
- After use, should be wiped clean.
- May be cleaned with routine soaps or detergents.
- May be autoclaved.

India Stones
Comments
- Fine or medium in coarseness.
- Used with oil.

Advantage
- Can sharpen excessively dull instruments.

Disadvantage
- May wear the instrument away excessively if used for routine sharpening.

Maintenance
- After use, should be wiped clean.
- May be cleaned with routine soaps or detergents.
- May be autoclaved.

Ceramic Stones
Comments
- Made from compressed glass.
- Used with water or dry.
- Fine to medium in coarseness.

Advantages
- Do not create mess, as does oil.
- Come in kits.*

Disadvantage
- Expensive.

Moving Flat Stone Technique
Advantages
- Easiest technique to learn.
- Good visibility of sharpening surface.
- Sharpens side of instrument, maintaining strength *(A)*.

Disadvantage
- Some operators prefer stationary stone technique.

Materials
- Stone oil.
- Sharpening stone.

Technique

Step 1—A drop of oil is placed on an India or Arkansas sharpening stone *(B)*.

Step 2—The oil is distributed over the face of the stone by wiping with a tissue *(C)*.

Step 3—The instrument is held vertically over the side of a table with the edge to be sharpened down *(D)* so that the face of the working end is parallel to the floor.

Step 4—The stone is placed so that the open angle between the face and stone is 110 degrees *(E)*. This creates a 70 degree angle between the face and side of the blade. The stone is drawn up and down to sharpen the blade while maintaining this angle.

Step 5—The sharpening sequence always ends on the down stroke so as not to leave a rough edge.

Step 6—The other side of the blade and the blades of the opposite tip are sharpened in a similar manner.

---

*Sharpen-Rite, P.O. Box 03371, Portland, OR 97203

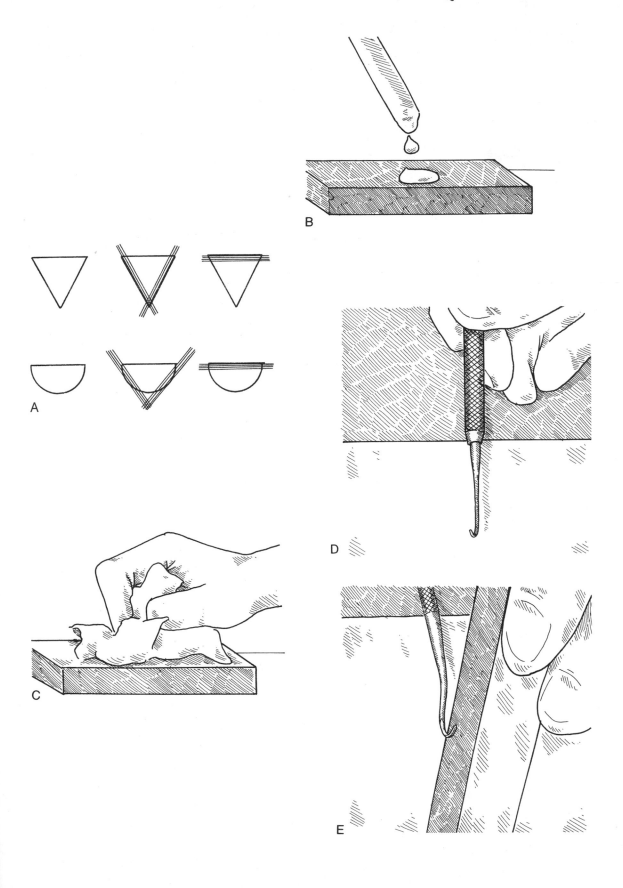

Moving Flat Stone/Sharpen-Rite Technique

Advantages
- Guides the inexperienced sharpener effectively.
- Helps achieve a sharp instrument.

Disadvantages
- Cumbersome and slow to use.
- Requires time to read instructions and understand.

Materials
- Sharpen-Rite kit.*
- Does not require stone oil.

---

*Sharpen-Rite, P.O. Box 03371, Portland, OR 97203

Technique
Step 1—The Sharpen-Rite Guide is taped to the edge of a counter *(A)*.

Step 2—The operator is sitting directly in front of the countertop *(B)*.

Step 3—The stone is placed parallel to one of the two black lines marked "stone."

Step 4—The instrument is held with the toe pointing directly toward the operator and the operator's hand rests firmly on the countertop *(C)*.

Step 5—The instrument is lined up in the area corresponding to the marking for that type of instrument *(D)*.

Step 6—Keeping the stone parallel to the stone line, the stone is moved up and down to sharpen the instrument.

Step 7—The toe of the instrument is sharpened by repositioning the instrument at a 45 degree angle between the stone and face of the blade.

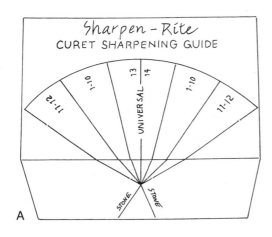

A

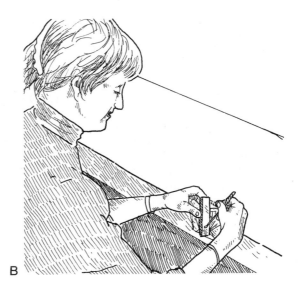

B

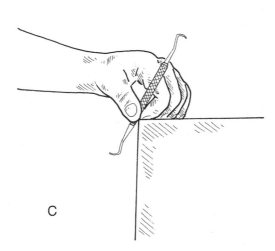

C

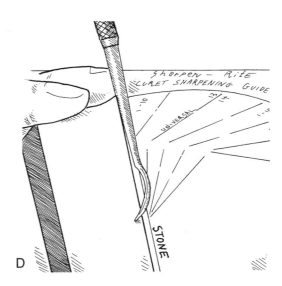

D

Stationary Flat Stone Technique
Advantage
- Once learned, may be the fastest technique to perform.

Disadvantage
- Takes time and practice to use this technique effectively.

Materials
- Stone oil.

Technique

Step 1—The stone is oiled as with other techniques.

Step 2—The stone is placed flat on a table and is held by hand *(A)*.

Step 3—The instrument is held in the opposite hand with a modified pencil grip *(B)*. The index finger and thumb hold the instrument while the middle, ring, and little fingers act as a guide and slide along the table. The blade to be sharpened is positioned with the face of the instrument opened at a 110 degree angle to the stone. The cutting edge is formed between the face and side of the blade, and that angle should be between 70 and 80 degrees. The instrument is moved back and forth on the stone while keeping the blade at this constant angle.

Conical Stone Technique
Advantage
- Less skill is involved in using a conical stone.

Disadvantages
- Decreases the strength of the instrument by decreasing the body of the blade, whereas the other techniques remove sides but keep the thickness *(C)*.
- Changes the angle between the face and side of the blade of a curette.

Materials
- Stone oil.

Technique

Step 1—A small amount of stone oil is placed on the stone *(D)*.

Step 2—The stone is wiped with a tissue *(E)*.

Step 3—The stone is placed on the face of the instrument and is rotated and, at the same time, rubbed along the face toward the tip *(F)*. One to three rotations over the face of the blade are made to remove excess flash or uneven edges.

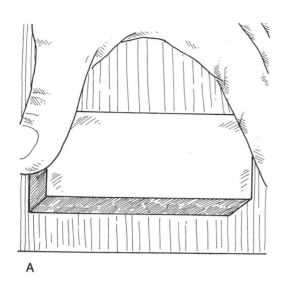

A

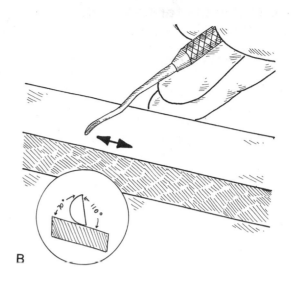

B

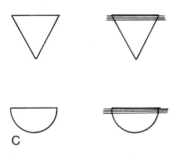

C

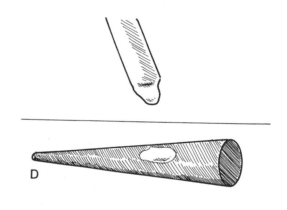

D

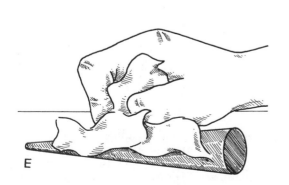

E

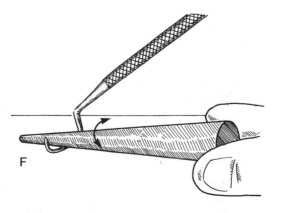

F

Instruments for Periodontal Diagnosis

Periodontal Probes

Comments

- Are either notched or color-coded and may be single-ended or double-ended in combination with another type of probe or explorer.
- May be contra-angled for more accurate reading on the distal side of teeth.

Use

- Measure gingival recession and periodontal pocket depth, allowing the evaluator to estimate epithelial attachment level.[5, 7]

Advantage

- Can be used to measure the degree of periodontal disease.

Disadvantage

- If used improperly, probes can damage epithelial attachment.

Types

Notched Probes
Comments
- Are generally notched in millimeters.
- Are either flat or round; flat probes are easier to fit into a thin sulcus; round probes are easier to see at different angles.
- Goldman Fox and Williams probes have notches at 1-2-3-(skips 4)-5-(skips 6)-7-8-9-10 mm *(A)*.

Advantage
- The notch is a clear indication of depth.

Disadvantage
- May not be as easy to read as color-coded probes.

Color-Coded Probes
Comments
- Have color-coded bands.
- Come in 10-, 11-, and 12 mm lengths.
- The 3-6-9-12 mm readings are popular markings *(B)*.

Advantages
- The longer probes may record deeper depths.

- The probes are longer and easier to see at different angles than are the flat probes.

Disadvantage
- Color coding may wear off in time or in ultrasonic cleaners; however, some manufacturers recoat probes for a reasonable cost.

World Health Organization Pressure Probe
- This probe mechanically closes a gap once 20 g of pressure in the gingival sulcus occurs. The closure of the gap on the head of the instrument can be visualized by the person charting the patient *(C)*. Twenty grams is the pressure that should be sustained in a healthy gingival sulcus before bleeding occurs. This probe comes color-coded in a variety of patterns.

Advantage
- Enables uniformity among staff members in measuring gingival bleeding indices.

Disadvantage
- Made of plastic and is more bulky than some of the metal instruments.

Periodontal Explorers

Comments

- Explorers are used to examine the tooth and detect abnormalities through the senses of touch and sound.[8]
- Of the several types of explorers available, the most common is the Shepherd hook (no. 23) *(D)*.
- The no. 17 explorer is shown in *(E)*. This explorer is particularly useful in determining the adequacy of a surface restoration preparation.
- The finer, more delicate tips allow greater tactile sensitivity.
- The more flexible steel helps tactility.

Use

- Explorers are used subgingivally to detect calculus and supra- and subgingival surface irregularities, to assess tooth mobility, to evaluate root smoothness,[9] and to probe for soundness.

Advantage

- Ability to easily detect decayed soft dental areas, open pulp chambers, subgingival calculus, and surface irregularities with minimal equipment.

Disadvantage

- May damage tissue.

Mirrors

Comments

- Dental mirrors are usually attached to handles for easier access and extension.

- Some mirrors come with light sources attached.
- Mirrors are supplied in several diameters, most commonly from ½ to ¾ inch.

Uses

- Mirrors are used for direct vision; retraction of lips, cheeks, and tongue; and illumination.
- Mirrors may be used for transillumination to detect caries.
- Large mirrors are used for intraoral photography.
- Saliva or warming the mirror may prevent fogging.

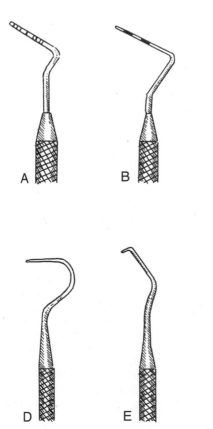

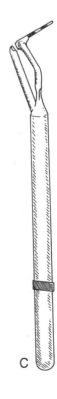

Instruments for Periodontal Surgery

- With a few additional instruments, the general veterinary surgical pack can be adapted for periodontal surgery.
- Necessary instruments are periodontal knives, periosteal elevators, curettes, and chisels.
- These instruments should be as fine as possible to allow delicate manipulation of tissues.

Scalpel Blades

Comments
- Generally, smaller blades are more useful for periodontal surgery.
- A no. 3 scalpel handle is used with these blades.

Types
No. 11
Comment
- The no. 11 blade has a sharp, triangular point *(A)*.

Uses
- Stab-type incisions.
- Delicate sulcular incisions, especially in extractions, to sever the epithelial attachment.

Advantage
- Sharp, pointed tip.

Disadvantage
- Pointed tip may not give as much control as other blades.

Nos. 12 and 12B "Hawk-Billed"
Comments
- Both have hooked-type tips
- No. 12 has a cutting surface on the inner side only *(B)*
- No. 12B has a cutting surface on both sides.

Uses
- Both may be used with a lifting (pulling) motion that places tension on the tissue, giving increased stability.
- Both provide interdental access.
- No. 12B may be used for pulling or pushing.
- Both may be used for flap, mucogingival, and graft operations; gingivoplasty; and gingivectomy.

Advantage
- Getting to distal surfaces that may not be reachable with no. 11 or no. 15C.

Disadvantage
- Tip may get locked in bone.
- Tip may break in osseous bone.

No. 15
Comment
- Thin blade *(C)*.

Advantages
- Finer blade than that of the larger small-animal veterinary blade (no. 10).
- Costs less than no. 10 blade.

Disadvantages
- May break if used for heavy-duty work.
- Becomes dull more quickly than no. 10 blade.

No. 15C
Comment
- Thinner, initially sharper blade than that of larger no. 15 *(D)*.

Advantages
- Allows for finer work.
- Costs less than no. 15 blade.

Disadvantages
- May break if used for heavy-duty work.
- Becomes dull more quickly than no. 15 blade.

Surgical Knives

Comment
- Various angles and shapes are available.

Use
- Periodontal surgery.

Advantages
- The angulation of the surgical knives gives flexibility and ease of cutting soft tissue.
- Thicker than scalpel blades; can be used for reflection.

Disadvantages
- The blades must be kept sharp, a skilled process that takes practice.
- Isolated storage must be provided for these delicate instruments.
- The blades can be easily damaged by inexperienced clinicians.

Types
Orban Knife
Advantage
- Good for interproximal removal of tissue *(E)*.

Kirkland Knife
Advantage
- Good for removal of large amounts of firm, fibrous tissue *(F)*.

Disadvantages
- Must be kept sharp.
- Cannot be used for fine, delicate procedures.

Maintenance: Sharpening Technique
Step 1—The sharpening stone is placed flat on a table and oiled as described in the earlier section titled Sharpening Scalers and Curettes.

Step 2—The edge of the blade is held at 15 to 25 degrees to the stone *(G)*. The wrist is rotated so the blade edge moves along the stone to sharpen the tip.

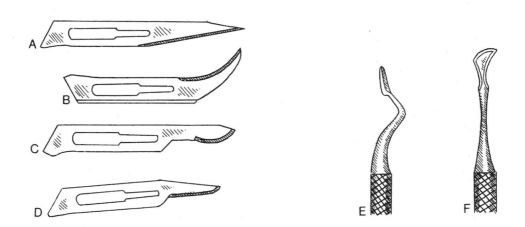

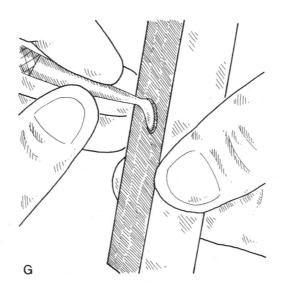

Periosteal Elevators

Comment
- The blade shapes include rounded, straight, and sharp points.

Uses
- Reflect and retract mucoperiosteum after initial incision of gingival tissue.
- Blade portion is used with the convex side against the soft tissue, reducing the chance for tearing or puncturing the gingiva.

Types
Molt No. 9 (A)
- No. 7 wax spatula looks similar to Molt No. 9 but is more delicate and achieves better access to the periodontal space.

Molt No. 4 (B)
Molt No. 2 (C)
Pritchard (D)
ST 7 (E)
No. 14 Goldman Fox
Maintenance
- Sharpening as with other sharp instruments.

Surgical Curettes

Comment
- Thicker and wider than other curettes, with a less flexible shank.

Use
- Removal of hard deposits, granulation tissue, necrotic cementum, and fibrous interdental tissue.

Advantage
- Stronger than other curettes; less likely to break.

Disadvantage
- Bulkier than other curettes; may not allow access into all areas.

Surgical Scissors

Goldman Fox No. 15
Comment
- Sharp-sharp scissors that have slightly curved blades, one being serrated *(F)*.

Use
- Enlarging initial incisions, trimming tissues, and incising muscle attachments.

LaGrange Scissors
Comment
- Sharp-sharp scissors that have S-shaped blade and handle *(G)*.

Advantage
- Better accessibility to osseous side of flap.

Minnesota Retractor
Comment
- Used for retraction of gingival tissue *(H)*.

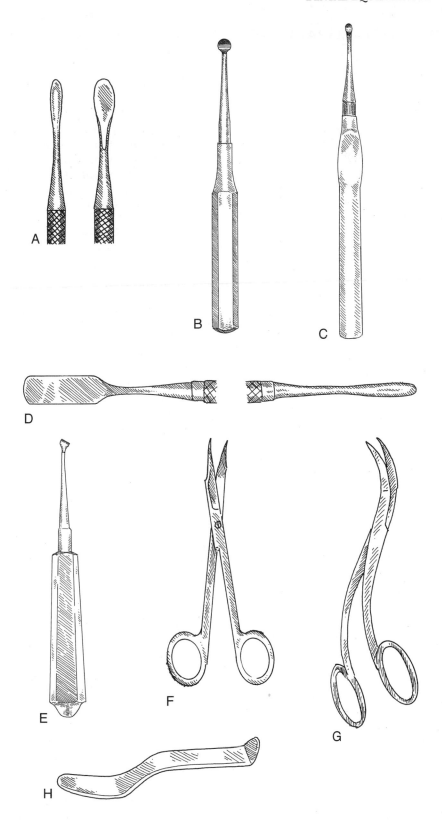

A

B

C

D

E

F

G

H

INSTRUMENTS FOR EXTRACTIONS

Surgical Elevator

Comment

- Surgical dental elevators are available in various sizes and shapes to fit different tooth sizes. Styles may vary, even within the same style of elevator. Some clinicians prefer serrations to be added either to the cutting edges of the tips or to the sides of the working end. Additionally, they may desire a diamond dust coating on the gouge surface. Dental instrument suppliers can provide these products.

Use

- As different types of levers or gouges to stretch and break the periodontal ligament and to displace the tooth root from its socket.

Disadvantage

- Because of these instruments' mechanical advantage, careful use is needed to avoid fracturing the crown, root, or alveolar bone.

Comment

- Handles are available in various sizes and shapes. More control is provided with handles of larger diameter. Likewise, the shaft should ideally be short enough to allow the index finger to be close to the working end.

Types

Manufacturers vary the appearance of each instrument, even though they may use the same number. The armamentarium should consist minimally of a thinner, short-shanked (no. 301s) *(A);* a small (no. 301) *(B);* a medium (no. 34) *(C);* a large (no. 3) *(D);* and a dog-leg style (no. E46) *(E)* elevator.

Modifications of the 301s Elevator

- Bent (No. 301s Bent*, EX-5E† *(F)*) has been modified with an 80 degree bend to make entering the periodontal ligament space easier and avoiding interference with the opposite jaw.
- Notched (No. 301s-Modified Fork*) (EX-5H†) *(G)* has been modified with a notch in the working tip. This notch creates a two-tipped fork that helps to prevent slippage on smaller dental alveolar ridges.
- Bent and Notched (No. 301s Bent Fork*)(EX-5EH†) *(H)* has been modified with an 80 degree bend and a notch.

Use

- Elevating very small teeth in crowded arches and loosening fractured retained roots.

---

*Dentalaire, 1820 S. Grand Ave., Santa Ana, CA 92705
†Cislak Manufacturing, Inc., 1866 Johns Dr., Glenview, IL 60025

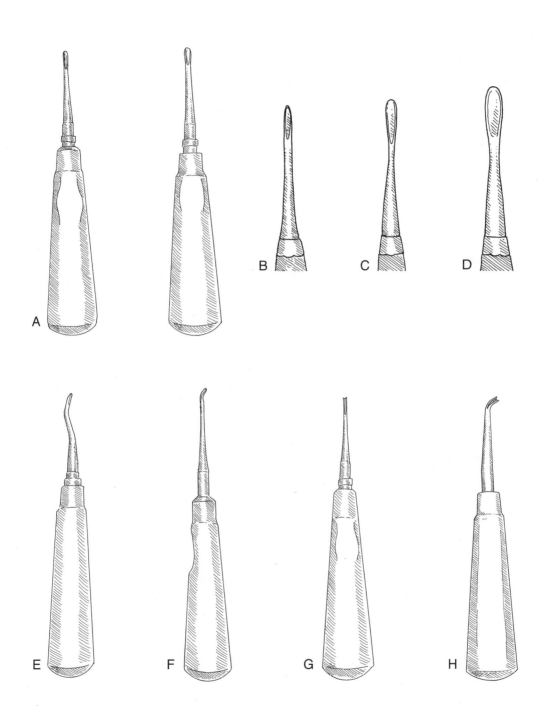

Cryer Elevators

Comment
- Triangular working tip *(A)*. They are supplied by numerous distributors.

Use
- Levering retained roots by an upward rotational motion, thus avoiding the risk of implosion fractures, which result in driving a root tip through a necrotic nasal plate and into the nasal passage.

Luxators*

Comment
- Are similar to surgical elevators but have a slimmer design *(B)*. They are used to stretch and separate the periodontal ligament and luxate the tooth.

Advantages
- Supplied in a variety of sizes and fit well into the periodontal space.
- Broader working ends to encompass more of the root tip's circumference than in the surgical elevator.
- Have thin, sharp edge for getting into the periodontal ligament space.
- Have a fat handle for a more comfortable grip.

---

*Whaledent, New York, NY 10001

Disadvantages
- They do not replace surgical elevators and break if too much torque is applied.
- Finer instrument tip can be damaged with misuse.

Maintenance
- The working edges of elevators should be kept sharp. A conical stone is used to sharpen inside edges of rounded elevators. Instrument longevity and effectiveness is further enhanced by periodic professional sharpening and reconditioning by a company experienced in servicing surgical instruments. Frequency of this service varies with the amount of use, but annual care is recommended.

Fahrenkug Elevators

- Designed to follow the curvature in curved rooted teeth *(C)*.
- Modified with a horizontal concavity that helps prevent elevator slipping *(D)*.
- Manufactured in 2, 3, and 4 mm size.

Advantage
- Curved to follow most curved roots (canine and incisors).

Disadvantages
- This elevator is a fine instrument, which must be used with care.
- The handle may be awkward for some.
- Concavity may not follow all teeth.

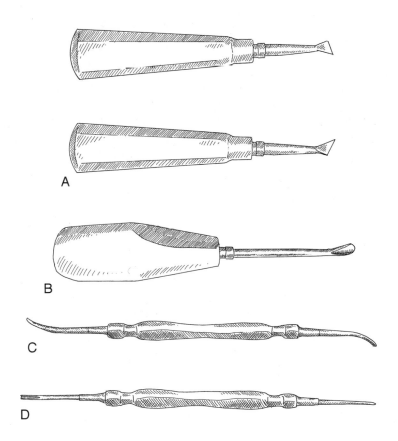

A

B

C

D

Heidbrink Root Tip Pick

Comment

- Have narrow, sharp points *(A)*.

Uses

- Stretching and breaking the periodontal ligament.
- Retrieving fractured root tips.

Advantage

- Small size to retrieve fractured root tips.

Disadvantages

- Requires light touch to avoid alveolar perforation.
- May break the tip of the instrument if too much force is applied.

ED10-11 Root Tip Pick

Comment

- Double-ended *(B)*.

Uses

- Stretching and breaking the periodontal ligament.
- Extraction of retained root tips.

Advantage

- Small size.

Disadvantage

- Requires light touch to avoid alveolus perforation/instrument fracture.

Bone Curette

Comment

- There are two styles. One style has a spoon-like end that comes straight or angled as a double-ended instrument. The working ends come in different sizes *(C)*. The other style has the more traditional "ice cream scoop" tip that is heavier and can also be used when gathering cancellous bone for grafting *(D)*.

Use

- Débride alveolus after extraction.

Advantages

- The spoon curette is a little more flexible to use and less expensive than the scoop-style bone curette.
- Both can easily remove granulation tissue and debris from the alveolus.
- The scoop curette size 5-0 is small enough for most alveolar débridement.

Disadvantage

- May be too large for cat teeth, except for canines (see the later section on excavator uses.)

Extraction Forceps

Comments

- Many different varieties are available.
- Human dental extraction forceps can be used, but available veterinary models fit the conical teeth better and provide better traction (have less rocking) when gripping the tooth.

Uses

- Gripping the tooth.
- Removing gross calculus (use caution).

Advantage

- Lifts a tooth out of alveolus.

Disadvantage

- Because of this instrument's mechanical advantage, careful use is required to avoid fracturing the crown, root, or alveolar bone.

Types

Small-Breed Extraction Forceps

Comments

- The veterinary instrument beaks are more parallel than are the human incisor forceps often used by veterinarians and therefore

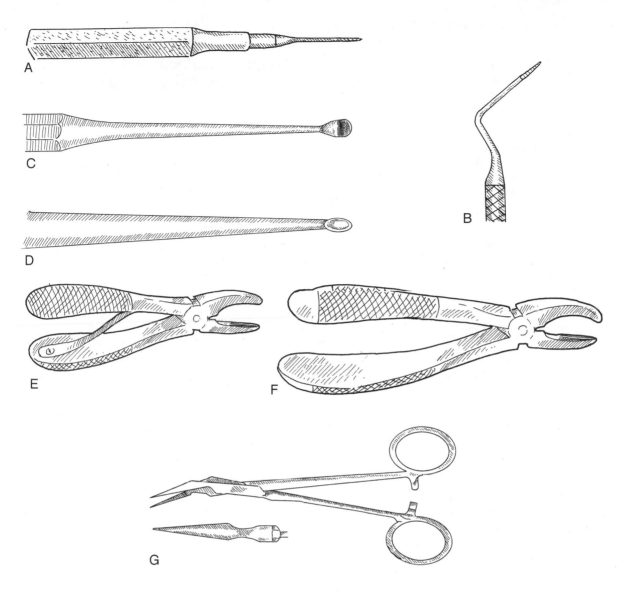

better adapted to conical carnivore teeth (*E*).

- Small forceps.

Advantage

- Small size fits most hands comfortably.

Veterinary Dog Forceps

Comments

- The beaks are more parallel than the human incisor forceps often used by veterinarians and therefore better adapted to the conical carnivore teeth (*F*).
- Large forceps.

Advantage

- May fit larger teeth better than human or cat extraction forceps.

Disadvantage

- May cause operator to "overpower" and fracture crown or root tip.

Human Extraction Forceps

Comment

- The grasping surfaces are concave to accommodate the bulge of the crown of human teeth and to grasp the crown down at the neck.

Disadvantage

- The concavity makes for poor contact with the conical teeth commonly encountered in veterinary dentistry. Grasping the tooth by the two points of the tips of the jaws only results in more pressure in small areas and creates intraoperative tooth fractures.

Root Tip/Fragment Forceps

Comment

- These forceps (*G*) have fine, pointed, serrated grasping tips at a 45 degree angle to the handle.

Use

- These forceps are invaluable for grasping and removing root tips or fragments as well as small delicate teeth such as feline incisors.

Advantages

- The fine tips allow them to reach deep into the alveolus to grasp and remove loosened root pieces.
- The 45 degree angle is more adaptable than right-angled forceps.

Disadvantage

- The fine tips can become damaged with misuse.

SUTURE MATERIAL

General Comments

- The choice of suture material should be based on factors such as procedure, length of time the material is to be in the oral cavity, and personal preference.
- Both absorbable and nonabsorbable materials may be used.
- There is no ideal suture material; all have advantages and disadvantages
- Absorbable materials include: coated polyglactin 910 (Vicryl),* polyglycolic acid (Dexon),† polydioxanone (PDS),* polyglyconate (Maxon),† and chromic gut.
- Nonabsorbable materials include nylon (Ethilon)* and polypropylene (Prolene)*

---

*Ethicon, Inc., Somerville, NJ 08878-0151
†Davis and Geck, Danbury, CT 06810

Coated Polyglactin 910, Polyglycolic Acid, Polyglyconate

Advantages

- Degradation by hydrolysis.
- Good for procedures in which healing is rapid and the suture does not need to be functional for long periods.
- Does not require removal.

Disadvantage

- Requires extra knots to tie, or will untie.

Chromic Gut

Advantages

- Good for procedures where healing will be rapid, and the suture does not need to be functional for long periods.
- Does not require removal.

Disadvantages

- Lasts a very short time in oral cavity.
- Degradation by proteolytic enzymes and phagocytic cells.

Nylon and Polypropylene

Advantages

- Good for surgeries requiring long-term attachment.
- Minimal tissue reaction.

Disadvantage

- Must be removed.

EQUIPMENT FOR ENDODONTICS

Cotton Pliers

Comment

- Cotton pliers (forceps) have two beaks and a handle; some are locking.

Uses

- Grasp materials to transfer them into and out of the oral cavity.
- Used in all phases of dentistry, including endodontics, orthodontics, and periodontics. Cotton pliers designed for endodontics have a longitudinal groove in each jaw to grasp absorbent points and gutta-percha points.
- Not intended to handle tissue.

Endodontic Broaches

Comment

- Broaches are manufactured by notching the walls of a round blank *(A)* and creating flared barbs.

Uses

- Bulk removal of pulp tissue and other debris from the pulp chamber and root canal.
- Have been used to retrieve absorbent points lodged in the root canal; occasionally, may aid in retrieval of a separated file tip.
- Should not be used to prepare the canal.
- Designed for single use only; however, may be cleaned intraoperatively by passing through rubber glove material.
- Made of soft iron and break easily when stressed.
- Should be used only in canals that have been instrumented at least to a size 25.

Endodontic Reamers and Files

Comments

- Reamers and files have two dimensions: length and diameter.
- Length is indicated by a millimeter notation.
- Typical lengths are 21, 25, 30, 31, 40, 49, 55, and 60 mm.

- The shorter files can be used for the incisors, premolars, and molars; the longer files are necessary for the canine teeth of dogs.
- Diameter is indicated by a number representing the diameter of the file at the working end (e.g., a no. 10 file is 0.1 mm; a no. 50 file is 0.5 mm; a no. 100 file is 1.0 mm at the working end).
- Standard (International Standards Organization (ISO)) sizes are 06, 08, 10, 15, 20, 25, 30, 35, 40, 45, 50, 60, 70, 80, 90, 100, 110, 120, 130, and 140.
- Series 29 file, a newer concept, is also available.*
- These files are designed to produce a tapered-funnel form, crown-down preparation quickly and efficiently without zipping, ledging, or perforating the canal. They conform to the new Series 29 standard, which maintains a constant 29% increase in tip diameters, thereby allowing a smooth, progressive enlargement of the canal from one file to the next.
- The rotary instruments come with a 0.04 or 0.06 taper as well as the constant 29% increase in tip diameter.

Advantages

- Offers fewer instruments, which are better spaced within the useful range (ISO no. 10 to no. 60). Usually, only three to five sizes of files are used in a root-canal preparation.
- The 0.04 taper files have twice the taper of ISO files. This creates a greater funnel form of the root canal for ease in obturating the canal.
- Available in a variety of sizes from 00–11 in 21 mm, 25 mm, 30 mm and 40 mm lengths.
- Available in either stainless steel or nickel titanium.
- Especially advantageous in curved canals when using the flexible nickel titanium files.
- Especially useful in retreatment cases requiring bypassing ledges and in removing gutta-percha.
- Supplied either as hand instruments or as rotary instruments used in a controlled low-speed, high-torque rotary handpiece.
- File will unravel before breaking.

---

*Profile 29 Variable Taper: Tulsa Dental Products, 5001 E. 68th St., Tulsa, OK 74136

Disadvantages

- Requires a 6:1 reduction gear handpiece if rotary pieces are to be used. Desired speed is 300 to 375 rpm.
- Must remember to fully depress rheostat foot pedal; do not adjust speed by foot pedal rheostat.
- If using rotary instruments, hand instruments are still needed initially and for measuring working length, larger-size canals, and longer canals. Hand instruments are often preferable at the apical end of the working length of the preparation.
- Does not reduce the need for irrigants during root-canal preparation or Gates Glidden drill for additional cleaning and shaping.
- Rotary instruments require a light touch.

Comment

- The clinician has better control and bends less files when using the shortest file possible.

Use

- Endodontics: root-canal preparation.

Types

Reamers

Comments

- Reamers are manufactured by twisting tapered and faceted wire to produce cutting edges, or flutes (B).
- Reamers are used for filing and reaming.
- Filing with a reamer is accomplished by pushing and pulling the instrument within the pulp chamber of the tooth.
- When filing, flutes scrape against the wall, gouging and removing dentin.
- Reaming is twisting the file in a clockwise direction. With this movement, the flutes scrape the walls and widen the canal and carry the debris coronally through the access site.
- Reaming creates a round canal. Reamers can be used well in any portion of the canal.

Advantage

- Reamers are stronger than other files of the same dimensions.

Disadvantages

- Do not have the cutting ability of most files.
- Should not be turned counterclockwise while filing.

Kerr Files (K-Files)

Comments

- K-files are manufactured in the same manner as reamers but are twisted to a greater degree (C).
- Because K-files cut when they are twisted as well as when they are pulled, they create a round canal apically and an oval canal coronally. They are best used to shape the apical third of the canal.
- The flutes are greater in number and more angulated than those of reamers.
- K-files may be used in reaming and filing.

Advantages

- They are stronger than Hedström files.
- K-files have a greater number of cutting edges and cut better than reamers.

Disadvantages

- K-files do not carry as much material out of the canal as reamers. This is called "carrier effect."
- If twisted clockwise with too much torque, they will become lodged and then break.
- Once trapped in the canal, they will break even more easily if twisted counterclockwise.
- With continued twisting they can penetrate the tooth apex.
- They are not as strong as reamers.

Hedström Files

Comments

- Hedström files are manufactured by cutting triangular pieces from tapered wire (D); as such, they are weaker than either K-files or reamers.
- Because of their push/pull use, they do not provide a round shape to the canal. Because of this and their weakness, they are best used to shape the coronal two thirds of the canal.

Advantage

- Very sharp when new and cut better than reamers or K-files.

Disadvantages

- Used only in filing; should never be used for reaming.
- More prone to breakage than are K-files or reamers.
- Less flexible than K-files.

Maintenance: Cleaning Files and Reamers

- Many manufacturers recommend single-use applications. These instruments should be disposed of in proper waste containers, according to regulations dealing with "sharps." Files tend to unravel with repeated use. If used more than once, files should be continually inspected. They should be discarded immediately when a shiny, weak spot is detected.

- Caution should be exercised when handling files and reamers not to stab oneself.

Step 1—Disinfect by soaking in chlorhexidine solution diluted as recommended on bottle.

Step 2—Scrub with a brush and submit to an ultrasonic cleaning cycle.

Step 3—Disinfect by soaking in chlorhexidine solution.

Step 4—Rinse. (An alternate approach is to use a bead sterilizer in place of steps 3 and 4.)

Step 5—Place in storage.

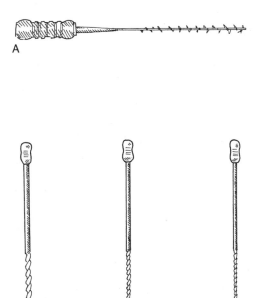

A

B   C   D

Accessories

File Organizers

Comments

- File organizers allow the orderly storage of endodontic files.
- Some organizers have containers for disinfectants *(A)*.
- Other models are autoclavable.

Advantage

- Allow an organized approach to file storage.

Disadvantages

- Vigilance must prevail to keep the organizer clean; it is difficult to keep sterile.
- The best system is to place only new files in the organizer when the file packages are opened. Files are destroyed after first use, thereby decreasing the incidence of file breakage in the canal.

*Endo-Ring**

Comment

- Endo-Ring is a plastic ring with ruler and replaceable sponge for intraoperative storage of files *(B)*.

---

*Almore International, Inc., Portland, OR 97225

Advantages

- Provides orderly storage of files and reamers in use as well as for pastes, such as RC Prep,* by placing on the sponge.
- Allows files that have been used to be separated from those in the organizer.
- Sponge on the Endo-Ring can be soaked in alcohol and used to clean files intraoperatively.

Disadvantage

- Care should be taken when placing file in the sponge not to stab one's fingers.

Maintenance

- The foam inserts are supplied in packs of 48 and are intended to be used once and destroyed.
- The Endo-Ring itself (exclusive of the foam insert) may be sterilized by steam, ethylene oxide, or cold sterilization.

---

*Premier Dental Products, 3600 Horizon Dr., King of Prussia, PA 19406

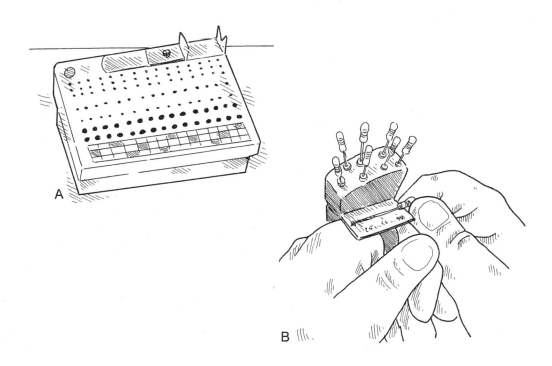

A

B

Bead Sterilizer

Comment

- Small sterilizer in which to place tips of instruments for sterilization *(A)*.

Advantage

- Allows relatively quick sterilization.

Disadvantage

- Only the tip of an instrument is sterilized.

Automated Files

Comments

- With the use of a special contra angle that oscillates at 90 degrees and files that fit into these contra angles, a canal can be filed with a low-speed handpiece.
- Automated files are best used in short canals.

Advantages

- Less physical strength required than filing with files manually.
- May speed filing of canal.

Disadvantages

- Time-consuming to change files.
- Less tactile sensitivity than hand files.
- Possible perforation of apex, flaring at the apical end of the canal, or "zipping" of canal wall.
- Risk of breaking files.

Instruments for Filling the Canal

High-Pressure Syringes

Comments

- A metal syringe with mechanical advantage that increases the pressure placed on the filling material to extrude it through a small opening.
- The pressure may be placed by a lever at the back of the plunger *(B)*.
- The pressure may be created by a screw at the back of the plunger *(C)*.

Advantage

- Material may be injected into small canals through a fine needle, as small as 30 gauge.

Disadvantages

- Special needles for these syringes have one-time use.
- Time is required to clean the syringe.

Maintenance

- E.L. Cor Solvent* cleaning solution is used to clean the zinc-oxide-eugenol compounds.

Plugger

Comment

- Has a blunt tip *(D)*.

Use

- Pushing gutta-percha into the root canal in the vertical condensation technique.

Advantage

- Helps gutta-percha reach the apex of the root canal.

Disadvantage

- Does not laterally condense gutta-percha.

Finger Plugger or Finger Spreader

Comment

- A short-shanked plugger or spreader with a handle similar to those of files or reamers *(E)*.

Use

- Reaching into canals when intraoral space is limited.

Advantage

- Better tactile sense.

Disadvantage

- Short, sometimes hard to hold.

---

*Lang Dental Manufacturing, 175 Messner Dr., P.O. Box 969, Wheeling, IL 60090

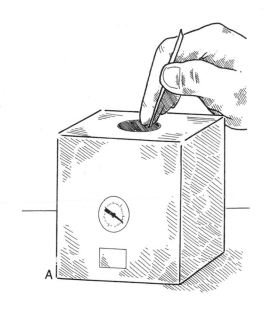

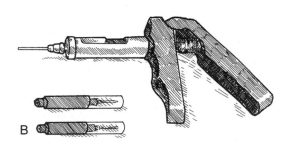

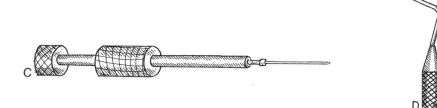

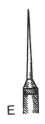

Spreaders

Comment

- Spreaders are tapered, pointed, and sized according to original standardized sizes of gutta-percha (A).

Advantage

- Condense gutta-percha laterally.

Disadvantage

- Slides along side of gutta-percha instead of pushing it deeper into canal toward apex.

Electrically Heated Spreaders*

Comments

- An electrical current passed through the spreader causes it to heat up (B).
- There are two mechanisms for heat control in the Touch and Heat. One mechanism uses a series of electrical pulses to heat the element. The more frequent the pulse, the hotter the tip. The second mechanism is a rheostat that varies the current passing through the spreader. The latter mechanism controls the temperature more accurately.

Uses

- Warming and condensing gutta-percha.
- Cutting gutta-percha.

Advantages

- Warming gutta-percha speeds up the process of placement, particularly in large canals.

---

*Touch and Heat, Analytic Technologies, 3301 181st Pl., Redwood, WA 98052

- When the spreader cools, it adheres to the gutta-percha and allows the gutta percha to be removed. This is helpful when a canal requires reinstrumentation.

Disadvantages

- There is a possibility of causing thermal damage to the tissue surrounding the tooth.
- Gutta-percha expands when warm and shrinks when cold.

Warmed Gutta-Percha Carriers,* Cannulas,† and Syringes‡

Comment

- Cannulas of gutta-percha are warmed in a heating unit and then placed into a special syringe for injection into the canal (C).

Use

- Plasticized root-canal filling.

Advantages

- Allows rapid filling of canals.
- Thermafil can be used in smaller canals than can Success-fil; obturators are supplied in sizes 20 to 100.

Disadvantages

- Thermafil comes in 25 mm length only.
- Warmed gutta-percha procedures are technique-sensitive and can be difficult to reinstrument.
- Cost of unit and cannulas.

---

*Thermafil: Tulsa Dental Products, 5001 E. 68th St., Tulsa, OK 74136
†Obtura II: Obtura Corp., 1727 Larkin Williams Rd., Fenton, MO 63026
‡Success-fil: Hygenic, 1245 Home Ave., Akron, OH 44310

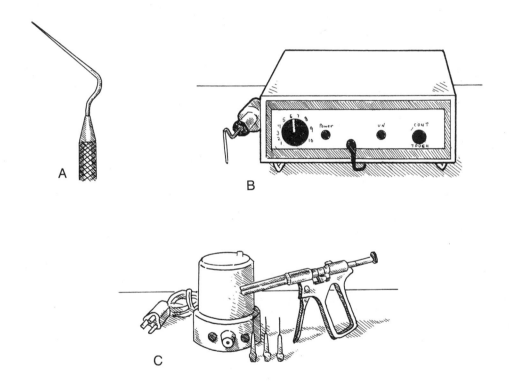

RESTORATIVE EQUIPMENT AND INSTRUMENTS

Chisels

Comments

- The cutting edge of a chisel forms a right angle to the long axis of the handle.
- When double-ended, one cutting edge is distal to the handle and is termed "reverse bevel." The other end is termed "standard bevel" *(A)*.
- The reverse bevel is indicated on the instrument shaft by an indented ring *(B)*.
- Chisels are straight-angle *(C)*, monangle *(D)*, biangle *(E)*, or triple-angle *(F)*.

Use

- Reshaping and smoothing dental tissue.

Hatchets

Comments

- The cutting edge is parallel to the angle of the handle (G).

Use

- Trimming and smoothing dental tissue— e.g., removing unsupported enamel rods, creating a bevel on cavity margins for composite restorations.

Excavators

Comment

- Double-ended instrument *(H)* with a flat, disc-like working end with fine, cutting edges; working tips come in different diameters.

Uses

- Removing carious dentin.
- Removing dental material from endodontic access sites.
- Débriding feline alveolar sockets after extraction.
- Excising gingival attachment around teeth of cats and small-breed dogs.

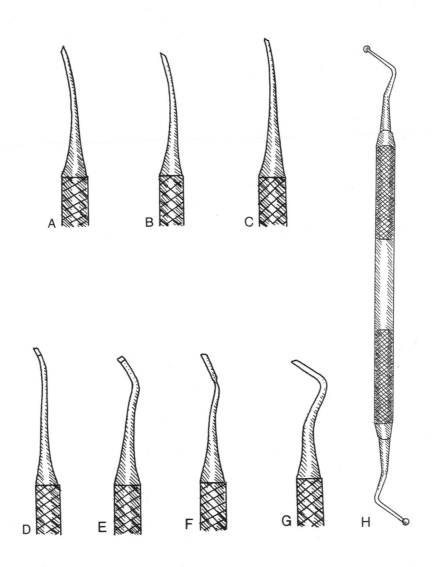

Light-Cure Gun

Comment

- The high-intensity light-cure gun is used to start the photochemical reaction that sets (hardens) the light-cure dental materials.

Uses

- Curing light-cure restorative materials.
- Curing light-cure periodontal packs.
- Curing light-cure orthodontic resins.
- Curing light-cure calcium hydroxide.
- Curing light-cure rubber dams.

Advantages

- Light-curing allows longer instrumentation time for easy shaping of the restoration and then rapid curing.
- Decreased polymerization shrinkage.

Disadvantages

- Cost of light-cure gun.
- Special eyeglasses or shields to protect the eyes from the intense light.

Options

"Continuous On"

Comment
- Many guns turn off automatically, slowing the procedure down.

Advantage
- A gun with "continuous on" allows long curing times.

Disadvantage
- May cause breakdown of light filter if used frequently for long periods.

High-Energy Output

Comment
- Light-curing guns are manufactured with different light intensities.

Advantage
- Brighter lights penetrate for a greater depth of cure.

Disadvantage
- Greater risk of eye damage.

Fiberoptic Cord versus Pistol

Comment
- Some light-cure guns have their light source in the control box and transmit the light via a long fiberoptic cord.

Advantage
- Having the light source in a box allows for larger fans than can be hand-held. This decreases the chance of bulb burn-out caused by overheating with long exposures.

Disadvantages
- Fiberoptic cords are very delicate; small breaks in the fibers may occur and decrease the output.
- Fiberoptic cords are thicker and harder to handle.

Accessories

Multiple Tips

Comment

- Some units come with several tips in different sizes and shapes.

Advantages

- Multiple tips allow greater range of uses (such as restorative, light-cure orthodontic materials, light-cure periopacks, light-cure rubber dams).
- Using larger-diameter tips reduces the chance of inadequate cure at the restoration margins.

Maintenance

- Inspect filter (with light turned off) on a regular basis (A).
- The filter should look like a blue-purple mirror (B).
- Holes in filter indicate that dangerous wavelengths of light may be escaping (C).
- Inspect the light bulb: black, discolored bulbs may need to be replaced.

Shield Tip

Comment

- Small plastic light shields fit over the fiberoptic tip *(D)*.

Advantage

- The shield is always with the light-curing gun.

Disadvantage

- Usually will not completely conform to shape of tooth; therefore, light shines out around the edges.

Light Analysis Tool

Comment

- For checking intensity of the light output.

Advantage

- Yearly monitoring of light ensures optimum curing.

Disadvantage

- Expense.

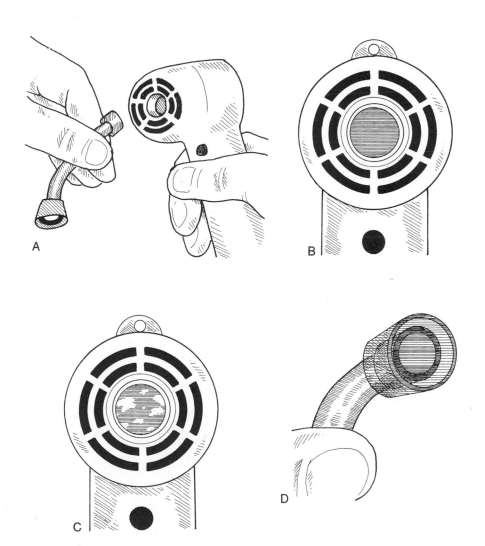

Amalgamators

Comment

* Amalgamators hold a capsule that contains amalgam or glass ionomer *(A)*.

Use

* Rapid mixing of glass ionomer and amalgam restorative material.

Advantages

* Thorough mixing of material.
* Helps prevent inconsistent mixing and environmental contamination.

Disadvantages

* Another piece of equipment to purchase.
* As with all equipment, instructions must be followed. Mixing the ingredients for an improper period produces an inadequate product.

Amalgam Wells

Comment

* Small metal bowl that holds amalgam mixture before mixture is transferred to cavity preparation.

Amalgam Carrier

Comments

* Transfers amalgam from amalgam well to restoration site *(B)*.
* Amalgam carriers and composite carriers look similar, but amalgam carriers have metal plungers that, if used with composite, will discolor it. Composite carriers have a nylon or plastic plunger.

Advantage

* Transfer amalgam to the restoration site quickly.

Disadvantage

* Training is required; the operator and assistant must know not to compact the amalgam into the carrier. If this occurs, the carrier will jam, and amalgam cannot be removed from the carrier.

Maintenance

* Periodic cleaning with paper points or cotton swabs.
* Once a carrier is jammed with amalgam, the barrel can be reamed clean with careful use of an appropriately sized cutting bur.
* Replacement of plastic tips.

Retrograde Amalgam Carriers

Comment

* Carry a smaller amount of amalgam and fit into smaller spaces *(C)*.

Uses

* Used in surgical root-canal treatments and for depositing restorative material into limited-access sites.
* Convenient for placing calcium hydroxide powder into pulpotomy access sites.

Advantages

* Small tip for placing amalgam into apical opening.
* One popular style* is supplied in two convenient barrel diameters, $\frac{3}{64}$ and $\frac{5}{64}$.

Disadvantage

* Limited to use in surgical root-canal therapy or very small fillings.

Amalgam Condensers (Pluggers)

Comments

* Condensers are used to pack (condense) amalgam into and within the surface defect restoration *(D)*.
* A variety of sizes are available for different-size restorations.

Use

* To condense the cold, molten amalgam into the undercut preparation so that it is a homogeneous, dense restoration without internal voids and with a tight seal at the surface margins.

Advantages

* By using different sizes and shapes, amalgam can be compacted into various sizes and shapes of cavity preparations.
* Performance can be improved over that of hand instruments by using an air-driven

---

*Retrograde Amalgam Carrier: Union Broach, 589 Davies Dr., York, PA 17402

vibrating handpiece that comes with a variety of tips that condense the amalgam and burnish its surface.*

Amalgam Carvers

Comments

- Various sizes and shapes have been designed to trim and shape amalgam (E).
- If working with amalgam, the practitioner will accumulate a variety of carvers. These should be kept separate from the com-

*Condensaire: Teledyne-Getz, 1550 Greenleaf Ave., Elk Grove Village, IL 60007

posite instruments and be used only for amalgam, both because of mercury contamination and to avoid discoloring the composite.

Advantage

- Rapid trimming of amalgam.

Amalgam Burnishers

Comments

- Smooth the surface of an amalgam restoration (F) and (G).
- Beneficial when mixing amalgam by hand.

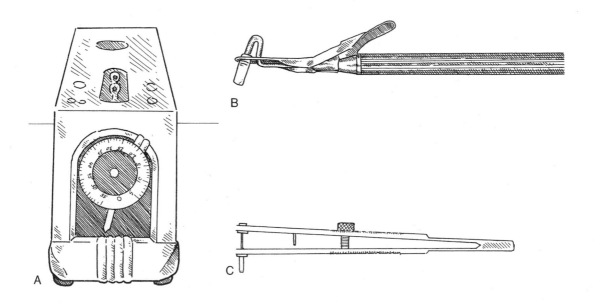

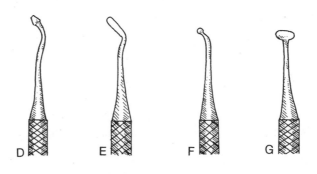

Plastic-Working (Filling) Instruments

Comments

- Plastic or metal instruments used to shape plastic restorative material before curing.
- Come in several sizes and shapes and are double-ended or single-ended. Double-ended instruments are often indicated as "de" or "D/E" in catalogs.

Advantage

- Made of a type of metal that does not leave a metal stain or discolor the restoration.

Mixing Spatula

Comment

- Thin-blade metal spatula.

Use

- Mixing filling and restorative materials.

Mixing Pads

Comment

- Glass slabs or waxed-paper pad slabs are used for mixing dental materials.

Uses

- Orthodontics.
- Restorations.
- Periodontics.

- Endodontics.

Types

Glass

Comments

- Glass slabs come in varying thicknesses and sizes.
- They may be cooled (e.g., stored in refrigerator) before use to provide longer working time for materials. This technique should not be performed in areas of high humidity.

Advantages

- Provides a smooth, sturdy working surface.
- Reusable.

Disadvantages

- Slab must be cleaned immediately after each mixing.
- Chemical residues may be present that could interfere with the mixing of the next chemical.

Paper

Comment

- Pad of wax-coated paper.

Advantage

- Disposable, one-time use; ease of cleaning: tear off and dispose of contaminated paper.

Disadvantages

- Must reorder and keep inventory.
- Some types of materials (glass ionomers) may pick up the wax coating on the paper pad.

Jiffy Tubes

Comments

- A jiffy tube is open wide at one end and drawn down to a fine delivery-tip point at the other end.
- The dental material is introduced into the open end, which is then pinched closed, forcing the material out of the fine delivery-tip point.

Use

- Restorative materials such as glass ionomers, liners.

Advantages

- Easy to use.
- Disposable; no clean-up after procedure.

Disadvantages

- Small size.
- A little messy in use.
- Less control and pressure than with other restorative placement methods.

Curved-Tip Syringes*

Comments

- Syringes with disposable curved tips of several sizes and rubber pluggers.
- The restorative material is pushed into the barrel of the curved tip.
- The rubber plugger is inserted.
- The syringe has a plunger on the shaft that

*Centrix, 770 River Rd., Shelton, CT 06484

advances the rubber plunger into one of various-size curved tips, forcing the material out of the tapered end.

Use

- Placing restorative.

Advantages

- Disposable delivery tips and rubber pluggers.
- Can inject under a fair amount of pressure.
- Creates a very fine and controlled flow of restorative material.

Disadvantage

- Small volume of material that can be accommodated by the tip.

Options

Plastic Syringe

Advantage
- Less expensive than metal.

Disadvantage
- May be stained by materials.

Metal Syringe

Advantages
- More resistant to staining.
- Easier to clean than plastic syringe.

Disadvantage
- Slightly greater initial cost than plastic syringe.

Maintenance
- Cleaning with alcohol or other solvent.

EQUIPMENT AND INSTRUMENTS FOR ORTHODONTICS

Impression Trays

Comments

- Because of the variety of sizes of veterinary patients, different-size impression trays are necessary *(A)*.
- Impression trays can be custom-made by the practitioner or purchased as pre-formed trays.
- Styrofoam or paper cups should not be used. They do not provide enough stability.

Uses

- Orthodontics.
- Restorative dentistry (crowns and bridges).

Options

Custom Trays

Comment
- The practitioner may need to make custom trays to fit an individual patient because of the variations in width and length of patients' mouths.

Disadvantages
- Time required to mix, shape, and cure the tray.
- Another skill to learn.
- For precision work (crowns and bridges), a tray should be made by the clinician and allowed to cure 24 hours before use to avoid distortion of the impression from polymerization (curing) of the impression tray.

Manufactured Trays

Comment
- Several companies manufacture trays that are shaped to fit dog and cat mouths.

Advantages
- Fit most patients.
- Fairly inexpensive.

Disadvantage
- Will not fit all patients; still need to have the ability to make custom trays, especially for the very large or wide mouth.

Maintenance
- Cleaning and disinfecting.

Trays Manufactured for Human Dentistry

Comment
- Trays of various sizes and shapes are available for human dentistry.

Advantages
- Less expensive than clinician version.
- Good when relatively small impression or an impression of only one tooth is required.

Disadvantage
- Will not fit the entire arch of most patients.

Accessories

Tray Adhesive
- Improves the ability of the material to stick to the tray.

Rubber Mixing Bowls

Comment
- Soft rubber bowls allow easy mixing and spatulation of alginate and dental laboratory stone materials *(B)*.

Advantages
- The flexibility of the bowl makes it easier to grasp and position material for mixing.
- The alginate is easy to clean up because it peels off the bowl once set up, and laboratory stone breaks free of rubber once dried.

Universal Cartridge Mixing and Delivery System

Comment
- A pistol-grip delivery system that holds twin cartridge barrels to which are attached a single mixing tip designed to consistently deliver the correctly mixed two-part vinyl

polysiloxane impression material into an impression tray.

Advantages

- Accurate mixture.
- Homogeneous mixture.
- Less mess.

Disadvantage

- Expensive.

Large Mixing Spatulas ("Buffalo" Spatulas)

Comment

- Made of plastic, nylon, or metal *(C)*.

Advantage

- Convenient mixing of a large volume of material with the use of a large spatula and rubber bowl.

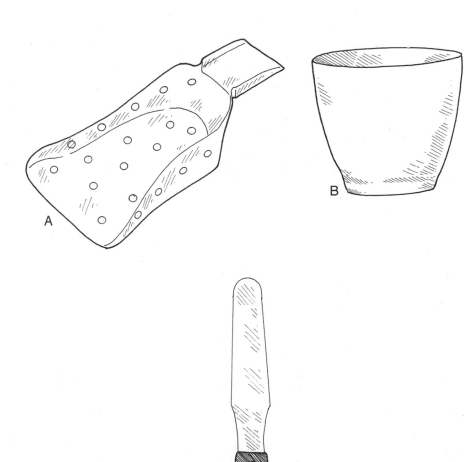

Vibrators

Comment

- Aid in working with dental plaster and stone by removing bubbles and facilitating flow of plaster or stone into the impression *(A)*.

Uses

- Formation of uniform, homogeneous dental models for orthodontics.
- Formation of cast for crown and bridge restoration.

Advantage

- Without a vibrator, air bubbles may be trapped in the dental stone, particularly for long, narrow canine teeth; these air bubbles may cause model fracture or distortion.

Maintenance

- The vibrator should be covered with a plastic bag or paper towel to prevent stone and plaster from getting inside the unit.

Accessories

Model Trimmer

Comment
- An electric motor drives a circular grinding disc; water is circulated to remove ground plaster *(B)*.

Use
- Trimming models for orthodontics and restorations.

Advantages
- Allows mounting of the model.
- Much more cosmetic appearance for client education.

Disadvantages
- Must be connected to plumbing and drain into sink or trap.
- Operation is very messy.
- Steps must be taken to prevent clogging of hospital plumbing. It is advisable to install a plaster trap at the bottom of the U-shaped portion of the sink drain.
- Expensive.

Plaster Trap

Comment
- A receptacle to collect solids flushed down the drain *(C)*.

Advantages
- Prevents plumbing blockage.
- Is supplied with disposable liners.
- Can be installed by a household plumber.
- Can be purchased through dental supply distributors.

Disadvantage
- Liner must be changed periodically, which is a messy chore.

Articulators

Comment

- Articulators are made of metal and plastic with two flanges hinged together.

Use

- Hold casts of jaws in proper alignment during stages of prosthodontics or orthodontics.

Welders

Comment

- Compact, miniature arc welders that weld or solder by electrical current.

Use

- Allow veterinarian to custom-make orthodontic appliances in the office.

Advantages

- Increased control of the quality and design style of the appliance.
- Ability to perform tableside adjustments.

Disadvantage

- Expense and time required to learn to use this equipment.

Maintenance

- Replacement of carbon electrodes.

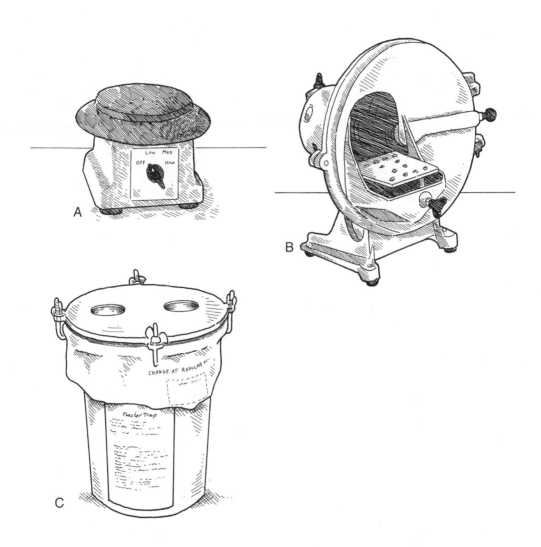

Pliers

Comment

- Bend wire for creation of orthodontic appliances.

Uses

- Orthodontics.
- Oral orthopedic surgery.

Types

Howe Pliers

Comment
- Holding wire and free-form wire bending (A).

Uses
- General-use orthodontic pliers: may be used for gripping wire during placement or removal, seating bands, making adjustments to appliances, and so on

Bird Beak (Loop-Forming) Pliers

Comment
- Have one round tip for round bends and one flat tip for sharp, angular bends (B).

Uses
- Bending orthodontic wire.
- Creating either a sharp or gradual curve.

Three-Prong (Triple-Beaked) Pliers

Comment
- Have a pair of prongs on one side and one prong on the other side (C). The single prong is centered to move between the paired prongs.

Uses
- Three-prong pliers bend by placing the pliers on the wire and squeezing.
- Three-prong pliers are useful in adjusting wire, bending heavier orthodontic wire, and activating appliances.

Tweed Arch-Adjusting Pliers

Comments
- Have heavy, nonslip beaks (D).
- Size limits use in the oral cavity; used mainly for laboratory work.

Use
- Holding and adjusting arch wires.

Tweed Loop-Forming Pliers

Comment
- Have various diameters at the tip (E).

Use
- Forming loops.

Band/Bracket-Removing Pliers

Comments
- Have a protective nylon cap over the longer beak; cap is placed on the crown of the tooth (F).
- Shorter beak is placed along the bracket or band to be removed.
- Pliers may be used to shear the remnants of the bonding cement off the tooth.

Maintenance
- The shorter beak may require sharpening to grasp fine bands.

Wire Cutters

Comment
- Can be purchased from dental suppliers or local hardware stores (G).

Accessories

Storage Trays

Comment
- For organization and visualization of instruments.

Boley Gauge

Comment
- A caliper that is calibrated in millimeters (H).

Use
- Measurement of size of teeth.

Iwanson Spring Caliper

Comment

- A caliper that is calibrated in millimeters (I).

Use

- Measurement of teeth prepared for an artificial crown.

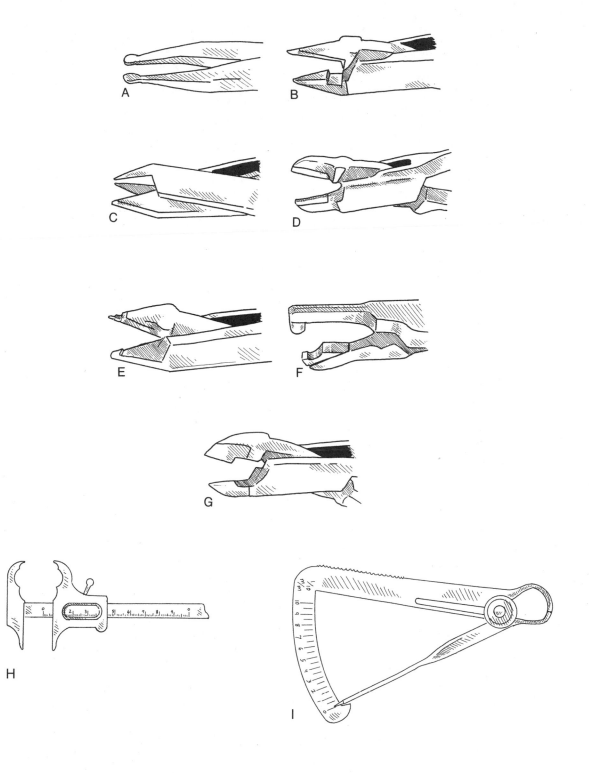

REFERENCES

1. Williams CA. Dental Equipment Needs. Las Vegas: Western Veterinary Conference, 1988:6–12.
2. Grove K. Periodontal Therapy. Compendium on Continuing Education 1983; 5:660–664.
3. Clinical Research Associates: Sonic and Ultrasonic Scalers. Provo, UT, 1982; 6:1.
4. Loose B, Kiger R. An evaluation of basic periodontal therapy using sonic and ultrasonic scalers. J Clin Periodontol Res 1987; 14:29–33.
5. Parr RW, Pipe P, Watts T. Periodontal Maintenance Therapy. Berkeley: Praxis Publishing Co., 1974:87.
6. Hu-Friedy. Smarten Up, Sharpen Up. Chicago: Hu-Friedy, 1982.
7. Tholen MA. Concepts in Veterinary Dentistry. Edwardsville, KS: Veterinary Medicine Publishing Co., 1983:164.
8. Finkbeiner BL. Periodontal instruments. In: Carter LM, Yaman P, eds. Dental Instruments. St Louis: C.V. Mosby Co., 1981:4.
9. Hawkins BJ. Periodontal Disease Therapy and Prevention. Philadelphia: W.B. Saunders Co., 1986:835–849.

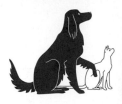

Chapter 3

DENTAL RADIOLOGY

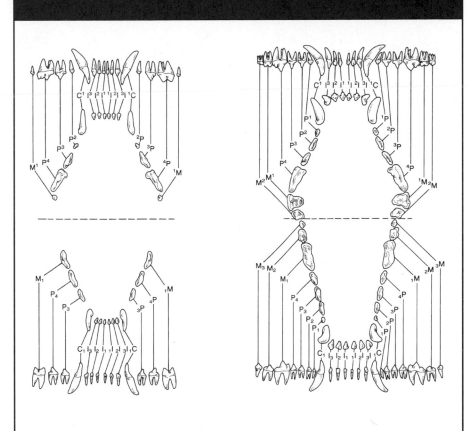

GENERAL COMMENT

- Dental radiology using intraoral film can be performed by all practitioners.

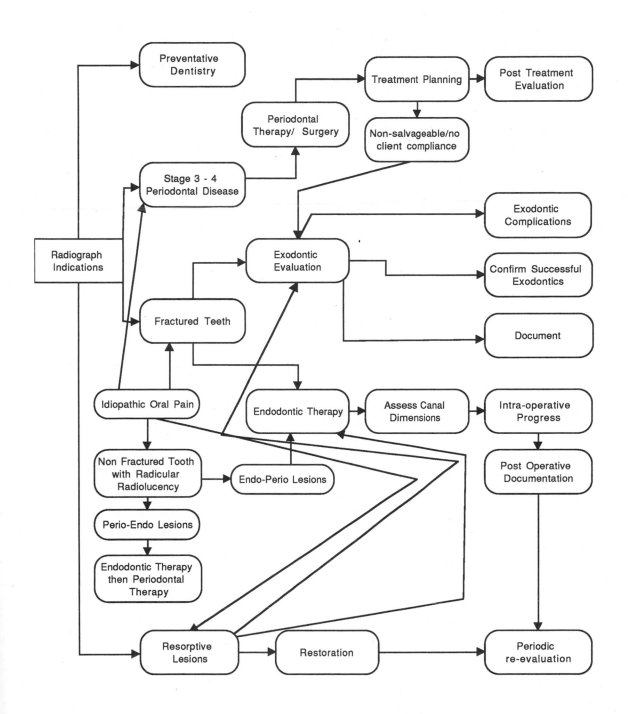

INDICATIONS

- In young patients, to evaluate the presence of unerupted or impacted teeth.
- During prophylactic or therapeutic teeth cleaning, to evaluate the extent of periodontal disease by measuring bone loss and to assist in treatment planning *(A) (B)*.
- In patients with oral stomas (fistulae), as a diagnostic tool *(C)*.
- In patients undergoing endodontic therapy, to allow the practitioner to evaluate therapy and to study radicular health and size before, during, and after endodontic therapy *(D)*.
- In patients with missing teeth, to ascertain the status of potentially impacted teeth or areas with resorbed roots or teeth *(E)*.
- In all types of dental/oral disease, to document and study the progress of therapeutic programs.
- In cases in which neoplasia or metabolic disease is suspected, to evaluate the involvement of teeth and bone.
- In oral trauma, to evaluate the injury in detail.
- Before or during extractions, to verify the complete removal of root tips or the location of retained root tips *(F)*.

CONTRAINDICATIONS

- Critically ill patients where the risk of anesthesia is so great that the risk of treatment is not justified.

OBJECTIVE

- To obtain a radiograph with fine detail that represents the patient's condition *(G)*.

RADIOGRAPHIC UNITS

Medical Radiographic Unit

- A medical radiographic unit can be used to obtain extraoral and intraoral films, but its use is limited due to the restricted movement of the radiographic head and because the unit is located distant from the dental operatory, thus requiring the patient to be brought to the machine for each film desired.
- A medical radiographic unit is used when having the ability to adjust the focal distance and angle of the head is preferred. A focal distance of approximately 12 cm is preferred, coning down as necessary to reduce scatter. The resultant focal film distance will have the collimator almost touching the patient's face.
- The parallel and bisecting angle techniques can be used with a medical radiographic unit. They require positioning the patient with foam wedges and sandbags to achieve the proper alignment with the primary beam.
- To achieve a bisecting angle technique of the maxillary teeth, the animal is placed in sternal recumbency, with the nose supported so that it is parallel to the table surface. The animal is then tilted obliquely 45 degrees, the film is placed intraorally, and the radiographic head is adjusted until the beam is directed appropriately over the area of interest (see the later section titled Bisecting Angle Technique).
- To obtain a rostral mandibular bisecting angle view, the animal is placed in dorsal recumbency with its top of the muzzle parallel to the table and then rotated obliquely 45 degrees. The film is placed intraorally, and the positioning is adjusted until the beam is directed appropriately.
- Each unit will have different technique ranges. A starting point is 100 mA, 65 kilovolt peak at $1/10$ second. When the kilovolt peak is too low, the result is low density with high contrast. When the kilovolt peak is too high, the result is high density and poor contrast. It is necessary to achieve a proper balance between kVp and mA. Practice with a skull to try several technique combinations until the most desirable exposure is achieved.

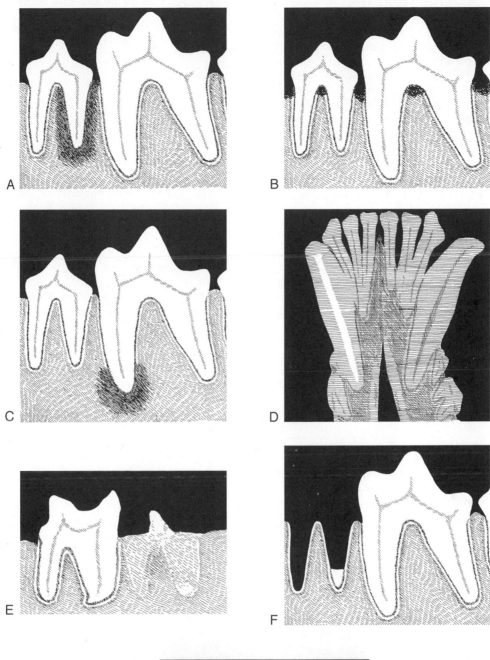

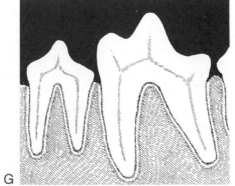

Dental Radiographic Unit

- A dental radiographic unit can be purchased new or sometimes used from human (not veterinary) dentists or dental supply warehouses. It can be wall-mounted in the dental area or mounted on a mobile floor stand. It has a compact tubehead with a multiple jointed arm for maneuverability.
- They are supplied with 70 kVp and 7, 10, or 15 mA with variable time-exposure capabilities. These units are very versatile and produce a more detailed image due to a smaller focal spot and a fixed focal distance.
- The newest dental radiograph machines are designed to use direct current (DC) instead of alternating current (AC) power to generate the x-ray beams. This gives greater contrast and less soft radiation to the tissues. These machines are digital and have a programmable keypad.
- Suggested technique chart using Ultraspeed (Type D) film with a 7 mA output and DC generator. If using AC, increase time slightly. Upper fourth premolar will use the same technique as the upper molar (Tables 3–1 and 3–2).
- The newer machines have lead-lined cones to reduce scatter radiation further. This is an important feature if purchasing a used machine because it enables compliance with present safety codes. The ease of using a dental radiographic unit will encourage taking more radiographs, thereby providing a better service to the client.

MATERIALS

Film

- Intraoral radiographic film is inexpensive, small, and flexible, fitting well into the oral cavity and conforming to the area placed

Table 3–1 • 60 KV (MAXIMUM IMAGE CONTRAST)

	Small Dog or Cat	Large Dog
Incisor	0.25 sec	0.4 sec
Canine	0.25 sec	0.4 sec
Premolar	0.32 sec	0.5 sec
Lower Molar	0.4 sec	0.63 sec
Upper Molar	0.5 sec	0.8 sec

Table 3–2 • 70 KV (MAXIMUM GRAY LEVEL DEFINITION)

	Small Dog or Cat	Large Dog
Incisor	0.125 sec	0.2 sec
Canine	0.16 sec	0.25 sec
Premolar	0.2 sec	0.32 sec
Lower Molar	0.25 sec	0.4 sec
Upper Molar	0.32 sec	0.5 sec

(Table 3–3). Intraoral film is nonscreen film, which provides greater detail than the larger cassettes used in most veterinary situations. Intraoral film can be processed in 1 to 2 minutes with rapid developer and fixer solutions, and there is minimal loss of detail. Using this film, small areas of interest can be isolated.
- Ultraspeed film is most commonly used because it provides greater detail and is less grainy, although it requires twice the exposure time as does Ektaspeed* to produce a comparable image. When taking radiographs of giant-breed dogs with a dental radiographic unit, it may be helpful to use Ektaspeed film to get the penetration of thicker bone without increasing the exposure time.

Film Identification

- When taking intraoral radiographs, it is important to be able to easily identify which patient they belong to. Several methods of film identification can be used, depending on the clinician's preferences.

Identification Methods

- Using an indelible ink pen to mark the client/patient identification directly on the radiograph.
- Using a radiograph marking pen that writes in white to mark the client/patient identification on the dry film.
- Placing on the outside of the film packet before exposure a small press-apply radiopaque number that correlates in a log to a specific client/patient.
- Placing processed films in plastic or cardboard film mounts that are made specifi-

---

*Eastman Kodak Co., Rochester, NY 14650

Table 3–3 • **FILM SIZES**

Size	Measurement	Ektaspeed (Type E)	Ultraspeed (Type I)
Periapical			
0	⅞ × 1⅜ in	EP-01	DF-54
1	¹⁵⁄₁₆ × 1⁹⁄₁₆ in	EP-11	DF-56
2	1¼ × 1⅝ in	EP-21	DF-58
Occlusal			
4	2¼ × 3 in	EO-41	DF-50

cally for the different film sizes and that are available through dental suppliers. Client/patient identification and other pertinent information can be written on the holder. Presized punches are available to make cutouts for these cardboard holders.

- Using small envelopes, with client/patient identification on the outside, to hold one or more films.
- Whole-mouth surveys can be placed in proper orientation (see the following sections titled Whole Mouth Survey) and taped in 8½ by 11 inch plastic cover sheets for easy viewing and storage.

Identifying Right and Left Sides

- All intraoral films have a small raised dimple present in one corner of the film. It is visible and palpable on both the film and film packet. The side with the raised dimple faces the x-ray beam when the film is placed in the mouth.
- One technique is to place the dimple on the radiograph on the animal's right in the mouth. When the radiograph is mounted in normal alignment (as when the teeth are radiographed with the raised dot facing you), it will be easy to tell whether the tooth is on the right or left.
- Identification is still possible for personnel who forget to be consistent on where they place the dimple. To do this, the raised side of the dot is found and oriented so that the convex side of the dimple faces the viewer while viewing the film. The film is placed in proper alignment with the maxilla or mandible (crown appropriately up or down). Next, the film is oriented with proper alignment of the teeth rostral to caudal. The orientation of the teeth on the film will match the patient as seen on the patient, thereby identifying the side.

- Placing processed films in plastic mounts or plastic sheets, with the dot facing the viewer and with the films of the patient's right side on the viewer's left and films of the patient's left on the viewer's right, with incisor views in the middle in proper orientation when whole-mouth surveys are taken, will provide easy viewing that corresponds to the dental chart.

Film Storage

- Individual film envelopes or envelopes holding film mounts can be placed in the patient record or stored in a separate radiographic filing system. Dental radiograph logs are helpful in retrieving past films with number identification placed in the chart. Due to their small size, it is best not to keep intraoral films together with large cassette–size radiographs of the same patient.

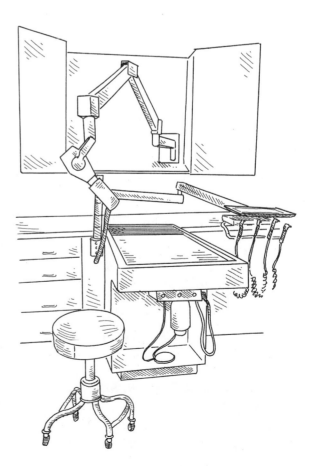

TAKING AN INTRAORAL RADIOGRAPH

- Keep the distance from the subject to the film as short as possible.
- Use a fine-grain or high-detail nonscreen film.
- The side of the film packet with the raised dot is placed facing the x-ray beam.
- Use a machine with as small a focal spot as possible.
- Collimate to the area of the subject needed.
- Process the film carefully after exposure.

Step 1—The patient is positioned appropriately for the radiograph to be taken.

Step 2—The intraoral film is placed in the proper position. As a supportive aid in positioning the film, a mouth gag, film wedge, gauze sponge, or other object can be placed behind the film.

Step 3—The head of the x-ray machine is placed as close as possible to the structure being evaluated and positioned for the study.

Step 4—The appropriate milliamperage, kilovolt peak, and time are selected.

Step 5—The film is exposed.

Step 6—The film is developed (see the later section entitled Radiographic Developing).

CAUTION: Personnel should wear exposure monitors or protective apparel or be at a safe distance from the x-ray machine or stand behind a protective screen.

Whole Mouth Survey: Large Dog

- Maxillary incisors and canines: anterior bisecting angle technique.
- Maxillary rostral premolars and canine tooth: lateral bisecting angle technique for each side.
- Maxillary caudal premolars and molar teeth: lateral bisecting angle technique for each side.
- Mandibular incisors and canines: anterior bisecting angle technique.
- Mandibular rostral premolars and canine tooth: lateral bisecting angle technique for each side.
- Mandibular caudal premolar and molar teeth: parallel technique for each side.

Whole Mouth Survey: Small Dog or Cat

- Maxillary incisors and canines: anterior bisecting angle technique.

- Maxillary premolars and molars: lateral bisecting angle technique for each side.
- Mandibular incisors and canines: anterior bisecting angle technique.
- Mandibular premolar and molar teeth: parallel technique for each side.
- Additional films may be required, depending on the disorder involved. It is often helpful to take multiple views when questioning whether a finding is valid or an artifact. Rostral, caudal oblique, and occlusal views can be taken in addition to a whole mouth survey or individual study.
- The parallel technique is the most accurate technique because it follows the principle of accurate shadow writing (in which the projected shadow of an object from a light source resembles the height of the object most accurately). If the angle between the film and the structure to be radiographed is greater than 15 degrees, then the x-ray beam should be directed according to the bisecting angle technique.

Specific Intraoral Radiographic Techniques

Parallel Technique

Indications

- Radiographs to evaluate the posterior mandibular teeth *(A)*.
- Evaluation of portions of the mandible *(B)*.
- Evaluation of the facial maxillary complex and nasal cavity *(C)*.

Contraindications

- Any location where the film cannot be placed parallel to the structure being radiographed. If the angle between the film and the long axis of the structure is greater than 15 degrees, a bisecting angle technique should be used.
- Any area where other structures would be superimposed onto the film.

Objective

- To take a radiograph where the long axis of the tooth or structure being evaluated and the radiographic film are parallel to each other and perpendicular to the x-ray beam. The parallel technique is the most accurate as it closely follows the principle of shadow writing.

Technique

Tubular collimator cones with filter are preferable and in some states are the only equipment allowed by law.

- The film packet is placed parallel to the structure being radiographed. The plane of the film should be parallel to the plane through the long axis of the structure *(D)*.

- The head of the machine is placed as close to the film as practical, and the x-ray beam should be perpendicular to the long axis of the structure being radiographed.

Complication

- In many areas of the mouth it is not possible to place a film parallel because other structures interfere.

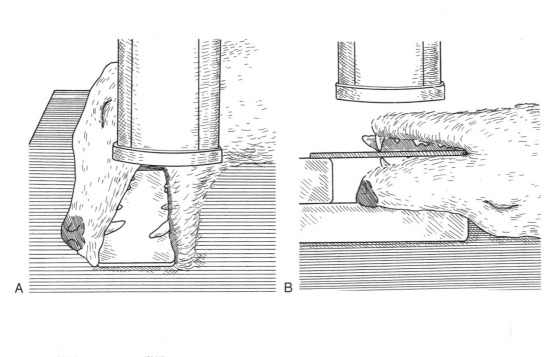

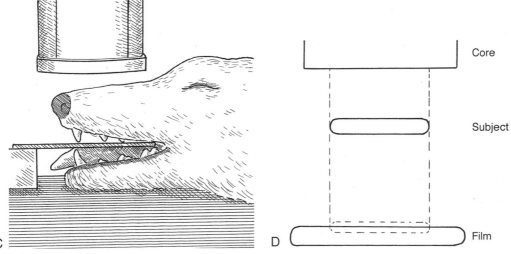

Bisecting Angle Technique

General Comments

- Ideally, all exposures should be made using the parallel technique. However, in the mouth, few areas physically accommodate this technique.
- The bisecting angle technique is an application of the geometric principle of equilateral triangles: in equilateral triangles, if two triangles share a side and both triangles have an equal angle at their apex, then the opposite sides are the same length.
- The caudal maxillary dentition is the most difficult to radiograph with intraoral techniques.

Indications

- Bisecting angle technique is used when parallel projections are not possible.

- Caudal portion of the maxilla *(A)*.
- Rostral portion of the maxilla, including canines *(B)*.
- Maxillary incisors and canines *(C)*.
- Mandibular incisors and canines *(D)*.
- Anterior portion of the mandible, including canines *(E)*.
- Posterior portion of the mandible may be radiographed with the bisecting angle technique if the parallel technique cannot be used.

Contraindication

- If parallel projections can be utilized, they are easier to produce and have less error.

Objective

- To obtain an accurate representation of the tooth.

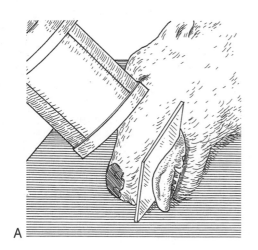

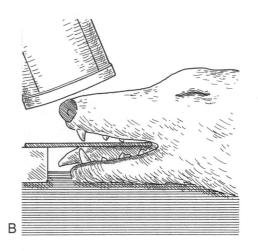

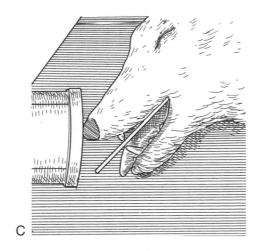

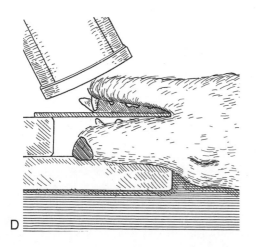

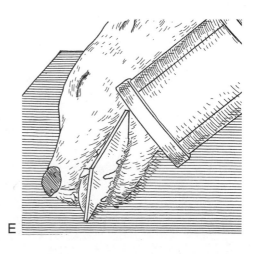

Technique

- The angle formed by the x-ray film and the structure is visualized, and an imaginary line bisecting this angle is visualized *(A) (B)*.
- The head of the x-ray machine is positioned so that the x-ray beam is perpendicular to the imaginary line. When learning this technique, it is often helpful to use props, such as sticks (e.g., cotton-tip applicators), to help visualize the angle and the bisected angle.

- As a general rule, aim the x-ray beam at a 45 degree angle to the hard palate on maxillary projections.

Complication

- The most common problems are not achieving a true bisecting angle and not aiming the x-ray beam perpendicular to the bisected angle. This may create foreshortening *(C) (D)* or elongation *(E) (F)*.

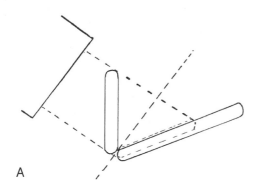

A

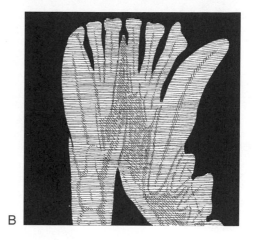

B

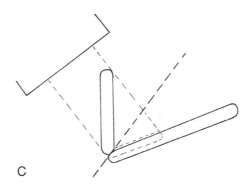

C

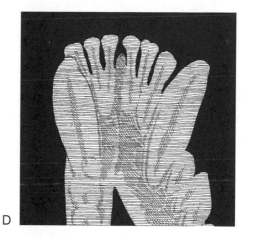

D

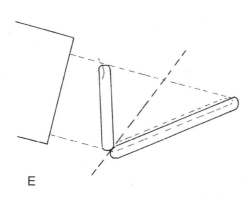

E

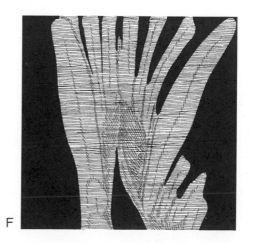

F

Extraoral Use of Intraoral Film

- This technique can be useful when obtaining a radiograph of the caudal maxillary teeth.
- Superimposition of the opposite arch can be avoided and greater detail is obtained by using nonscreen intraoral film instead of using screened film in a cassette *(A)*.

Technique

- The patient is placed in a dorsolateral recumbency position, with the side of interest closest to the table.

- The mouth is held open as wide as possible with a radiolucent foam block or other object, such as a syringe case.
- The intraoral film is placed on the table beneath the area of interest.
- The head is tilted until the long axis of the tooth is at a 45 degree angle to the table.
- The x-ray beam is directed perpendicular to the film *(B)*. Films must be marked "right" or "left" because the raised-dot rule of right and left is now reversed.

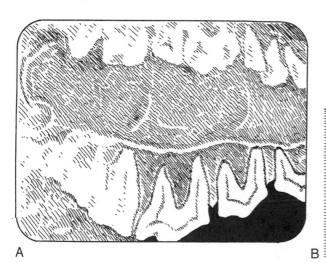

A

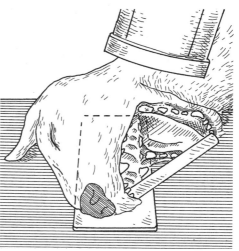

B

Complications of Radiographic Technique

- Improper exposure settings on the x-ray machine.
- Limitations imposed by the x-ray machine.
- Placing the film incorrectly in the patient's mouth. The raised-dot side placed away from the beam will result in exposure through the lead barrier, creating a lighter exposure with a stippled appearance.
- Inability to identify structures accurately, particularly when evaluating maxillary fourth premolar palatal and mesial buccal roots. A second film is then taken, with the x-ray beam moved either anterior or posterior. This creates an anterior oblique or posterior oblique position. The structure that is more lingual (palatal root) will be shadowed on the film closest to the direction the x-ray beam is coming from. The structure that is more buccal (mesial buccal root) will be shadowed the farthest from the x-ray cone. This phenomenon can be remembered by the "SLOB rule" (*S*ame *L*ingual *O*pposite *B*uccal). Another word device is Facial Farthest, Lingual Least. Diagrammed are lateral *(C)*, anterior oblique *(B)*, and posterior oblique *(D)* views of the maxillary fourth premolar *(A)*.

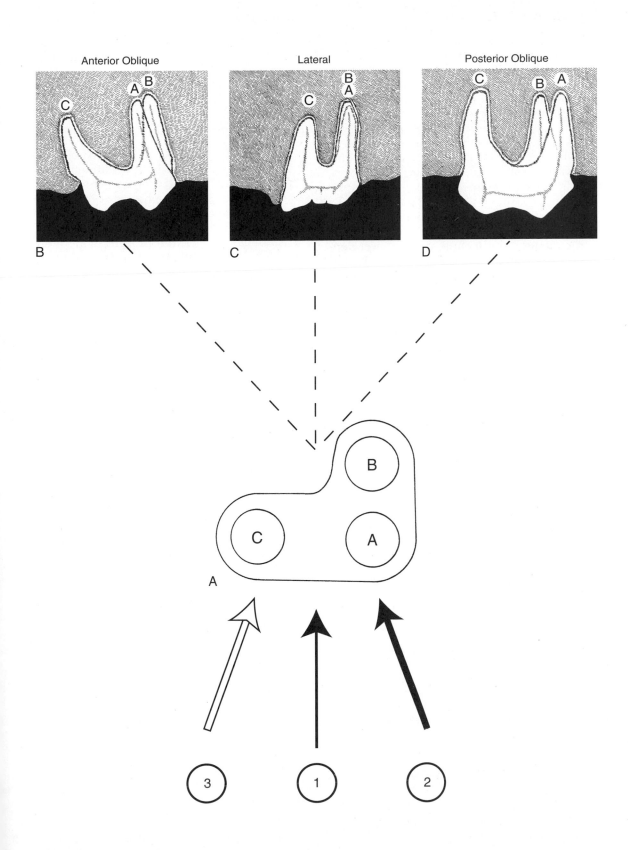

Anterior Oblique

Lateral

Posterior Oblique

Radiation Safety

- To minimize radiographic exposure to personnel, it is best if the patient is anesthetized or heavily sedated so it can be positioned and the dental worker can leave the area or be a safe distance (usually 6 feet) from the tube head.
- If there is a need to take a radiograph of an awake patient, personnel should wear full protective covering, including aprons, thyroid protectors, eye shields, and gloves. A hemostat clamped to the film can be used to position the film in the patient's mouth if normal bite positioners are ineffective. The authors of this text do not recommend this technique, but newer dental radiographic units with lead-lined cylinders make awake radiograph positioning safer with less scattered radiation. A dosimeter badge and ring should be worn by personnel and monitored routinely.

Radiographic Developing

- There are four methods of developing the exposed film: standard manual developing, rapid-processor developing, one-step rapid processing, and two-step rapid processing.

Standard Manual Developing

Comments

- The procedure is the same as for cassette radiographic film.
- Specialized racks or holders may be used to hold the film(s) during the developing process (A).

Advantage

- Additional equipment and materials are not required.

Disadvantage

- The biggest disadvantage is the slow developing time.

Rapid-Processor Developing

Comment

- An automatic processor is used to develop, fix, and dry the film.

Advantages

- Automatic processors establish constant developing and fixing, eliminating human error.
- This method decreases operator time.
- A dry film is produced for viewing.

Disadvantages

- Unless the processor is designed to transport small films, there will be difficulty with this method. Some veterinary medical automatic processors will process occlusal-sized dental radiographic film. Approximate developing time for each film is 4 minutes.
- Automatic dental film processors are available, with a developing time of 1 to 8 minutes, which may take even longer than automatic processing.
- Automatic dental film processors are expensive.
- Large 10 × 12 or 14 × 17 inch radiographic film can be used as a "leader" by taping the smaller dental film to it with a specific tape for this purpose. The large film is used to transport the dental film through the processors normally used in veterinary practices. This technique is discouraged because it is impractical and, if the dental film becomes dislodged, potentially damaging to the film processor. Films to be developed can also be placed in film mounts specially designed with tape around the edge of the film opening to secure the film as it passes through the processor attached to the mount.

One-Step Rapid Processing

Comment

- A special combination developing/fixing solution is used for this procedure.

Disadvantage

- Because developing and fixing are done by the same solution, detail is compromised; therefore, this process is not recommended.

Two-Step Rapid Processing

Comments

- This is the recommended processing technique for veterinary dentistry.

- Separate solutions are designed for rapid developing and fixing of intraoral film.
- Single film clips are used to dip the film in each container. Multiple film hangers can be used to hold a single patient's radiographs during the final rinse so single clips can be used for additional films.
- At least three or four small containers are used.
- The containers are arranged as follows: one for developing solution, one for water rinse, one or two for fixing solution, and one or two for the final rinse. The number of containers advisable depends directly on the size of the container and the volume of films being processed.
- Small dip tanks may either be bought for this purpose, or empty, clean plastic or glass containers may be used. Tight-fitting lids are needed for the developer and fixer containers. Rinse water should be replaced during breaks in film developing, and the chemicals should be replaced weekly.
- The dip tanks or containers may be housed in a darkroom or in a "chairside darkroom" *(B)* (see Chapter 2).
- Chemicals must be changed frequently; 6 oz of developer will develop 10 to 15 occlusal films or a greater number of smaller films.
- Disposal of chemicals after use should be done according to state health requirements. The lead packet insert can be saved for recycling.

Technique

Step 1—The solutions are stirred to mix.

Step 2—In a dark environment, the film packet is opened, and the film is removed from the packet and attached to a film clip *(C)*.

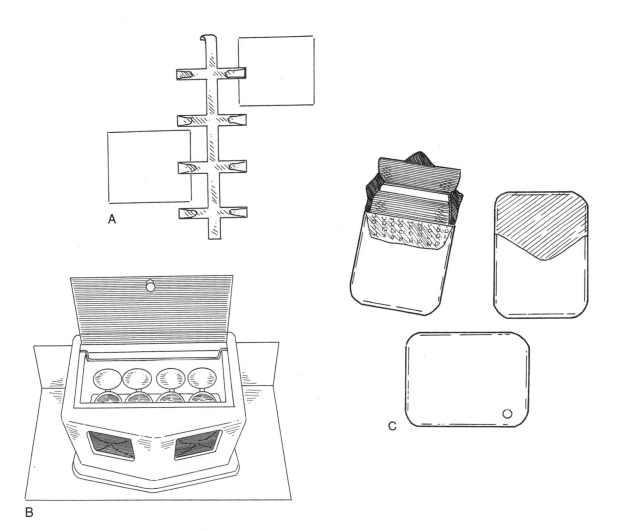

A

B

C

Step 3—The film is immersed in the water rinse for at least 5 seconds to hydrate the emulsion on the film.

Step 4—The film is immersed in the developer, agitated to remove bubbles, and then no longer agitated. The amount of time depends on the solution used, the temperature, and the exhaustion state of the chemicals. The manufacturer's recommendations should be followed. The film is removed from the developing solution, with minimal drip-back into the developing tank.

Step 5—The film is placed into the water rinse, with continuous agitation for 30 seconds.

Step 6—The film is transferred to the fixing solution and intermittently agitated during its fixing. Generally, fixing time is twice the developing time. For archival-quality films, 10 minutes is recommended.

Step 7—After the time prescribed for fixing by the manufacturer passes, the film is transferred into the final rinse. The fixing solution is allowed to drip back into the fixing tank. The film may be read at any time; however, it should be returned for a minimum of 10 minutes in a freshwater rinse (longer rinse time gives more assurance of removing all fixer from the emulsion). For archival quality, 30 minutes is recommended.

Step 8—The film can be air-dried by hanging it from a single or multiple film hanger so that it will not touch adjacent films. Hair driers at low heat or specially designed film driers can be used to speed the drying process. (Be sure to identify multiple cases during the drying process to avoid misidentification later.)

Complications

- Once the film is removed from the protective packet, processing should begin as soon as possible.
- Resist the temptation for prolonged viewing of the film between the developing and fixing stages.
- If Ektaspeed film is used, or if the unit is below a bright light source, a red filter should be placed over the amber filter.
- Old developing solution gives a "washed-out" background and fogs the film. Developing solution oxidizes rapidly in open containers. Storage of solution in a container with a tight lid will prolong its life.
- If the films are not rinsed for a long enough time, they will turn brown as the remaining fixing solution oxidizes with age.
- The film should be removed from the protective paper. If the paper is left attached to the film, the film will not develop properly.
- Accidental exposure to light in the darkroom after the film is removed from the packet during developing creates an overall fogging or darkening of the film.
- Films touching during developing or fixing, films sticking together during processing, films being handled by fingers contaminated with solution, or film clips and fixing solution splashing together before developing will all cause artifacts on the processed film and should be avoided.
- Nail or tooth indentations on film before processing will create dark line artifacts on the processed film.
- Insufficient fixing time will produce a yellowish-brown film.
- Silver jewelry should not come in contact with processing solutions.

DUPLICATING DENTAL RADIOGRAPHS

General Comments

- Radiographs are a record. They belong to the veterinary hospital and not to the client. Written medical records also belong to the veterinary hospital. The client has the right to request copies of the medical record, but a potential problem arises when duplicate radiographs are requested.
- The nature of the problem varies, depending on the circumstances. Clients often claim they own the radiographs; in fact, they do not—they own the information gained by the interpretation. The ill will that occurs between clients and clinics when clients are denied "their radiographs" may damage public relations.
- The clinic can send the original radiographs to a veterinarian of the client's choice, requesting return of the film at an appropriate time. However, if the clinic wants to maintain possession of the films, several alternative approaches are available.
- It is appropriate to charge a fee for duplicate films.

Duplicating Techniques

Double-Loaded Film Packets

Comment

- This is the least expensive method of obtaining a duplicate radiograph. Radiograph film with two films per packet is available in ultraspeed and Ektaspeed film (Table 3–4).

Table 3–4 • DESIGNATION

Type	Size	Ultraspeed/Ektaspeed
Periapical 0	DF-53	EP-02P
Periapical 1	DF-55	EP-12P
Periapical 2	DF-57	EP-22P
Occlusal 4	DF-49	EO-42P

Advantages

- Results in a nearly perfect duplicate film.
- Easy to use.

Disadvantages

- Additional dental film must be kept in inventory.

- Clinician must know ahead of time that duplicate film is desired.
- Film may be wasted, especially if repositioning and additional exposures are required to obtain diagnostic films.

Single-Film Duplicator

- Single radiographs may be duplicated by means of a relatively inexpensive single-film duplicator (Mini-Ray Duplicator: Rinn, Model 72-1220) (A), or Henry Schein, Catalog No. 100-7268). The duplicator costs slightly less than $100.
- Duplicating film is also required (e.g., Kodak X-Omat: Catalog No. 158-6460).
- This system works well for duplicating individual dental radiographs, one at a time. The duplicator will accept size no. 0, 1, 2, and 3 films (not size no. 4 [occlusal] film).

Technique

- The duplicator holds one 9 V battery. In the darkroom, the lid is lifted, the film to be duplicated is placed on the small light table inside the duplicator, and the duplicating film is placed on top of the duplicator.
- The lid is closed, and the activating button is pushed. The button turns on a light beneath the small light table and turns it off automatically after the film has been duplicated.
- The exposed duplicating film can then be developed in the usual manner. If using a chairside darkroom, the exposed film must first be brought into the darkroom (B).

Advantages

- Quick and easy for single films of sizes 0 to 3.
- Relatively inexpensive.

Disadvantages

- Tedious process if a radiographic survey of 6 to 12 films needs to be duplicated.
- Occlusal film, which is too large for the duplicator, is used with regularity in veterinary practice.

Panoramic Film Duplicator

- A system similar to that of the single-film duplicator, but larger, made by Rinn *(C)*. Kodak film can be used: X-Omat: Catalog No. 121-582I.

Technique

- Similar to that of single-film duplicator, but several films can be duplicated at the same time.

Advantages

- Reproduces film up to 5⅞ inches × 12⅝ inches.
- Accommodates five no. 2 films or three no. 4 (occlusal) films.

Disadvantage

- Cost is more than $200.

Professional Medical Film Duplicating System

- If duplicating larger cassette radiographs is desired, a radiographic duplicating system for large-cassette medical radiographic film is available.

Technique

- Similar to those of single-film and panoramic duplicating systems, with ability for several dental films to be placed on the glass at one time.

Advantages

- The system works very well.
- Multiple dental films can be duplicated at the same time.

Disadvantage

- Cost is more than $300.

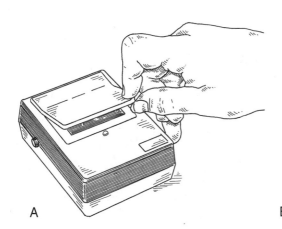

A

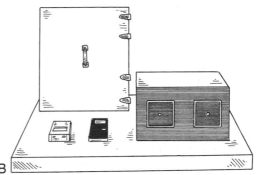

B

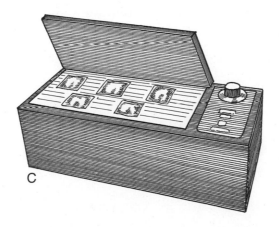

C

Economy Duplicating System Using a Printer/Proofer

- There is an additional way to duplicate either large-cassette or dental radiographs satisfactorily and relatively inexpensively.

Uses in Veterinary Dental Department

- Diplomates sending duplicated films to referring source or in matters of dispute.
- Marketing: providing duplicates for client, relieving a source of contention with clients who want films.
- Serving as an additional client service and source of revenue for general practices and dental departments.

Materials

- 18 inch ultraviolet light (blacklight) wall-mounted 42 inches from the working surface.
- Electrical hook-up with pull string or wall switch.
- 10 × 12 inch printer/proofer (a 10 × 12 inch glass hinged to cover a soft parallel surface of similar size) available at photographic supply stores.
- Duplicating film (e.g., Agfa Curix Duplicating Film; Kodak Omat: Catalog No. 161-8909, both from radiographic supply distributors).
- Darkroom with film safe and flat working space.

Setup

- The blacklight tube is mounted horizontally 42 inches above the flat working space.
- The printer/proofer is positioned in front of the technician.
- The films to be duplicated are laid out in order, to one side, with all the lights off.
- The closed box of duplicating film is placed for easy access.

Technique

Step 1—In the darkroom, the printer/proofer glass is lifted so that a piece of 10 ×

12 inch duplicating film can be placed with its emulsion side (lighter, pinker, shinier) facing up on the soft bottom surface of the printer/proofer.

Step 2—Dental film(s), or the portion of a 14 × 17 inch film to be duplicated, is laid directly on top of the sheet of duplicating film because, in this case, the light source is above the unit (D).

Step 3—The glass cover is brought down atop the two layers of film, and the blacklight is turned on to expose the film for exactly 5 seconds.

Step 4—The glass is lifted, and the exposed duplicating film is developed, either manually or in an automatic processor in the usual manner.

Advantages of the Printer/Proofer

- Duplicating 6 to 12 films in 5 seconds is more efficient than duplicating the films individually.
- The system can duplicate the larger medical radiographs routinely taken in veterinary hospitals.
- The system can be installed for approximately $100 and requires little equipment.
- The detail is quite adequate for useful communications with other veterinarians.
- The duplicating service creates goodwill.
- It is to the clinician's advantage to be able to duplicate large-cassette film for referral cases or for clients seeking second opinions.
- It is appropriate to charge a fee for duplicate films.
- The service removes the question of whether the distributed film will be returned to the hospital of origin.

Disadvantage

- Duplicated (second-generation) films are not quite as high in quality as first-generation films.

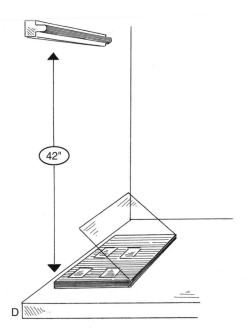

D

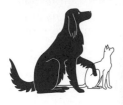

Chapter 4

DENTAL PROPHYLAXIS

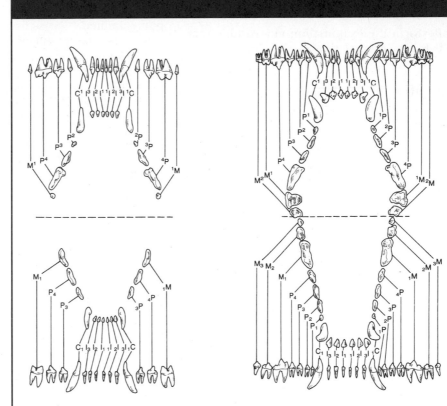

GENERAL COMMENTS

- The deleterious effects of untreated dental disease on the rest of the body have long been recognized.
- The oral examination and prophylaxis are basic to good dentistry.

ORAL EXAMINATION

General Comment

- Perform the examination in a routine that is followed every time.[1]

Indications

- Cooperative patients receiving a physical examination.
- All patients undergoing general anesthesia.

Contraindication

- Uncooperative patients that will not allow examination without risk to the examiner.

Objective

- Thorough examination of all oral and dental structures for evidence of abnormality or disease.

Materials

- Periodontal probe/explorer.
- Mouth gag.

Technique

Step 1—The head, muzzle, and nostrils are observed and examined. Check for asymmetry and lymph node enlargement. In the awake patient, note any pain on palpation.

Step 2—The lips are lifted; starting rostrally, buccal and labial surfaces of the teeth and gingiva are examined.

Step 3—Working caudally, the mandibular and maxillary teeth, cheek tissues, and salivary gland ducts are evaluated.

Step 4—The contralateral side of the mouth is examined in a similar fashion.

Step 5—Once the external examination of the lips and the buccal surface of the teeth and gingiva is completed and the clinician has gained familiarity with the patient, the mouth is opened.

Step 6—The lingual and palatal gingival tissues are examined. The lingual, palatal, interproximal, and occlusal surfaces of the teeth are evaluated. The examiner's thumb can be placed in the diastema behind the maxillary canine tooth so that the thumb pushes on the hard palate as an aid in keeping the mouth open. In the awake patient, thorough visualization is limited.

Step 7—The tongue and floor of the mouth are examined. This area may be visualized more easily by pushing on the skin beneath the tongue on the ventral portion of the mandible posterior to the symphysis.

Step 8—The hard and soft palates are examined.

Step 9—The pharyngeal area and tonsils are examined. In tolerant animals, a finger can be placed over the base of the tongue for better visualization of the oral pharynx.

Complications

- The patient may require general anesthesia if it will not submit to examination.
- A mouth gag should be used only for a short time to prevent undue tension on the temporomandibular joint.
- The clinician should use caution to prevent being bitten.

Aftercare: Follow-Up

- An initial treatment plan is formed after the oral examination.

PERIODONTAL DISEASE

Cause of Periodontal Disease

- The tissue degradation process appears to be driven by subgingivally advancing plaque, acute inflammation, and prostaglandin-induced bone resorption.[2]
- The host response, bacterial actions, and bacterial endotoxins destroy the periodontium.
- Page[3] likened the area of periodontal disease to a battleground destroyed in the process of the battle.

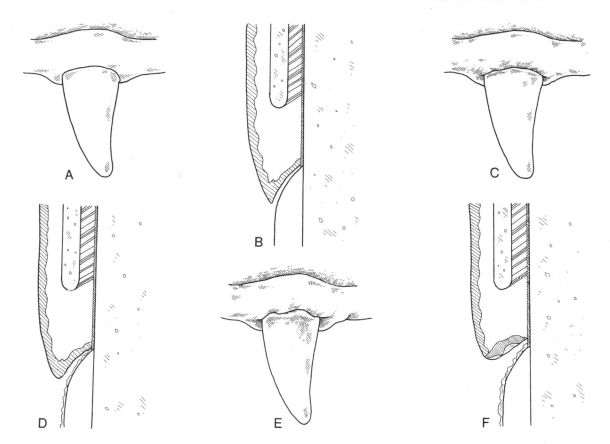

Stages of Periodontal Disease
Comments

- Periodontal disease is divided into grades for the purpose of treatment planning and evaluation of patient progress. In reality, a given stage of periodontal disease is fairly subjective; what matters is the overall evaluation of a combination of factors that includes plaque, calculus, gingival inflammation, gingival recession, and bone loss. One treatment schedule was based on the predominant cell types in the connective tissue of the marginal gingiva.[4] Periodontal pocket measurement[5] was used in another. Harvey and Emily proposed a six-stage system.[6]
- This text uses a system with a clinical approach. "Healthy" is defined as the absence of disease and therefore is not assigned a grade. Likewise, once a tooth is extracted, although disease may be present, the intact periodontium is missing. Therefore, the missing tooth is not graded. As well, a great variance in size exists among veterinary patients.

A Healthy Periodontium

- The healthy gingiva has a knife-like margin *(A) (B)*. The gingiva flows smoothly from tooth to tooth, called "smooth topography."
- Radiographically, alveolar crestal bone is seen close to the neck of the tooth.

Stage 1: Early Gingivitis

- There is a redness of the gingiva at the crest of the gingiva and a mild amount of plaque *(C) (D)*. There is loss of visualization of the fine blood vessels at the gingival margins.
- Radiographically, there is no change from a healthy periodontium.
- The condition is reversible with treatment.

Stage 2: Advanced Gingivitis

- Stage 2 is similar to the stage 1, but there is an increase in inflammation, including edema and subgingival plaque development. Amounts of supragingival plaque and calculus are increased *(E) (F)*. The gingival topography has started to become irregular but is still good. Root exposure has not yet occurred.
- Radiographically, there is little noticeable change.
- The condition is reversible with treatment.

Stage 3: Early Periodontitis

• Stage 3 is an incipient periodontal-disease stage, with gingivitis, edema, beginning pocket formation, and increasing amounts of plaque and calculus. The gingiva bleeds on gentle probing *(A) (B)*. The gingival topography no longer flows smoothly from tooth to tooth.
• Radiographically, subgingival calculus may be noted, and a rounding of the alveolar crestal bone at the cervical portion of the tooth can be seen on careful examination.

Stage 4: Established Periodontitis

• Some of the signs that may be associated with stage 4 are severe inflammation, deep pocket formation, gingival recession, bone loss, pus, and tooth mobility. The gingiva usually bleeds easily on probing *(C) (D)*.
• Radiographically, subgingival calculus and bone loss are noted.

Prevention and Treatment of Periodontal Disease

• Different areas of the mouth can be affected with different stages of periodontal disease at the same time. Each area should be treated accordingly.
• Patients with early gingivitis (stage 1) should receive home-care instruction and polishing supra- and subgingivally (above and below the gum line).
• Advanced gingivitis (stage 2) should be treated with supra- and subgingival scaling, teeth polishing, fluoride treatment, and regular home care.
• Early periodontal disease (stage 3) should be treated with thorough calculus removal supra- and subgingivally, polishing, antimicrobial treatment, root planing, gingival curettage, sulcular irrigation with fluoride or chlorhexidine, and home care on a regular basis.
• Established periodontal disease (stage 4) should be treated with thorough scaling, subgingival curettage, root planing, polishing, sulcular irrigation with fluoride or chlorhexidine, antimicrobial treatment, gingival flap surgery, and other periodontal procedures as indicated. An intensive home-care program is necessary.
• Once periodontal disease reaches stage 3 or 4, a simple dentistry, dental, or prophy treatment as commonly perceived in many veterinary practices will not be enough to stabilize the infectious disease (Table 4–1).

Table 4–1 • **TREATMENT AND PREVENTION PROTOCOLS FOR PERIODONTAL DISEASE**

Procedure	Healthy	Stage 1	Stage 2	Stage 3	Stage 4
Scaling*	No	Possible	Yes	Yes	Yes
Polishing	Yes	Yes	Yes	Yes	Yes
Irrigation†	Yes	Yes	Yes	Yes	Yes
Gingival curettage	No	No	No	Yes	Yes
Root planing	No	No	No	Yes	Yes
Flap surgery	No	No	No	Rare	Yes
Splinting	No	No	No	No	Possible
Extraction‡	No	No	No	Possible	Yes

* Sub- and supragingival scaling
† Chemical irrigation with chlorhexidine or fluoride
‡ Extraction for periodontal disease

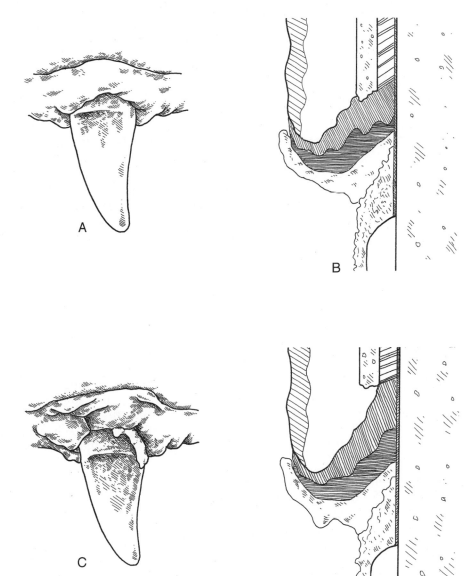

DENTAL PROPHYLAXIS

General Comments

- A thorough dental prophylaxis consists of supra- and subgingival gross calculus removal, fine-hand scaling, polishing, diagnostics, irrigation, and home-care instruction.
- The procedure is performed properly with the patient under general anesthesia and intubated.
- Steps for a thorough prophylaxis are presented below in order of application.
- Time needed for a thorough prophylaxis for an uncomplicated case is 30 to 45 minutes. Procedure time increases as patient size increases.

Step 1: Gross Calculus Removal

General Comments

- Gross calculus is removed by using scalers and curettes, calculus-removing forceps, ultrasonic scalers, sonic scalers, or rotary scalers.
- Large accumulations of supragingival calculus are removed from the buccal, lingual, palatal, and interproximal surfaces of the teeth.
- Removal of gross calculus alone is not a complete prophylactic dental procedure and is of minimal therapeutic value. It is, however, an important step in providing visualization and access to the smaller deposits and stains.

Objective

- To prepare for the subsequent steps of removing smaller accumulations of calculus and plaque.

Scalers and Curettes

Indications

- Scalers are used for removal of gross calculus above the gumline.
- Curettes are used for the same purpose above and below the gumline.
- Scalers and curettes are useful in areas that may be difficult to reach with power instrumentation.
- Hand instrumentation is necessary in all prophylactic procedures to remove all sizes of dental deposits.

Materials

Scalers and Curettes of Choice

Techniques
- Instrument-holding techniques, use of finger rests, and proper instrumentation.

Instrument-Holding Techniques
- Scalers are designed to be used with a modified pencil grasp for greater control of the working end *(A)*.
- A pencil grasp should be avoided *(B)*.
- The modified pencil grasp is achieved by first holding the instrument between the thumb and index finger, with the remaining fingers held straight *(C)*.
- The remaining fingers are then moved over so that they are to the side and slightly on top of the index finger. The instrument remains in the front part of the hand *(D)*.

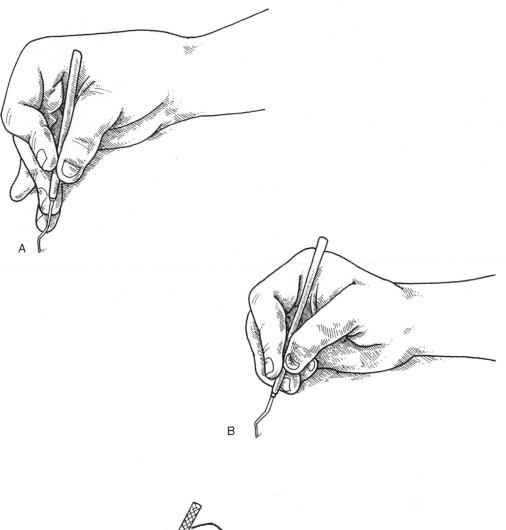

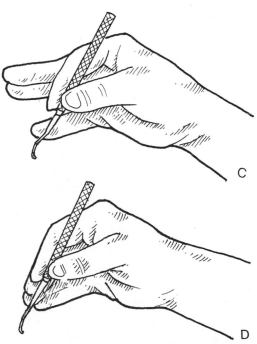

Finger Rests

- Fine-instrument control is necessary for cleaning teeth without causing tissue injury.
- A large variety of finger rests may be used in each situation.
- Hand size, position of operator in relation to patient, and type of instrument affect the selected finger rest.

Standard Position

- The middle or the ring finger is placed against the tooth being instrumented or the proximal (adjacent) tooth. This finger becomes the fulcrum to effect power for the working stroke.
- The instrument is placed on the tooth to be scaled *(A)*.
- The wrist is rotated while keeping the fingers straight; as the blade of the instrument moves, it is made to follow the contour of the tooth *(B)*.

Cross-Arch Rest

- The fulcrum finger is placed on a tooth in the opposite arch *(C)*. This is often done when working in smaller areas.

Open or Extended Grasp

- The middle and ring fingers are allowed to separate *(D)*.
- This technique is used when the finger rest (fulcrum) cannot be near the work area.

Long Reach

- The instrument is grasped farther toward the middle of the handle *(E)*.
- This technique reduces the amount of instrument control at the working end.
- A fulcrum is still used to provide as much stability as possible.

Secondary Rest

- The hand not holding the instrument is used as a rest for the fulcrum *(F)*.

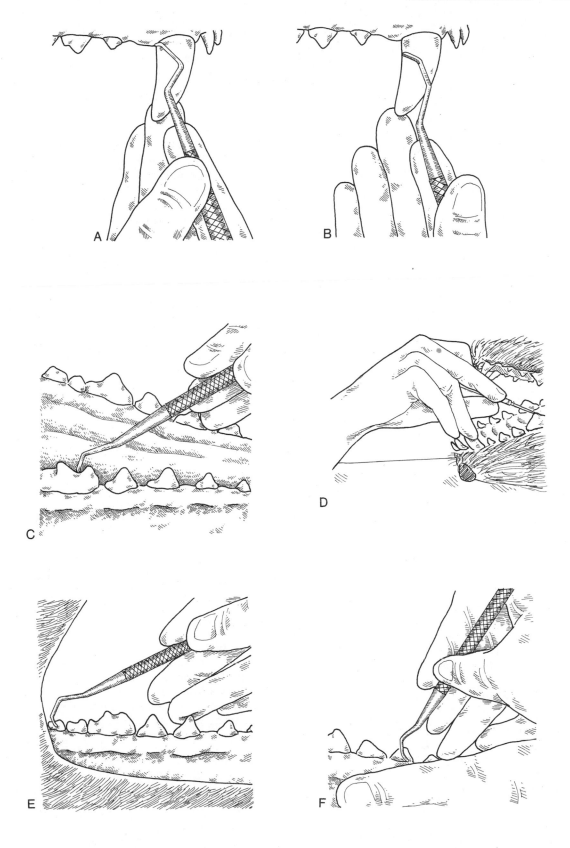

Working Techniques

- When using a scaler or curette, the blade of the instrument is placed so that the face of the working end is at a 70 to 80 degree angle to the tooth surface *(A)(B)*.
- The instrument should follow the contour of the tooth and should maintain the 70 to 80 degree angle as the pull stroke is made toward the cusp of the tooth from the gingival margin.
- The tip of the instrument may be used for removing calculus from pits and fissures; the maxillary fourth premolar is a site where these deposits frequently occur.
- Scalers should not be used subgingivally because they distend and lacerate tissues.
- Curettes may be used supragingivally in a manner similar to that of scalers.

Complications

- Scratching the enamel or dentin.
- Removing restorative material from previously filled teeth.
- Risking gingival lacerations, abrasions, tears, and damage to the sulcus.

Calculus-Removing Forceps

Indication
- Removal of large pieces of calculus.

Contraindication
- Fractured teeth with unstable fragments.

Basic Principle
- Rapid but uncontrolled removal of calculus.

Materials
- Calculus-removal forceps.
- Needle holders.
- Extraction forceps.

Technique
- One jaw of the forceps is placed on the cusp of the crown, the other jaw below the calculus to be removed.
- The handle is squeezed, and the calculus is loosened from the tooth.
- Extraction forceps may also be used in this manner *(C)*.

Complications
- Fracturing the crown.
- Tearing gingival tissue.
- Luxating or extracting the tooth.
- Damaging enamel.

Power Instrumentation: Ultrasonic

General Comments
- Ultrasonic instrumentation: magnetostrictive (with stack).
- If done properly, ultrasonic scaling is a safe method for removing large amounts of calculus rapidly.
- The pot (stack) should be inspected at regular intervals for fractures in the metal leaves (see Chapter 2, Dental Equipment and Care).
- The correct angulation of the working end of the scaler is necessary for efficiency and safety.
- The side of the tip is most effective and least likely to cause damage if the handle is held parallel to the tooth surface *(D)*, rather than perpendicular to it *(E)*.[7]
- To avoid damaging the tooth surface, the pressure applied should be less than approximately 50 g (the weight of two aspirin tablets).

Indication
- Removal of gross calculus from supragingival surfaces.

Materials
- Ultrasonic scaler with water source.
- Universal tip.

Technique
Substep 1—Handpiece is grasped with a modified pencil grip with fulcrum for control.

Substep 2—The terminal 1 to 2 mm on the side of the tip of the instrument is used *(F)*.

Substep 3—Rapid, overlapping short strokes are made over the tooth surface. The strokes should start at the edge of the calculus to free it more readily.

Complications
- Either an inadequate water spray or lingering at one spot on the tooth may result in thermal injury to the pulp.
- Etching the enamel with excessive pressure or using the instrument tip rather than the side of the working end.

Aftercare: Follow-Up
- Polish and use other techniques to ensure complete removal of plaque and calculus.

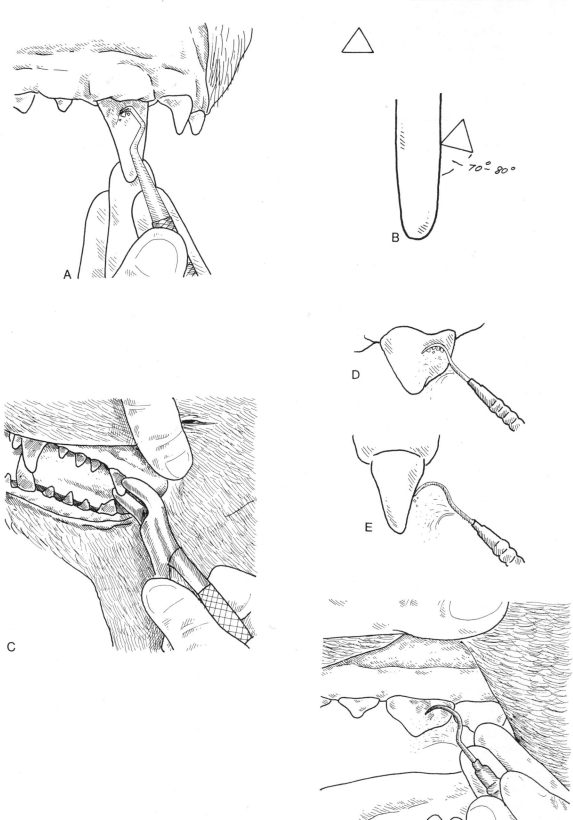

70°–80°

Ultrasonic Instrumentation: Magnetostrictive with Ferrite Ceramic Transducer (rod)*

General Comments

- The instrument is used in a manner similar to that of other ultrasonic handpieces.
- The properties that are similar to those of a piezo transducer allow the ferrite ceramic unit to generate an exceptionally high frequency of 42,000 cps.
- The ferrite ceramic rod should be periodically inspected for tightness at its attachment to the working end. If the performance of the handpiece appears reduced, the transducer may have become loosened.
- The scaler tip moves in a circular fashion so any side of the tip is active.

Technique

- The unit is supplied with an external pump, flexible tubing, and wand. During routine use, the wand remains resting at the bottom of a beaker filled with tap water. This is the source of water for cooling the working end and irrigating the sulcus.
- Because of the design of the scaler tip, the water is delivered directly down the tip of the working end.
- The wand may be immersed in another beaker filled with an antimicrobial solution, and the scaler tip may be used to administer deep-root therapy.
- The external irrigation system and pump are built to ensure an easy, safe, sterile flow of irrigant from the source to the treatment site.
- The external tubing and scaler tips may be sterilized to reduce the risk of cross contamination.
- The on/off switch is in the handpiece, which has the ergonomic benefit of allowing the operator to place both feet up at a restful height on a foot rest. This relieves the lower back by reducing the fatigue that is caused when one reaches a foot to the foot pedal, resulting in a less than horizontal plane of the upper leg (see Chapter 12, Ergonomics in Veterinary Dental Practice).

Complications

- Similar to those of other ultrasonic scalers.
- Fragile ferrite rods.

---

*Odontoson: Periogiene, P.O. Box 9, Fort Collins, CO 80522

Maintenance

- All removable parts are autoclavable: tips, handpiece and cord, irrigation lines.

Ultrasonic Instrumentation: Piezo Electric

General Comments

- The unit operates with an electromagnetic transducer that allows it to operate at 40,000 cps, thus reducing the operator time. The scaler tip moves in a linear manner (back and forth), rather than in a figure-of-eight motion as do magnetostrictive stack units, and is less damaging to the enamel.
- The unit utilizes a water spray, either from an independent source or from the hospital main water supply, to supply irrigation and to act as a coolant (although the coolant effect is claimed by the manufacturer not to be necessary because the electromagnetic transducer produces little heat).

Technique

- The handpiece is held and used in a manner similar to that of the stack model of magnetostrictive ultrasonic scalers.

Complications

- Because of their high frequency, the tips suffer metal fatigue fractures and need replacement approximately twice as often as do the magnetostrictive stacks, but tips are generally half the cost.

Power Instrumentation: Sonic

Basic Principles

- Less heat is created by sonic scalers than by ultrasonic scalers.
- Sonic scalers require compressed air to operate.
- Sonic scalers produce minimal heat, decreasing the chance of thermal damage to the pulp.
- Sonic scalers can be used subgingivally.

Indication

- Removal of gross calculus from supragingival and (with caution) subgingival surfaces.

Materials

- Dental station with compressed air.
- Sonic scaler.

Technique

- A systematic approach is recommended.
- The finger rest will vary from tooth to tooth and operator to operator.

Step 1—The labial surface of the maxillary canine tooth is scaled with a sonic scaler and using extended-reach finger rests *(A)*.

Step 2—The buccal surface of the maxillary premolars is scaled using standard finger rests *(B)*.

Step 3—The palatal surface of the maxillary incisors is scaled using extended-reach finger rests *(C)*.

Step 4—The palatal surface of the maxillary canine is scaled using standard finger rests *(D)*.

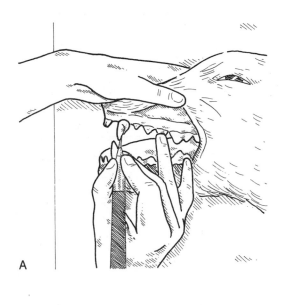

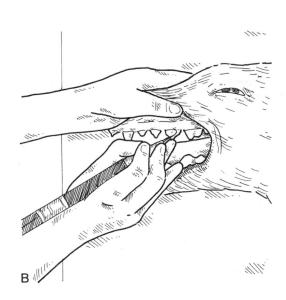

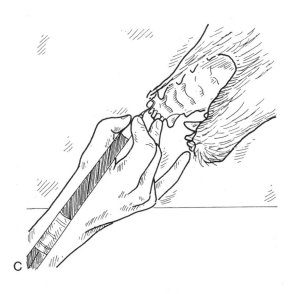

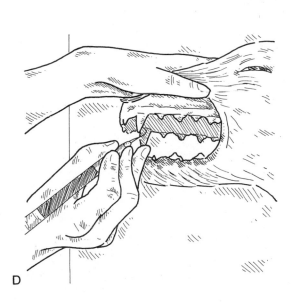

Step 5—The palatal surface of the maxillary premolars is scaled using cross-arch finger rests *(A)*.

Step 6—The labial surface of the mandibular canine is scaled using standard rests on the incisor *(B)*.

Step 7—The lingual surface of the mandibular incisor is scaled using standard rests *(C)*.

Step 8—The lingual surface of the mandibular molar is scaled using extended rests *(D)*.

Complication
- Etching enamel.

Aftercare: Follow-Up
- Same as that of ultrasonic.

Power Instrumentation: Rotary Scaler (Rotosonic Scaling)

General Comment
- There is a limited place for this type of instrumentation in veterinary dentistry. When performed, it must be used carefully by trained and skilled personnel.

Indications
- Removal of gross calculus from supragingival surfaces.
- Subgingival root planing (with caution).

Contraindication
- Inadequate user training.

Basic Principle
- A high-speed bur is used to remove calculus.

Materials
- High-speed handpiece.
- Cleaning bur.*

---

*Rotopro: Ellman Dental Manufacturing Co., 1135 Railroad Ave., Hewlett, NY 11557

Technique
- With very light pressure, the bur is moved over the surface of the tooth.

Complications
- Etching tooth enamel or dentin. The bur is six-sided. At 300,000 rpm at the handpiece, each edge will make contact with the deposit 10,000 times/second (see Table 4–2). If the contact is with the enamel, traumatic injury may result.

Table 4–2 • APPROXIMATE RELATIVE SPEEDS OF POWER SCALING

Pot/stack	25,000, 30,000 cps
Piezoelectric	40,000–45,000 cps
Ferrite ceramic transducer	42,000 cps
Sonic	8000–18,000 cps
Rotary highspeed	10,000 contacts per sec at 300,000 rpm

- Damaging the tooth thermally. The instrument is a soft metal and is designed to be replaced often. If not replaced frequently, the dulled working end will burnish the dental deposits onto the tooth's surface.
- Burning bone.
- Removing calculus incompletely.
- If a burning smell is noted, the instrument is being used incorrectly.
- If used subgingivally, the angle required to accomplish root planing will likely result either in soft tissue damage to the wall of the gingival sulcus or gouging (ledging) of the root surface.

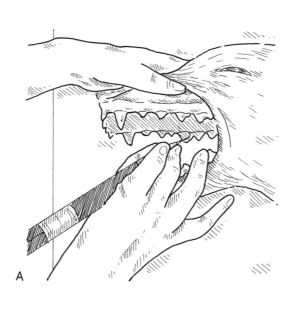

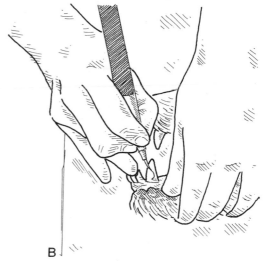

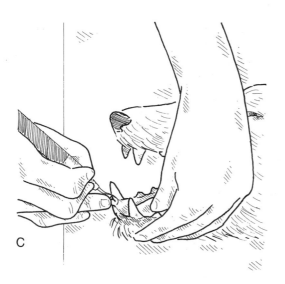

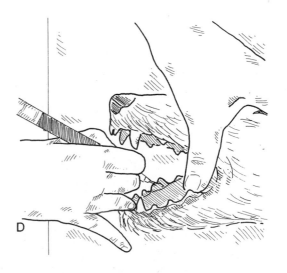

Step 2: Closed Subgingival Plaque and Calculus Removal

General Comments

- If subgingival calculus remains, only a cosmetic benefit and no health benefits have been accomplished.
- Sharp instruments are necessary for this procedure.
- Pocket depth, pocket epithelium, rough tooth surface, and necrotic cementum may necessitate root planing, subgingival curettage, and/or periodontal surgery.

Indications

- Removal of calculus below the gingiva when pocket depth is less than 5 mm.
- If periodontal pocket depth is greater than 5 mm, surgical treatment may be indicated.

Contraindications

- Severe systemic disease.
- Increased bleeding time.

Objective

- Removal of all subgingival calculus and plaque.

Materials

- Curettes of operator's choice.

Technique

Step 1—The angle of the face is nearly parallel to the tooth surface (closed position) (A). The curette is held with a modified pencil grip and gently introduced to the bottom of the sulcus or pocket (B).

Step 2—The bottom of the sulcus or pocket is encountered and should feel soft and resilient (in contrast to the hard and firm feeling of calculus on the tooth surface) (C).

Step 3—Once the bottom is reached, the curette is rotated so the face of the working end is at a 70 to 80 degree angle to the tooth surface. Plaque and calculus are removed, by the cutting edge, with a pulling stroke (D).

Step 4—Repeated strokes are taken in different directions—vertical stroke (E), oblique stroke distad (F), oblique stroke mesiad (G), and horizontal stroke (H)—until the sulcus/pocket is clean.

- It may be necessary to start at an edge of the subgingival calculus and chip away at the calculus until the sulcus is clean.

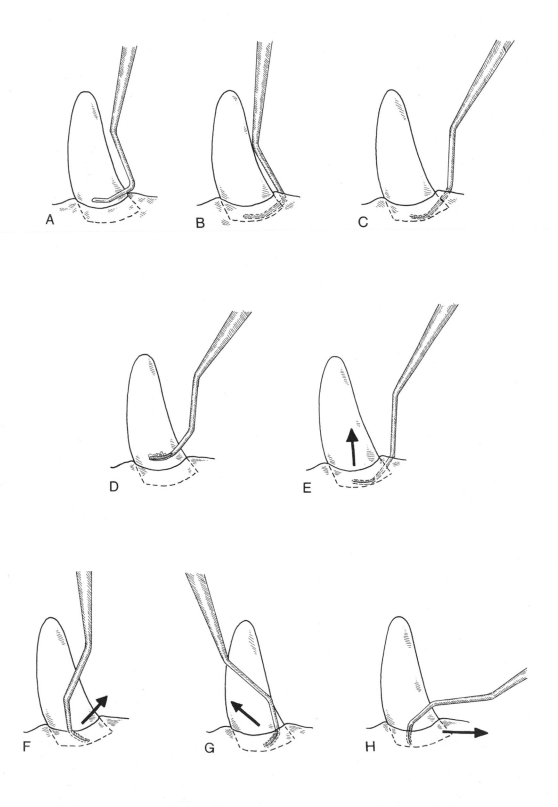

Complications

- The gingiva may become lacerated *(A)*.
- The epithelial attachment may be torn *(B)*.
- The tooth surface may be roughened *(C)*.

Aftercare: Follow-Up

- Routine home care; see pp. 160 to 166.
- Re-examination in 14 to 21 days.
- Evaluation under general anesthetic in 3 to 6 months.

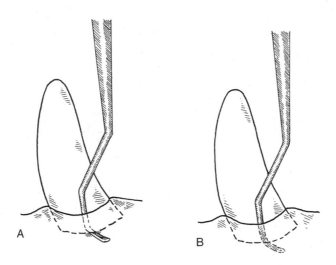

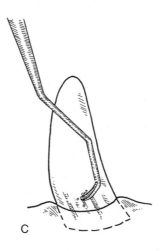

Step 3: Detection of Missed Calculus and Plaque

Objective

- Ensure removal of all calculus and plaque.

Techniques

- Air-drying and using disclosing solutions, explorers, and periodontal probes.

Air-Drying

General Comments

- Calculus is more visible when dry.
- Calculus appears chalky on the dental surface after it is air-dried.
- This method is good to use during the prophylactic procedure on a tooth-by-tooth inspection after scaling. For examining the entire mouth, the staining techniques are preferable.

Indication

- Rapid detection of calculus and plaque that may not be visible to the eye.

Contraindication

- May not be as thorough as using a disclosing solution.

Materials

- Compressed air from a three-way syringe or other air source.

Technique

- Air is directed toward the gingival sulcus to lift the free gingival margin gently and to dry the tooth surface (A).

Disclosing Solutions

General Comment

- Stains are not retained on the surfaces of clean teeth.

Indication

- Disclosing solution can help detect plaque that may otherwise be unnoticed.

Contraindication

- White or light-colored dogs because overflow may temporarily stain the haircoat.

Materials

- One-stage disclosing solution, which stains plaque and calculus one color.
- Two-stage disclosing solution, which stains recently formed plaque a different color from long-standing plaque and calculus.
- Fluorescein stain, which may be observed in light or ultraviolet light.

Technique

Step 1—A small amount of disclosing solution is applied to a cotton-tipped applicator.

Step 2—The disclosing solution is applied to the teeth (B).

Step 3—The oral cavity is rinsed with water to remove nonadhering disclosing solution from enamel (C).

Step 4—The disclosing solution stains the plaque and calculus. The stain does not absorb to normal enamel or dentin (D).

- Stained calculus and plaque are then visualized and removed using techniques described above.

Complications

- Staining gingiva and hairs. Because disclosing solutions are water-soluble, they are washed away in several days by eating and drinking.

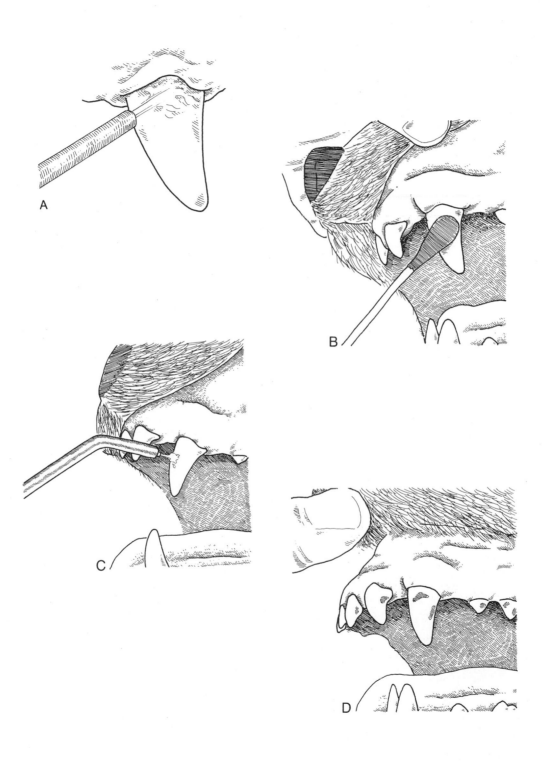

Step 4: Polishing

General Comments

- Slow speed should be used.
- The polisher should spend only a short time on each tooth to avoid thermal injury to the tooth.
- Adequate supply of prophy paste is used for lubrication and polishing.
- A light pressure minimizes thermal injury and tooth damage.
- If the teeth are not polished, the slightly irregular roughened surface is perfect for bacterial plaque formation to recur promptly.

Indication

- After every tooth scaling.

Contraindications

- With some restorative materials, alternative prophy pastes should be used.
- With some restorative materials, polishing should be avoided until curing is complete.

Objective

- Smoothing the tooth surface and removing residual plaque.

Materials

- Dental delivery system (electrical or air-powered).
- Prophy angle (the oscillating prophy angle (Prophy-matic*) creates less heat, does not tangle hair, and does not sling paste).
- Prophy cup.

---

*Medidentia, 39–23 62nd St., Woodside, NY 11377

- Prophy paste supplied in bulk or individual containers.
- Prophy paste dish.

Technique

Step 1—A small amount (½ teaspoon) of prophy paste is placed into a prophy paste dish (A).

Step 2—A rubber prophy cup is dipped into the prophy paste dish (B).

Step 3—The prophy paste is transferred to the surface of the teeth to be polished (C).

Step 4—A liberal amount of prophy paste is used on each tooth surface to act as a lubricating as well as a polishing compound (D).

Step 5—The rubber prophy cup is lightly applied to the tooth surface and turned at a slow speed (2000 to 4000 rpm) (E). The edge of the cup can be slightly flared to move subgingivally.

Step 6—The tooth surface and sulcus are thoroughly rinsed (F).

- Coarse or supercoarse ("stain-remover") prophy paste is available to assist in cleaning hard-to-clean enamel. When using coarse prophy paste, more enamel is removed. A fine prophy paste should be used after the coarse paste in order to make the surface as smooth as possible.

Complications

- Thermal injury to the pulp.
- Wrapping patient's hair in the cup with the rotating prophy cup. Children's "banana" hair clips can be used to keep hair out of the operating field. The patient's face may be toweled-in to prevent hair entanglement and prophy paste from being splattered into the eyes. Reciprocating prophy angles rather than rotating prophy angles, although more expensive, are also available.

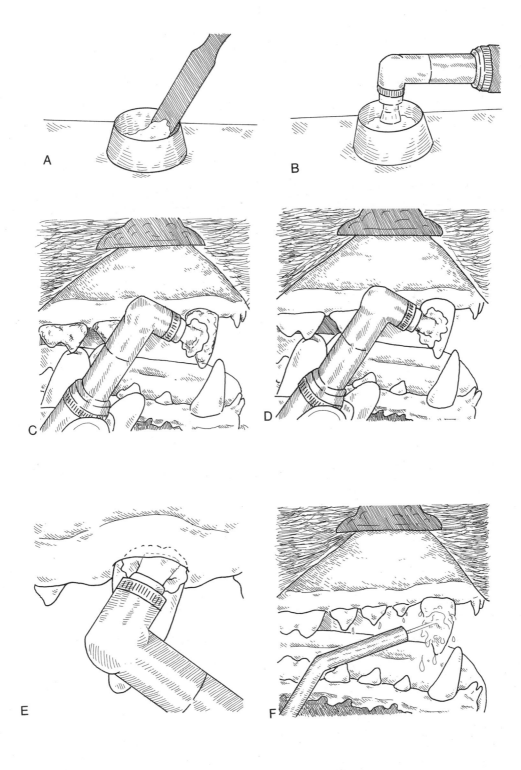

Step 5: Diagnostics

Periodontal Probing/Exploring

General Comments

- Periodontal probing and exploring are important diagnostic procedures.
- Thorough treatment of any pocket more than 5 mm in depth requires periodontal surgery.
- The periodontal probe/explorer is one of the most important diagnostic instruments for the veterinary dentist.
- The delicate, blunt tip of an explorer may be moved along the tooth surface at the gingival margin to detect tooth irregularities and deposits. It can be used to detect dentinal softening of carious lesions and to percuss and test the sensitivity of pulp chambers in fractured or worn teeth.

Indications

- To examine dental structures.
- To detect periodontal pockets, roughened tooth surfaces, and calculus deposits.

Objective

- To assess periodontal health and periodically monitor and evaluate the progress of therapy.

Materials

- Periodontal probe of operator's choice (see pp. 70 to 71.)

Technique

Step 1—The probe is gently inserted parallel to the long axis of the tooth to the bottom of the sulcus or pocket *(A)*. Deep pockets are detected *(B)*.

Step 2—The probe is "walked" along the entire wall of the tooth (do not drag the probe), measuring the depth of the sulcus or pocket, testing in at least six places around the tooth *(C)*.

Step 3—The pocket depth is recorded in the dental record.

Complication

- Perforation of floor of gingival sulcus from too much pressure. This can happen easily because in the fundus of an unhealthy sulcus, the tissue is weaker than in the fundus of healthy tissue.

Dental Radiology

Indications

- Radiographs are taken to evaluate the dental and bony structure for evidence of periodontal disease, endodontic pathology, traumatic injury, or metabolic imbalance.
- Intraoral dental radiology enables the clinician to find dental disease that can be easily missed during physical examination or that is detectable only by radiographic means.
- See Chapter 3 for further information.

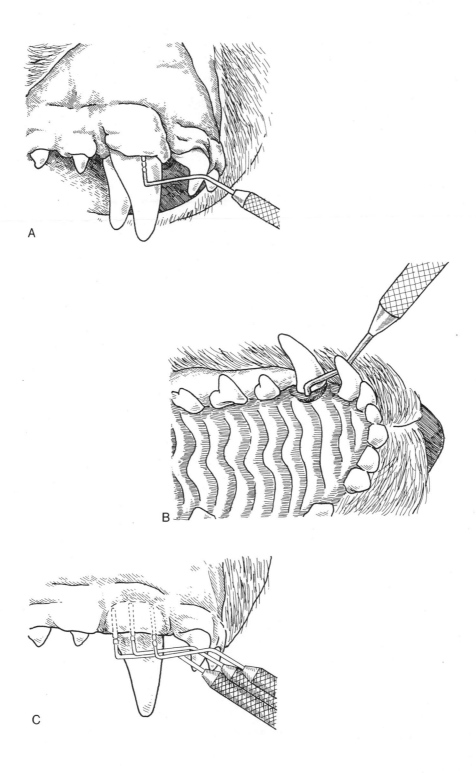

A

B

C

Step 6: Sulcus/Pocket Irrigation

General Comments

- Irrigation cleanses the subgingival sulcus or pocket of loose calculus, prophy paste, and miscellaneous debris and decreases bacterial counts.[8]
- A 0.12% chlorhexidine solution administered by sulcular irrigation has been shown to decrease the periodontal microbial count.
- A 1.64% stannous fluoride treatment administered by sulcular irrigation may be beneficial in causing a dramatic and sustained decrease of subgingival motile bacteria and spirochetes following irrigation.[8]

Indication

- To remove debris after every scaling, curetting, and polishing.

Contraindications

- Drug sensitivity.
- Mobile teeth.

Objective

- Flushing all debris from the sulcus or pocket and coating the clean sulcus surfaces with antimicrobial substance.

Materials

- Blunted, 23-gauge needles with a 6 or 12 ml syringe.
- Curved-tip syringes.
- Alternative rinsing solutions may include water, 0.02% chlorhexidine, stannous fluoride gel, or sodium fluoride foam.

Technique

Step 1—The blunted tip is gently introduced into the pocket or sulcus, and the irrigating solution is infused (A). Alternatively, a curved-tip syringe may be used (B).

Step 2—Rinsing is continued until clear solution is noted.

Step 3—Some irrigants should be rinsed off the tooth structures.

Complications

- Tearing the gingival tissues caused by excessive pressure or by rough instrumentation with the tip.
- Failing to clean thoroughly.

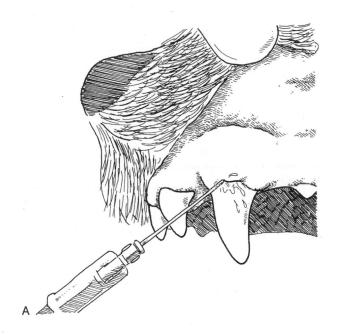

A

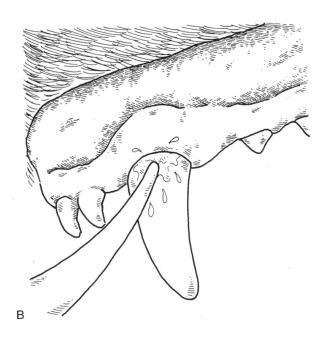

B

Step 7: Home-Care Instruction
General Comments

- The veterinarian has traditionally assumed complete responsibility for managing the dental patient. Currently, more clients are willing to assume responsibility for the daily dental hygiene of their pet(s) in order to increase the interval necessary to maintain good oral health and to decrease the number and frequency of costly anesthetic procedures and professional care. At the time of the physical examination, a frank discussion to evaluate client commitment and patient cooperation in home-care procedure will help the practitioner create a successful treatment plan. If the client is unwilling, or if the patient will not allow dental home care, extraction of diseased teeth is indicated rather than advanced dental procedures. Home care is most often successful when started as a pup or kitten, before dental disease starts.
- The client's commitment should be determined. Then the client should be shown appropriate techniques to be able to provide the adequate home care necessary to maintain clean teeth and a healthy mouth. After prophylaxis, teeth stay clean only for a short time without such care.
- Not all patients are willing to submit to nor are clients capable of providing home care. Overexuberance in the presentation of the home-care procedure can drive a client away from the clinic or hospital and can actually decrease the bonding between owner and pet.
- Another equally important consideration is the patient's temperament. Clients and handlers should be advised of the potential risks involved in home care. If the owner is injured by the pet, the veterinarian may be vulnerable for litigation.
- A member of the staff should spend time reviewing brushing and home-care techniques with the client. Time spent in staff training will aid client rapport and increase the chances of successful therapy.
- Clients should be educated regarding the early signs of oral infection and be encouraged to return for further instruction as often as necessary. Some clients may assume they are doing a great job, giving them a false sense of security, which can lead to unintentional damage; it is therefore advisable to schedule periodic recall appointments for oral examination and evaluation.
- Client handouts are also beneficial in reinforcing the need for brushing and home care.
- A release consultation is important. The consultation may be conducted either by the doctor or by a trained staff member.
- The client should be informed of the extent of dental disease, the type of home care necessary, and the need for future professional follow-up. It is helpful to review the patient's dental chart and radiographs with the client at this time.
- Visual aids such as wall charts, models, case radiographs, and photo albums enable staff members to be more effective in communicating with the client.
- A written evaluation with suggestions and a maintenance plan should be sent home as the patient is released from the clinic. The primary care-giver at home may not be the person who arrives for the pet and pays the bill; the veterinarian's advice needs to reach the primary care-giver.
- Home care can be either active or passive; that is, the client can perform such activities as brushing or can rely on other methods such as feeding treats and foods that decrease the formation of plaque and calculus.

Active Home Care

Indication

- To remove and prevent formation of plaque and prevent formation of calculus.

Contraindications

- Unruly or dangerous patient.
- Inability of client to perform.

Materials

- For demonstrations, the patient, a demonstrator dog/cat, or plastic/plaster models can be used to show brushing techniques.

Technique

- The two major methods of plaque control are mechanical and chemical.
  Mechanical Devices
- Toothbrush.
- Various sizes and designs of toothbrushes are available in the veterinary market for dogs and cats.
- Toothbrushes designed for human use are also available in supermarkets and vary from neonatal to adult size.

Advantages
- Readily available.
- Most effective method of removing plaque.

Disadvantage
- Some clients lack the manual dexterity required to brush animal teeth effectively.

Mechanically Powered Toothbrush*

Advantage
- Easy to use.

Disadvantage
- Noise and mechanical action may frighten the patient.

Gauze Sponge
- Pumice-impregnated gauze sponges.
- May be wrapped around a cotton-tip swab for ease of application.

Advantage
- Easy client use.

Disadvantages
- Greater risk to client of being bitten.
- Greater expense.
- May not be as thorough as a brush beneath the gumline.

Water Pick
- Water picks should be used on low power.

Advantages
- Can be directed toward problem areas or areas that are hard to reach.
- May not be as painful as the application of a brush or gauze immediately following periodontal therapy.
- Useful in cases of sensitive gingiva or before or until gingival pain is decreased.

Disadvantages
- Messy.
- Patient may not tolerate it.
- Do not introduce directly into sulcus; can cause transient bacteremia.

Types of Dentifrices
- Various chemical agents have been proposed for the removal and prevention of plaque in humans and animals. Generally, dentifrices operate in one of three ways: (1) by abrasion—these products contain either a calcium or a silicate ingredient; (2) by oxidation—these products contain an oxidizing agent designed to be inhospitable to anaerobic bacteria; (3) by various chemical ingredients designed to promote gingival health—e.g., zinc ascorbate.

---

*Rotoplus: Interplaque, Rota-dent Professional Dental Technologies, P.O. Box 4129, Batesville, AR 72503

Powders

Advantages
- Powders have an abrasive quality that can vary with size, structure, and composition of the powder.
- Powders can be made into a paste.
- Patients help to distribute the powder to the palatal and lingual surfaces of their teeth with their tongue.

Disadvantages
- Powders are messy.
- Particles may be accidentally inhaled.
- Particles can accidentally contaminate the eyes and cause irritation.

Liquids

Advantages
- Have a variety of delivery systems ranging from spray to water-pick–type reservoirs.
- Can irrigate hard-to-reach areas.

Disadvantages
- Messy.
- Cannot be used easily with toothbrushes unless fairly viscous.

Sprays

Advantage
- Sprays are quick and easy to use.

Disadvantages
- The hissing noise may startle the patient.
- Sprays may accidentally contaminate the eyes, causing irritation.

Pastes

Advantages
- Carried well by toothbrushes to the surface of the teeth.
- Provide good abrasive action.
- Adhere well for application.
- Often flavored for better acceptance.
- Can be distributed to the palatal and lingual surfaces of the teeth by the tongue.

Disadvantages
- Products designed for people will be swallowed and may cause gastric irritation in the pet.
- May stick to muzzle hairs or vibrissae.

Gels

Advantages
- Carried well by toothbrushes to the surface of the teeth.
- Adhere well for application.
- Often flavored for better acceptance.

Disadvantage
- May stick to muzzle hairs or vibrissae.

Products

Na or K Pyrophosphate

- When present in dog biscuits, may inhibit plaque and supragingival calculus formation.

Saliva Substitutes*

- Helpful in patients with xerostomia.
- Has some fluoride in formulation.

Enzymatic†

- Marketed in pastes, spray, and impregnated pads.

Advantages

- Antiplaque; augments salivary peroxidase system.
- Flavored products available for pets.

Disadvantage

- Not as effective in plaque inhibition as chlorhexidine or fluoride.

Sanguinaria-Based‡

- Marketed as paste and rinse.

Advantage

- Possible antiplaque agent.

Disadvantage

- Flavoring.

Chlorhexidine

- Marketed as a rinse§ and gel‖.

Advantages

- A premixed solution of chlorhexidine is recommended over dilution of a concentrated chlorhexidine.
- True antimicrobial.
- Antiplaque.
- Chlorhexidine adheres very well to the tissues, prolonging the contact time.

Disadvantages

- Bad aftertaste.
- Hampers ability to taste for a short time.
- Black or brown staining of protein pellicle may become noticeable after prolonged use (can be polished clean).

Zinc Ascorbate*

- Marketed as a spray and as a viscous solution.

Advantages

- Supports collagen synthesis.
- Reduces odor.

Disadvantage

- Some patients object to the spray.

Stabilized Chlorine-Dioxide Based (Oxygene)†

Advantages

- Easy to use.
- Oxidizes volatile sulfur compounds that cause malodor.
- Inhospitable to anaerobes.
- Neutral flavor is particularly acceptable to cats.
- Supplied as a solution, may be added to drinking water for dogs or cats.
- Supplied as a gel, may be brushed onto the teeth.
- Gel form also contains aloe vera as a soothing agent and to support healing of oral tissues; can be applied immediately after periodontal procedures or oral surgery for a soothing effect.

Disadvantage

- Less effective plaque control agent.

Fluoride-Based‡

- Marketed as gel or liquid.

Advantages

- Antibacterial.
- Inhibits plaque formation.
- Reduces surface tension of tooth surfaces.
- Reduces dental hypersensitivity.

Disadvantages

- May be toxic in large doses.
- May combine with other fluoride sources to cause toxicity.

Types of Fluoride

- Stannous.
- Monofluorophosphate.
- Sodium fluoride.

---

*Xero-lube Scherer: GelKam International, P.O. Box 80004, Dallas, TX 75380

†CET: St. Jon Laboratories, 1656 West 240th St., Harbor City, CA 90710

‡Viadent: Vipont Pharmaceuticals, 1 Colgate Way, Canton, MA 02021

§Nolvadent: Fort Dodge Laboratories, 800 Fifth St. NW, Fort Dodge, IA 50501

‖CHX, CHX-Guard, CHX Gel, CHX-Guard LA: St. Jon Laboratories, 1656 West 240th St., Harbor City, CA 90710

---

*Maxiguard, Oral Hygiene Gel: Addison Laboratories, 507 N. Cleveland Ave., Fayette, MO 65248

†Oxyfresh Products: Oxyfresh Worldwide, Inc., East 12928 Indiana Ave., Spokane, WA 99220

‡GelKam International, P.O. Box 80004, Dallas, TX 75380

Brushing Technique

- It may be helpful to hold the muzzle with the free hand to control head movement and chewing while brushing the teeth.

Step 1—Dentifrice is applied to the brush or sponge (A).

Step 2—The brush is placed at a 45 degree angle to the tooth (B).

Step 3—A circular, sweeping motion, with the emphasis on the stroke away from the gumline, is used to brush plaque from the sulcus (C).

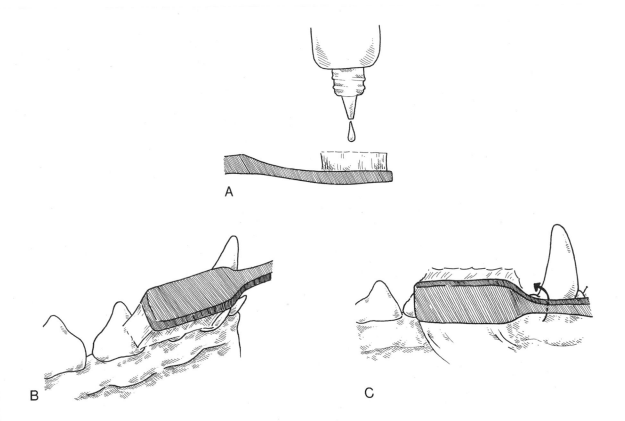

A

B

C

Wiping Technique

Step 1—The dentifrice may be placed on a cotton-tipped applicator (D), the teeth may be wiped with a gauze sponge (E), or the teeth may be wiped with a gauze sponge wrapped around a cotton-tipped applicator (F) if gingiva is sensitive or bleeds easily.

Step 2—To brush or wipe the lingual or palatal surface, a hard rubber toy is placed in the patient's mouth, and the mouth is held closed onto the toy with the opposite hand while the teeth are brushed (G).

Complications

- The client should be advised of the dangers of being bitten or scratched.
- Client-caused iatrogenic oral trauma may occur because of poor technique.
- Failure to respond to conventional therapy may be a sign of: (1) a systemic disease such as diabetes; (2) hyperparathyroidism; (3) low calcium intake; (4) chronic nephritis; (5) leukemia; (6) leptospirosis; (7) deficiency of the vitamin B complex;[9] and (8) feline immunodeficiency virus infection.
- Calculus left subgingivally may lead to periodontal abscess.

Passive Home Care

Indications

- Patient will not allow brushing.
- Client unable or unwilling to brush or to use active home care techniques.

Products

- Dental Diets*

Comments

- Studies have been performed comparing food formulated to reduce the accumulation of dental substrates with commercially available dry foods.[10–12] These studies conclude that dogs and cats consuming a diet formulated to reduce plaque and calculus had less plaque and calculus at 6 months. This resulted in significantly less plaque accumulation and gingival inflammation and improved maintenance of gingival health.

Advantages

- Proven reduction in plaque and calculus formation.
- Patient acceptance.
- Does not rely on client compliance, which may be a significant problem with many clients and patients.[13]

Disadvantage

- Patient may not chew on all surfaces; areas will be missed. Plaque and calculus will still form and periodic professional care will still be necessary.

Rawhide Chewing Products

- Chew-eez*
- C.E.T.†

Comments

- Studies have shown that chewing rawhide reduces plaque and rate of calculus formation in dogs.[14, 15] There was an improvement in the gingival indices, and the animals had improved oral health.
- An additional study has shown that the addition of sodium hexametaphosphate, a calcium sequestrant, to the rawhide resulted in a reduction in calculus formation of about 42%.[16]

Advantage

- May be beneficial for clients/patients who will not brush.

Disadvantages

- The client must be cautioned that the patient must be closely monitored for ingestion of the product with little or no chewing (could result in a foreign body gastrointestinal tract obstruction).
- Patients may not chew on all surfaces; professional care and monitoring is necessary.

---

*Prescription Diet Canine t/d, Prescription Diet Feline t/d: Hills Pet Nutrition, Inc., Topeka, KS 66601

*Friskies Petcare, Glendale, CA 91203
†Chews Veterinary Prescription, 1656 West 240th St., Harbor City, CA 90710

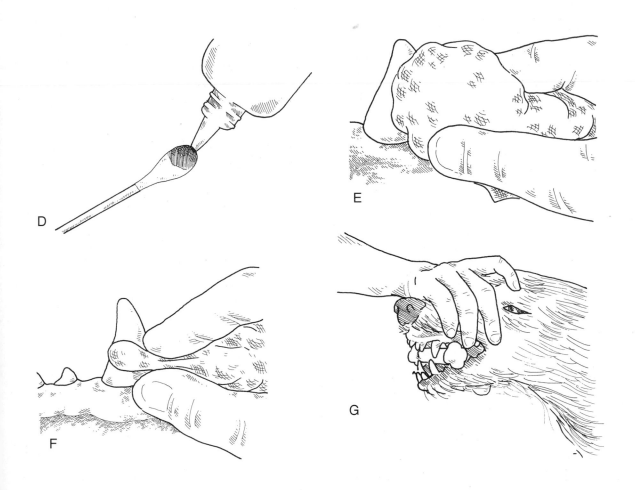

D

E

F

G

Home-Care Plans by Condition/ Ability

Noncritical Patient

- These patients, who are not critically ill, should be started on a toothbrushing routine.
- Starting with flavored water or flavored toothpaste is fine.
- Once the routine is accepted, fluoride gel may be recommended.
- In young adult patients, treatment should be performed at least twice weekly along with chewing activity on rawhide-like chewies.

Intermediate Care Category

- These patients have had chronic gingivitis and need to have plaque prevention more intensively than noncritical patients.
- They should begin with flavored water or flavored toothpastes.
- Home care should be performed at least every other day to be effective.
- Additionally, fluoride may be recommended at least twice a week.

Dental Intensive Care Category

- These patients are periodontal patients that have lost tooth-supporting bone. They often have just had some type of periodontal therapy.
- These patients are put on a routine of twice-daily rinses or brushings with a chlorhexidine solution.
- After 2 weeks, the patient switches at least once a day to a fluoride gel, fluoride animal toothpaste, or some product that promotes gingival health.
- Advanced periodontal disease patients may require daily brushing products to be alternated monthly between an antimicrobial product and a wellness product.
- Additionally, monthly pulse antibiotic therapy may be indicated to support overall medical health.[17]

REFERENCES

1. Fagan DA. Diagnosis and Treatment Planning. Philadelphia: W.B. Saunders Co., 1986:785–799.
2. Page RC, Schroeder HE. Periodontitis in Man and Other Animals. New York: Karger, 1982:158.
3. Page RC. Keynote Speech to the Academy of Veterinary Dentistry. Cincinnati, 1987.
4. Suzuki JB. Diagnosis and Classification of the Periodontal Diseases. Philadelphia: W.B. Saunders Co., 1988:195–216.
5. Tholen MA. Concepts in Veterinary Dentistry. Edwardsville, KS: Veterinary Medicine Publishing Company, 1983:102.
6. Harvey CE, Emily PP. Small Animal Dentistry. St Louis: Mosby, 1993:102–103.
7. Parr RW, Green E, Madsen L, et al. Subgingival Scaling and Root Planing. San Francisco: University of California, 1975:90.
8. Mazza JE, Newman MG, Sims TN. Clinical and antimicrobial effect of stannous fluoride on periodontitis. J Clin Periodontol 1981; 8:203–212.
9. Bojrab MJ, Tholen M. Small Animal Medicine and Surgery. Philadelphia: Lea & Febiger, 1989:51.
10. Logan EI. Oral Cleansing by Dietary Means: Results of Six-Month Studies. In: Proceedings of a Conference on Companion Animal Oral Health. Lawrence, KS, 1996.
11. Harvey CE, Anderson JG, Miller BR. Longitudinal Study of Periodontal Health in Cats. In: Proceedings of a Conference on Companion Animal Oral Health. Lawrence, KS, 1996.
12. Logan, EI. Oral Cleansing by Dietary Means: Feline Methodology and Study Results. In: Proceedings of a Conference on Companion Animal Oral Health. Lawrence, KS, 1996.
13. Miller BR, Harvey CE. Compliance with oral hygiene recommendations following periodontal treatment in client-owned dogs. J Vet Dent 1994; 11:18–19.
14. Lage AL, Lausen N, Tracy R, et al. Effect of chewing rawhide and cereal biscuit on removal of dental calculus in dogs. J Am Vet Med Assoc 1990; 197:213–219.
15. Goldstein GS, Czarnecki-Maulden GL, Vener ML. Beefhide Strips in the Maintenance of Dental Health. In: Proceedings of Veterinary Dentistry 94, Philadelphia, 1994:81.
16. Stookey GK, Warrick JM, Miller LL, et al. Reducing Calculus Formation in Dogs with HMP-Coated Rawhide. In: Proceedings of Veterinary Dentistry 95, Vancouver, 1995:65.
17. Hamlin RL. A Theory for the Genesis of Certain Chronic Degenerative Diseases of the Aged Dog. Small Animal Scope. Kalamazoo, MI: Upjohn Co., 1991:1.

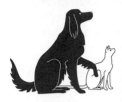

Chapter 5

PERIODONTAL THERAPY AND SURGERY

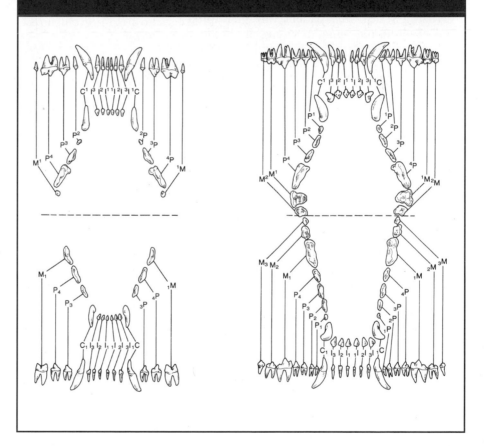

PERIODONTAL THERAPY AND SURGERY ALGORITHM

General Comments

- Patients with advanced periodontal disease are often presented for teeth cleaning. In these cases, more than dental prophylaxis or a simple cleaning is necessary to restore gingival health. The additional treatment may be broadly termed "periodontal therapy." Client communication in this case is important: the client should understand that the patient's condition has progressed beyond gingivitis to periodontitis. Treatment for this patient will therefore take additional time, resulting in higher fees. Because of this, it is advisable to perform a preliminary examination. In this way a tentative treatment plan can be communicated to the client. The information presented to the client should also include the need for possible extraction of nonsalvageable teeth.
- Antibiotics should be started before periodontal therapy or surgery[1, 2] to establish a blood level. Preferred treatment is an antibiotic by injection 1 hour before surgery.
- A broad-spectrum bactericidal antibiotic such as ampicillin or amoxicillin may be used in most cases. Some cases require treatment with antibiotics selective for gram-negative organisms such as cephalosporin-based agents, enrofloxacin, or combinations of antibiotics. Clindamycin hydrochloride (Antirobe) and amoxicillin trihydrate/clavulanate potassium (Clavamox) have been used successfully in the oral cavity.
- Antibiotics are an adjunct to treatment and prevention of secondary infections, not a cure for periodontitis, although it is often a disease associated with infection.
- Periodontal bacterial plaque is the leading cause of periodontal disease (gingivitis/periodontitis). Plaque-retentive areas (the periodontal pocket) should be eliminated to help prevent further periodontal breakdown.

Objectives

- Periodontal therapy has three principal objectives: (1) pocket reduction and/or elimination of the soft and bony lesions, (2) eradication or arrest of the periodontal lesion, with correction or cure of the deformity created by it, and (3) alteration in the mouth of the periodontal climate that was conducive or contributory to allowing periodontal disease to become established, creating a more biologically sound environment.[3]

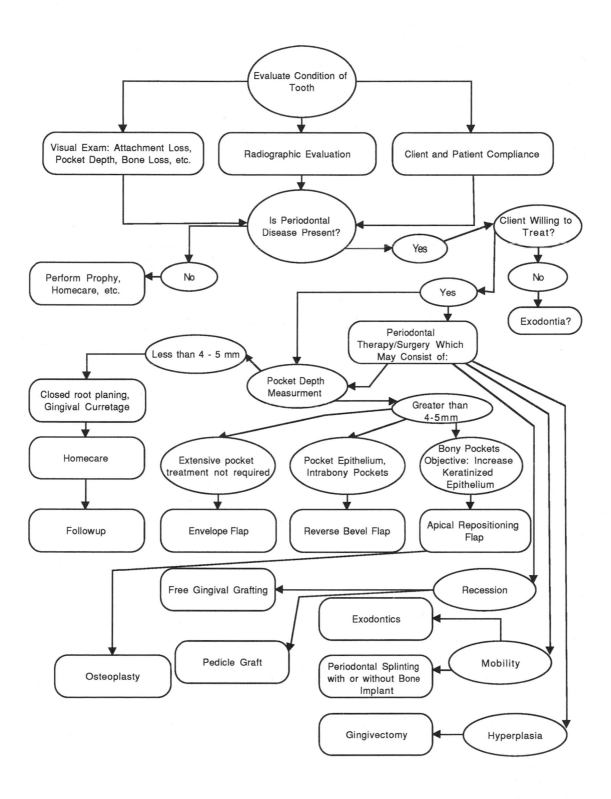

ROOT PLANING: CLOSED TECHNIQUE

General Comments

- Root planing is the process whereby residual embedded calculus and portions of the necrotic cementum are removed from the roots to produce a clean, hard, smooth surface that is free of endotoxin.[4]
- The objective of this hand instrumentation is to render the root surface biologically acceptable to the soft tissue wall of the periodontal pocket without causing unnecessary loss or damage to hard or soft tissues.

Indications

- Calculus on root surface.
- Gingival recession with calculus on root surface.
- Roughening of root surface.
- Presence of periodontal pocket of less than 4 to 5 mm. This depends on relative tooth size.
- Root planing can be performed in patients with pocket depths greater than 5 mm, but it is better to perform open techniques so that treatment can be more definitive.

Contraindications

- Pockets deeper than 4 to 5 mm; because of the inability to access the base of the pocket, the subgingival bacterial plaque cannot be removed. When this is the case, open flap surgery should be considered.
- Nonsalvageable teeth.
- General health considerations (systemic disease, patient's overall health).

Equipment

- Curette (a sharp instrument is important). Often, it is necessary to sharpen the instrument during the procedure to ensure a sharp edge at all times in order to prevent burnishing the calculus, which creates a greater nidus for periodontal disease.
- Hoes.
- Periodontal files.

Technique

- The patient should receive a preoperative antibiotic if pus is present in the pocket or if the patient has any other systemic disease.
- A routine, systematic approach should be used on each quadrant and on each tooth.
- The blade of the instrument is gently inserted in the closed position; that is, the face of the instrument moves parallel to the tooth (A). This allows the positioning of the curette apical to the calculus (often called the exploratory stroke).
- The blade of the curette is positioned against the root surface (adaptation) and opened (B).
- The opened blade of the curette is withdrawn from the pocket in an oblique manner while applying pressure (known as the working stroke) (C).
- Root planing is performed using a curette with overlapping strokes in horizontal, vertical, and oblique directions (also known as cross hatching) (see the later section on gingival scaling technique). This may require additional cleaning strokes after all calculus has been removed to obtain a smooth surface, being careful not to gouge the root surface.
- Cross hatching creates an optimally smooth surface while maintaining root anatomy.
- As root planing is being performed, an assessment must be made regarding the nature of the dental deposits and tooth surface. This evaluation determines how much pressure and in what direction the working strokes should be made.
- The object of calculus removal is to fracture it cleanly away from the tooth surface, not to shave, wear down, or smooth out the deposit (referred to as burnishing).

Complications

- Deposit cannot be removed. The solution is to reposition the blade to remove less calculus per stroke, change the angle and direction of pull of the instrument, change instrument, or sharpen the instrument. Too little pressure can cause the instrument to glance over the deposits and, in fact, to smooth down the deposits rather than to remove them. As these deposits become smoother, they also become harder to detect and remove.

- The surface is still rough after planing. The solution is to check the instrument for sharpness and replane, or if too much force has been applied, causing "ruffling," to use light, smooth strokes.
- Failure to root plane the apical portion of the pocket leaves bacterial plaque and causes an increase in periodontal pocketing and subsequent periodontitis and bone loss.
- Some root surfaces do not lend themselves to thorough root planing, e.g., the maxillary first and second molar. In this case, careful instrument selection and adaptation is important. Failing to do this, it is better to perform a periodontal flap procedure or extract the tooth.
- Hemorrhage may limit visibility. Limited visibility may require the use of pressure, water irrigation, and/or suctioning during the procedure.

- It may be difficult to access the root surface, particularly in areas of exposed furcations that may be large enough to allow accumulation of plaque and calculus but too small and inaccessible to permit thorough root planing. Micro-ultrasonic instruments may be the solution, due to their thinner tips and type of movement.
- Overinstrumentation and aggressive instrumentation cause damage to the gingival fibers (periodontal ligament) at the apical edge of the pocket.

Aftercare: Follow-Up

- Follow routine home-care instructions (see the section titled Home-Care Instruction in Chapter 4, Dental Prophylaxis).
- Antibiotics.

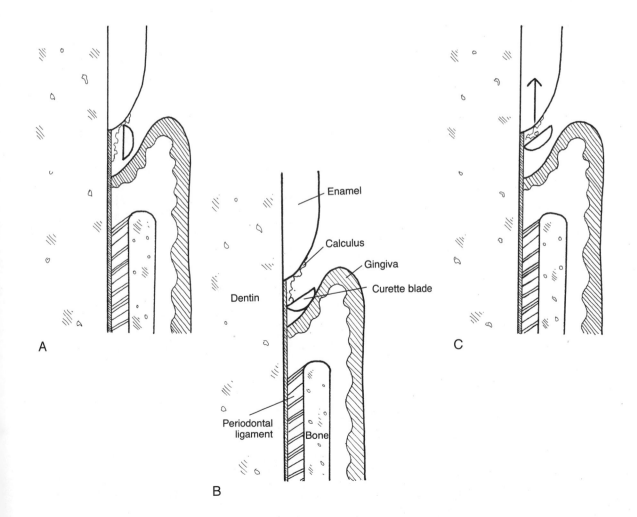

GINGIVAL CURETTAGE

General Comments

- Treatment of the gingival soft tissues.
- Allows optimal reattachment and shrinking of the periodontal pocket.
- Usually performed in conjunction with root planing; called coincidental curettage when performed adjacent to teeth being root planed.
- Pocket epithelium and infiltrated subepithelial connective tissues are removed without reflecting flaps, i.e., without direct vision of the surfaces to be treated.

Indications

- Removal of sulcular epithelium, inflammatory infiltrate, subgingival bacteria, and invasive bacteria.
- Débridement of a periodontal abscess.

Contraindications

- Pockets more than 4 mm deep and furcation areas may not be accessible.
- Nonsalvageable teeth.
- General health considerations.

Objective

- Elimination of the microorganisms that elicit inflammation and of diseased or infiltrated tissues.[4]

Equipment

- Curette (sharp instruments are important).

Technique

- Performed after root planing.
- Performed with the curette held in the reverse position from normal scaling; this places the blade against the soft tissue for epithelial removal (A).
- A finger against the gingiva may be used to support gingival tissue during curettage (B).
- Curette is pulled along the tissues and around the pocket wall, débriding pocket epithelium.
- Gingival tissues are irrigated with a chlorhexidine or fluoride solution.
- Gentle compression applied for several minutes to aid readaptation of tissues to the teeth and to control hemorrhage.

Complications

- Excessive destruction of the gingiva.
- Deepening of the periodontal pocket—may be caused by placing the curette too deeply into the pocket and tearing or cutting the periodontal ligament or perforating the junctional epithelium at the base of the pocket (C).
- Plaque or calculus left in the pockets—the superficial and coronal tissue heals, and the pocket shrinks and tightens, trapping mineralized bacterial plaque/calculus and resulting in increased chronic lysosomal release, tissue breakdown, increased bone loss (periodontitis), and possible abscess, which further prevents healing (D). As part of the process, the tissues should be irrigated with water or an antimicrobial irrigant to cleanse the area further.
- Formation of a thick blood clot, which may hinder the adaptation of the gingival tissues to the teeth. Applying gentle pressure until hemorrhage stops may help avoid this.

Aftercare: Follow-Up

- Re-examination in 7 to 14 days; possible open surgical techniques.
- Open surgical techniques will be necessary if the gingiva does not respond to this conservative treatment.

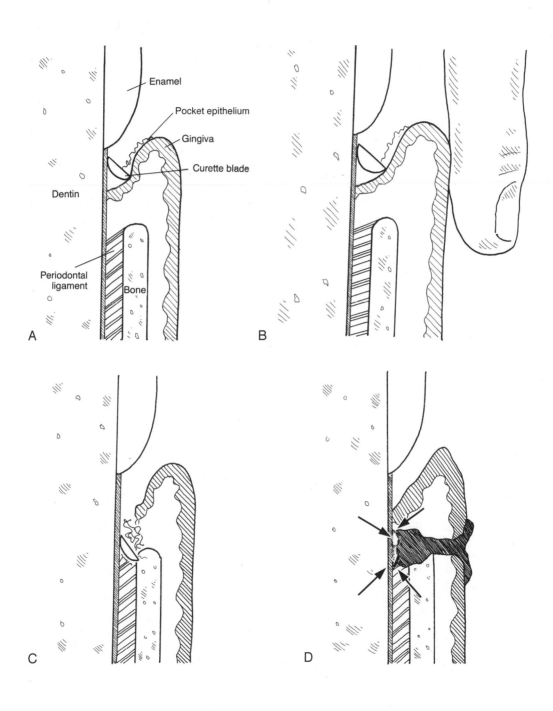

A

Enamel

Pocket epithelium

Gingiva

Curette blade

Dentin

Periodontal ligament

Bone

B

C

D

ULTRASONIC PERIODONTAL DÉBRIDEMENT

General Comments

- There has been a paradigm shift from the traditional emphasis on treatment of the tooth and root surface in periodontal therapy to a focus on establishing and maintaining healthy periodontal tissues.
- Removing bacterial plaque and endotoxins and removing plaque-retentive deposits and surfaces are the main goals of periodontal débridement.[5]
- If plaque is thoroughly removed, periodontal tissues have been found to heal in the face of residual deposits of calculus.
- This procedure may involve three phases: supragingival débridement, subgingival débridement, and deplaquing.
- This procedure removes less cementum than manual root planing with curettes; this creates less dentinal hypersensitivity and less chance of overinstrumentation and gouging of tooth/root surfaces.
- The long slender tips allow removal of bacteria to the apical limit of the pocket.
- Specialized tips can be used in and around furcations to improve removal of bacterial colonies and calculus, especially in the dome areas of furcations, previously inaccessible.
- This procedure can be performed in pockets greater than 4 mm in a closed fashion.
- This procedure can be performed as an adjunct to open procedures.
- This procedure can be performed more quickly, with less anesthesia time and with less effort, than manual root planing.
- Antimicrobial irrigants (dilute chlorhexidine or betadine solutions) can be added to the water source of some ultrasonic scalers to aid in plaque reduction and reduction of bacterial aerosolization.
- Ultrasonic bactericidal débridement combines the cavitational effect of the instruments destroying or lysing bacterial cell walls with their antimicrobial lavage.

Indication

- All patients with dental plaque and calculus.

Contraindications

- Nonsalveageable teeth.
- General health considerations of the patient (systemic disease, patient's overall health).

Equipment

- Sonic scaler with long, thin perio-tip.
- Ultrasonic scaler with specialized probe-like tip: Slim-line (Dentsply) or Odontoson (see Chapter 2, Dental Equipment and Care).
- Probe.
- Explorer.
- Curettes.

Technique

- The patient's mouth is lavaged with a dilute chlorhexidine solution to reduce external bacterial counts.
- Supragingival calculus and plaque are removed with the broad tips and with light, rapid sweeping motions over the surface of the crown.
- The ultrasonic or sonic scaler is fitted with the long, thin perio-tip, tuned properly; the water spray is adjusted.
- The instrument tip is used similarly to a probe, placed into the sulcus or pocket parallel to the long axis of the tooth surface.
- The side of the tip of the instrument is used with a paintbrush-like motion over the root surface in diagonal strokes. The pressure is very light and rapid strokes are used (also referred to as feather-light touch).
- Removal of subgingival calculus starts coronally and works apically, using the end of the tip in a gentle tapping motion against the calculus to shatter and remove it.
- After calculus removal, the tip is used in a broad sweeping motion in the sulcus or pocket to remove bacteria from the tooth surface. The instrument tip must touch every square millimeter of root surface; therefore, overlapping or cross-hatching strokes are most desirable.
- High-speed suction should be used, if available, to remove water build-up and reduce aerosolization. If suction is unavailable, the patient's head should be tipped down over a grate or laid on a towel to keep water from collecting under the patient.

Aftercare

- Follow routine home-care instructions (see Chapter 4, Dental Prophylaxis).

PERIOCEUTIC TREATMENT

General Comments

- A perioceutic is a medication designed to be delivered into a periodontal pocket for the treatment of periodontal disease.
- Doxycycline has been found to provide local control of the microorganisms responsible for causing periodontal disease.
- The need for continued home care must be stressed to the client.

Indication

- Patients with periodontal pockets equal to or greater than 4 mm; for treatment after root planing and/or periodontal débridement therapy.

Contraindications

- Patients who have not had thorough periodontal therapy.
- Patients younger than 1 year of age as tetracycline products may cause discoloration of teeth.

Objective

- To infuse the material into the periodontal pocket to allow for a 2–4 week release of antibiotic into the periodontal pocket.

Materials

- 8.5% Doxycycline.* This product comes in a packaged pouch with two syringes and a

---

*Heska Periodontal Disease Therapeutic, Heska Corporation, 1825 Sharp Point Dr., Fort Collins, CO 80525

23 gauge, 1-inch blunt cannula. Once mixed, the product becomes a flowable solution of doxycycline hyclate equivalent to 8.5% doxycycline activity.
- Plastic working instrument.

Technique

Periodontal therapy with root planing and/or periodontal débridement should be performed. The root surface and pocket should be completely free of calculus, plaque, and other debris. The product should be applied only after the teeth and pocket are clean.

Step 1—The two syringes are locked together.

Step 2—Beginning with syringe A, express the contents into syringe B, mixing the product by pushing the syringes back and forth approximately 100 times until the contents are completely mixed.

Step 3—Deliver all of the contents of the syringes, and remove syringe B from A and replace with the supplied 23 gauge cannula.

Step 4—Gently place the cannula 1–2 mm below the gingival margin of the tooth to be treated, and inject the mixture while moving the cannula in the pocket. The pockets should be filled to the gingival margin.

Step 5—Lavage with a few drops of water supragingivally to hasten the solidification of the material.

Step 6—As the material hardens, the product that is exposed supragingivally may be pressed into the pocket with a plastic working instrument or back of a curette.

Complication

- Loss of the material out of the pocket; in this case, the material may be tapped into place with a plastic working instrument.

Aftercare: Follow-Up

- As the product is biodegradable, removal is not required.
- Continued home care is important.

PERIODONTAL SURGERY

Mandibular Frenoplasty (Frenectomy/Frenotomy)

Indications

- Gingival recession or pocket formation and decreased attached gingiva on the distal side of the canine teeth, enhanced by the presence of the frenulum.
- As an aid to treatment of tight lip in the Shar Pei dog.
- As an aid to treatment of cheilitis adjacent to the canine teeth.

Contraindication

- Bleeding disorders.

Objective

- To minimize food accumulation in the anterior portion of the mouth and to improve self-cleaning of this area.

Equipment

- No. 10, 15, or 15C scalpel blade and handle.
- Sharp-sharp scissors.
- 4-0 or 5-0 absorbable suture.
- Needle holder, thumb forceps.

Technique

Step 1—The attachment of the frenulum to the mandibular gingiva near the first premolar is cut horizontally with scissors or scalpel (A).

Step 2—The incision is extended with sharp or blunt dissection into the frenulum to relieve the pull of the muscular attachments. The lip will relax laterally when the attachments have been completely severed (B). A diamond shape is created by the cut surfaces.

Step 3—A suture is placed to bring the mesial and distal edges together (C). Several simple interrupted, absorbable sutures are placed to prevent reattachment (D).

Step 4—The root surfaces of the canines should be planed smooth and polished.

Postsurgical Care

- Twice daily oral flushing with 0.2% chlorhexidine to keep the area clean for 2 weeks.
- Home oral hygiene to minimize progression of periodontitis.

Complications

- Hemorrhage (usually limited) caused by transection of the mental artery or vein; may be avoided by careful blunt dissection after the initial incision.
- Reattachment of frenulum if not sutured.
- Infection.

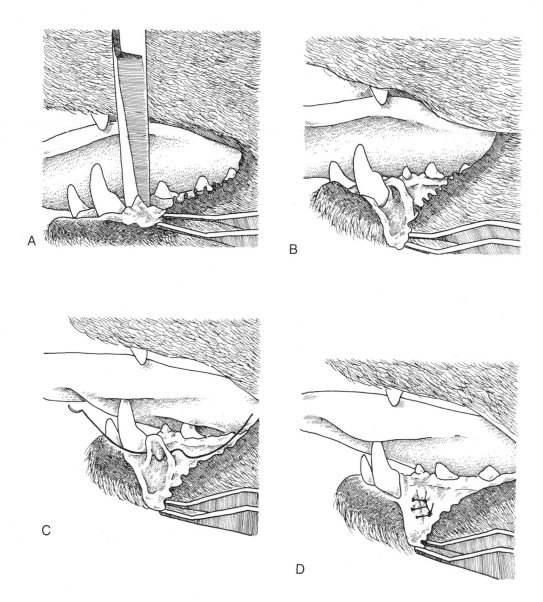

Gingivectomy

General Comments

- Careful case selection is necessary. Gingivectomy is performed only in patients that have at least 2 mm of attached gingiva.
- This procedure is not used for treatment of deep periodontal pockets or as part of routine prophylaxis.
- Reepithelialization takes place at the rate of 1 mm/d.

Indications

- Removal of excessive gingival tissue in cases with hyperplastic tissue.
- Incisional or excisional gingival biopsy.
- Reduction of suprabony periodontal pockets.

Contraindications

- Minimal or absent attached gingiva.
- Horizontal or vertical bone loss apical to the mucogingival junction.

Objective

- To remove excessive gingival tissue to achieve a clean tooth/root surface and a thin beveled gingival margin with pyramid-shaped or knife-like interdental tissue (papilla).

Equipment

- No. 15 or 15C scalpel blade with handle and/or:
- Gingivectomy knives, such as Kirkland or Orban.
- Periodontal probe.
- Electrosurgery/radiosurgery equipment (see p. 183).
- Wet compresses to control hemorrhage.
- Hemostatic agents.
- Cone-shaped rough diamond bur.

Technique

Step 1—The pocket's depth and contour are determined by inserting either a probe or a bleeding point forceps to the depth of the pocket at several areas around the tooth *(A)*. The probe can be walked around the tooth, providing six pocket readings. Use caution so as not to perforate the junctional epithelium.

Step 2—The corresponding depth is measured on the outside of the gingiva using the probe *(B)*.

Step 3—A bleeding point is made by closing the gingivectomy marking forceps (bleeding point forceps), with the tip of a probe by placing the probe perpendicular to the gingiva and applying slight pressure to make a small hole *(C)*, or by using a small-gauge needle to create the bleeding point. These points are made along the contour of the pocket and are used as a guide for the gingivectomy. The gingivectomy is made at an angle apical to the bleeding point to create a beveled margin. At least 1 mm of healthy, attached gingiva must be present apical to the base of the incision.

Step 4—Using the scalpel blade or electrosurgery blade, the gingiva is excised by cutting below the bleeding points with the blade held at approximately a 45 degree angle, with the tip of the blade toward the tooth crown *(D)*.

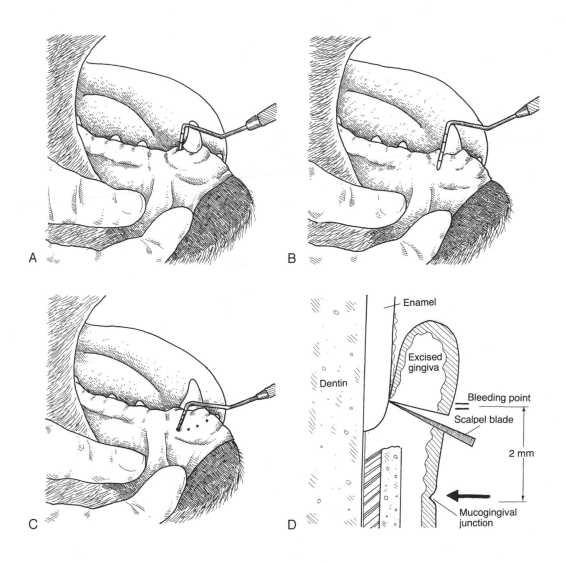

A

B

C

D

Enamel

Excised gingiva

Dentin

Bleeding point

Scalpel blade

2 mm

Mucogingival junction

Step 5—The ends of the excision should be tapered into the surrounding gingiva to create the normal scalloped contour, particularly if several adjacent teeth are treated *(A)*.

Step 6—Gingival tags can be removed with the blade or a sharp curette. An Orban Interproximal Gingivectomy Knife can be used to incise through the papilla between the lingual and buccal/labial aspects.

Step 7—The exposed tooth/root surface can now be scaled and planed smooth *(B)*. Even when thorough root planing has been performed before surgery, a surprising amount of calculus may be discovered after the gingivectomy procedure.

Step 8—Hemorrhage is controlled by applying pressure with wet gauze pads or hemostatic agents. The authors of this text have had little luck maintaining periodontal dressings on canine and feline patients. Properly used, electrosurgery may simplify the procedure by controlling hemorrhage more quickly, allowing a better visualization of the surgical field.

Postsurgical Care

- Most patients eat normally following surgery. Soft food can be fed initially, if necessary.
- Twice daily oral rinses with a 0.2% chlorhexidine solution for 2 weeks by the client at home to keep the oral cavity clean.
- Broad-spectrum oral antibiotics for 1 week.
- Re-examination in 14 to 21 days.
- Follow-up with home oral hygiene and periodic professional dental prophylaxis or periodontal therapy, as appropriate, for the stage of periodontal disease present.

Complications

- Inadequate beveling of the gingival margin, leaving a blunted gingival margin.
- Burning the gingival tissue by using too high a setting on an electrosurgery unit. Anticipate a 1 mm sloughing of tissue even with a normal setting.
- Poor healing, if electrosurgery is performed on unhealthy tissue.
- Not leaving a 1 mm margin of attached gingiva. This promotes potential cleft formation or further gingival retraction. Less keratinized gingival tissue potentiates subsequent bone and/or root exposure.
- Tip of electrosurgery unit touching root surface, especially in small breeds and cats. This can lead to necrosis or thermal injury to the pulp.

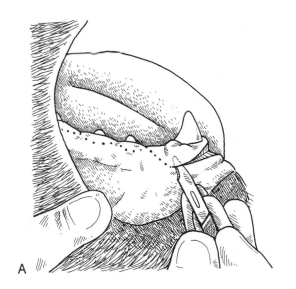

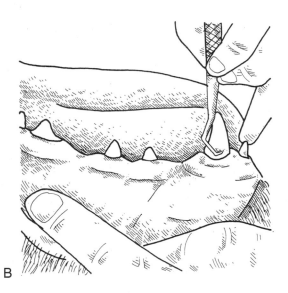

Gingivoplasty

General Comments

- Gingivoplasty is the procedure of surgically recontouring or remodeling the gingival surface.[4]
- Gingivectomy is one form of gingivoplasty. Gingivoplasty usually refers to procedures performed on hyperplastic areas without pseudopockets, whereas gingivectomy refers to procedures performed on hyperplastic areas with pseudopockets.

Indication

- Gingival hyperplasia in interdental areas.

Contraindication

- Narrow or absent attached gingiva.

Objective

- To create a physiologic contour of the gingiva.

Equipment

- Same as for gingivectomy.

Technique

- Gingivoplasty is often performed at the same time as gingivectomy.

Step 1—Using the scalpel blade or electrosurgery blade or loop, the gingiva is excised by cutting with the blade held at approximately a 45 degree angle, with the tip of the blade toward the crown.

Step 2—The marginal edge of the excision should be tapered into the surrounding gingiva to create the normal scalloped contour, particularly if several adjacent teeth are treated. An electrosurgery loop is used in a light superficial sweeping motion on the surface of hyperplastic gingiva, much as a sculptor would use a knife to gradually reduce the surface bulk of a clay model.

Step 3—Gingival tags can be removed with the blade or a sharp curette.

Step 4—Hemorrhage is controlled by applying pressure with wet gauze pads or hemostatic agents.

Complications

* See the preceding section, Gingivectomy.

Aftercare: Follow-Up

* See the preceding section, Gingivectomy.

Electro- (Radio-) Surgery

* Electrocautery uses low frequency, low wattage, and low heat, which creates incandescent heat, causing a third-degree burn that is harmful to tissues and can cause bone loss.
* Electrosurgery/radiocautery uses high frequency (2 to 4 MHz) and is relatively atraumatic.

Advantages

* Permits any degree of rapid hemorrhage control.
* Prevents seeding of bacteria into the incision site.
* Controls hemorrhage during incision.
* Flexible electrodes are available to conform to surgical site.
* Activated electrodes are sterile.
* Improved field of view with hemorrhage control.

Disadvantages

* Unpleasant odor.
* May disturb other electrical devices, e.g., electrocardiogram, radio, pacemaker.
* Caution required near volatile chemicals and gases.
* May cause skin burns.
* Bone loss.

Periodontal Flap Techniques

Open Flap Curettage/Envelope Flap

General Comments

- Open flap curettage can provide pocket reduction and reattachment by creating access to subgingival calculus and removal of fibrotic pocket epithelium.
- Generally, it is performed after evaluation of initial therapy.

Indications

- Local areas with suprabony pocket depths greater than 4 mm where extensive removal of pocket tissue is not required.
- To create better visualization and access for a restorative procedure.

Contraindications

- Poor health status of patient.
- Extensive periodontitis requiring additional exposure and visualization.
- Deep periodontal pockets requiring osteoplasty.

Objective

- To gain access to root surfaces for removal of subgingival calculus and necrotic cementum.

Equipment

- No. 11, 12, 15, or 15C scalpel blade and handle.
- Molt No. 9 periosteal elevator or number 7 wax spatula.
- 4-0 or 5-0 absorbable suture.
- Needle holder, thumb forceps, and scissors.
- Sharp curettes.

Technique

Step 1—The blade is inserted into the pocket with the tip directed toward the alveolar bone *(A)*, and the epithelial attachments are cut *(B)*. (The arrow points to the mucogingival junction.) This is a reverse bevel incision with the intent of removing sulcular epithelium.

Step 2—The gingiva is elevated with the periosteal elevator positioned lingually/palatally and labially/buccally *(C)* without exposing the crestal alveolar bone *(D)*.

Step 3—The exposed root surfaces are planed until they are smooth and hard *(E)*.

Step 4—The area is flushed with 0.2% chlorhexidine solution.

Step 5—The flap is repositioned and sutured with interrupted sutures placed interdentally *(F)*.

Postsurgical Care

- Twice daily oral flushing with 0.2% chlorhexidine solution for 2 weeks.
- Antibiotics as necessary.
- Home oral hygiene after healing, to minimize future plaque accumulation.
- Follow-up examinations, as necessary, to monitor healing.

Complications

- Inadequate treatment in areas of more extensive periodontitis.
- Bone loss with bony lesions that need osteoplasty.

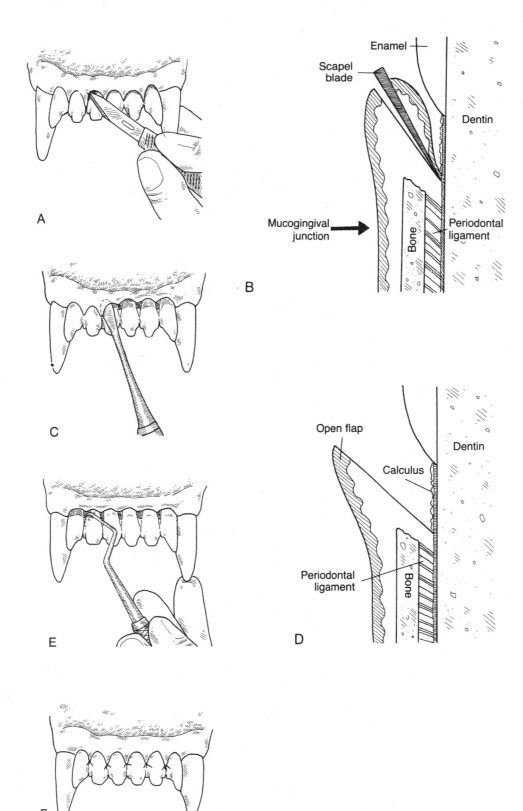

Canine Teeth: Palatal or Lingual Surface Flap Technique

General Comments

- Periodontal disease is often found on the palatal or lingual surface of the canine teeth.
- This area may be difficult to clean with closed techniques.

Indications

- Periodontal pockets greater than 4 mm on the palatal or lingual surface of canine teeth.
- To provide access for correction of osseous defects with or without grafting.

Contraindications

- Loose teeth where salvage is not desired.
- Signs of severe oronasal fistulation (nasal discharge, sneezing, nasal penetration of probe or presence of solution in nares after irrigation of pocket).
- Secondary mandibular osteomyelitis.

Objective

- To allow access to the palatal or lingual root surface of canine teeth for planing, removal of granulation tissue, and bony correction.

Equipment

- No. 11, 12, 15, or 15C scalpel blade and handle.
- Molt No. 9 periosteal elevator or number 7 wax spatula.
- 4-0 or 5-0 absorbable suture.
- Needle holders, thumb forceps, scissors.
- Curettes.
- No. 2, 4 round burs.

Technique

Step 1—The gingiva mesial and distal to the canine tooth is incised to the bone (A). To gain more access, the incision is extended palatally and then caudally in a U-shaped exposure (B).

Step 2—A reverse bevel incision is made to the level of the alveolar crest on the palatal or lingual surface (C).

Step 3—The periosteal elevator is used to elevate the full-thickness gingival flap off the bone to expose the depth of the pocket (D). (The collar of tissue is removed if a reverse bevel incision was made.)

Step 4—Hemorrhage is controlled with wet compresses and direct pressure.

Step 5—Subgingival calculus, granulation tissue, and debris are removed with a curette (E).

Step 6—The exposed root surface is planed smooth, and adjacent bone is curetted.

Step 7—The area is flushed with 0.2% chlorhexidine solution.

Step 8—The desired bony corrections are made as indicated (see the sections on Osteoplasty and Guided Tissue Regeneration and Bone Grafting).

Step 9—The gingiva is apically repositioned to the crest of bone and tooth junction tightly against the tooth surface and sutured with interrupted sutures to the buccal gingiva (F).

Postsurgical Care

- Oral antibiotics as necessary.
- Initially, oral flushing and swabbing; later, gentle brushing of the palatal or lingual tooth surface to prevent plaque buildup.
- Recheck in 3 months, with the patient under general anesthesia, including a follow-up radiograph. Periodic periodontal treatment as required.

Complications

- Puncturing into the nasal cavity during instrumentation. If only a small opening is created, it may be possible to continue with the procedure and allow the defect to granulate and ossify as periodontitis heals.
- Inadequate healing of tissue, with progression of periodontitis and oronasal fistula formation or mandibular bone loss and infection.

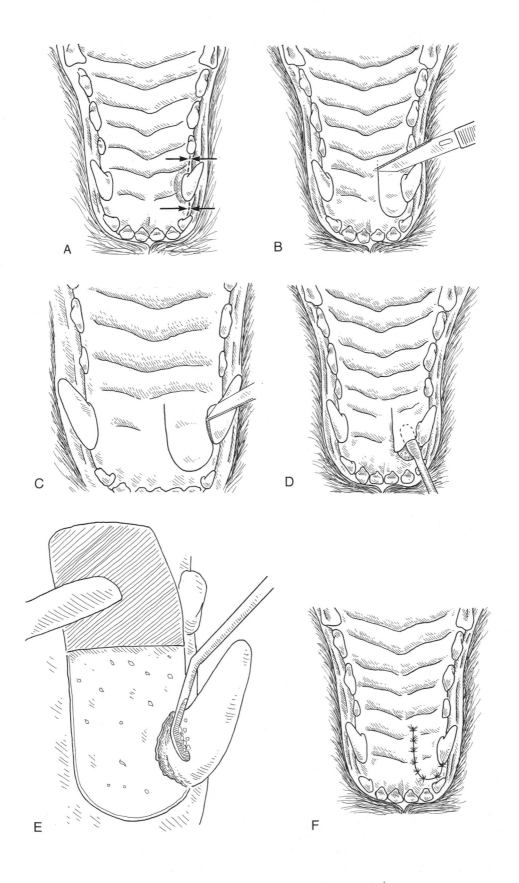

Reverse Bevel Releasing Flap Surgery

General Comments

- Reverse bevel releasing flap surgery is performed to remove diseased pocket epithelium and to gain access for root planing.
- Reverse bevel releasing flap surgery is performed when it is desired to maintain all of the keratinized tissue of the free pocket margin and to position the free pocket margin apically to have an adequate margin of attached gingiva postsurgically.
- As with all gingival surgery, the surgery is performed from line angle to line angle. The line angle is an anatomic landmark on the tooth that represents the corner where two vertical walls of the tooth meet. In *A,* "a" shows an inter-radicular incision and is incorrect; "b" shows a midfacial (radicular) incision and is incorrect; "c" shows an interproximal incision and is incorrect; "d" shows a line angle incision and is correct *(A).*
- Releasing incisions are not always necessary and should not be used indiscriminately.

Indications

- Teeth that have pocket depths greater than 4 mm.
- Periodontal pockets that have not responded to conservative treatment.
- Intrabony pocket formation with vertical bone loss and osseous defects in areas with sufficient attached gingiva.
- To reposition keratinized tissue apically for pocket reduction and increase the zone of attached gingiva.

Contraindications

- Deep pockets with minimal attached gingiva.

- Poor client compliance with home oral hygiene and recall dental prophylaxis.
- Brittle health status of patient.

Objective

- To gain access to root surfaces of teeth with deep periodontal pockets (>4 mm) to remove subgingival calculus and diseased cementum, to remove diseased pocket epithelium and inflammatory infiltrate, and to correct osseous defects.

Equipment

- A no. 11, 12B, 15, or 15C scalpel blade and handle.
- Sharp curette or scaler.
- 4-0 or 5-0 absorbable suture.
- No. 2 or 4 round bur for osteoplasty.
- Needle holder, tissue forceps, scissors.
- Molt No. 9 periosteal elevator or number 7 wax spatula.

Technique

Step 1—Starting at the line angle of the healthy tooth mesial or distal to the operative area,[6] a reverse bevel incision is made, extending through the top of the free gingival margin *(B),* with the blade directed toward the alveolar bone leaving the pocket epithelium and thin collar of marginal tissue around the teeth starting and ending at healthy gingiva. A scalloped incision is made, following the contour of the roots with the highest point of contour at the interproximal area *(C).*

Step 2—Vertical releasing incisions can be made if necessary on one or both sides of the affected area to permit better access to the root surface and alveolar bone *(D).*

Step 3—The flap is elevated with a periosteal elevator *(E).* If minimal bony correction is needed, the flap can be elevated just to expose that portion of the alveolar crest.

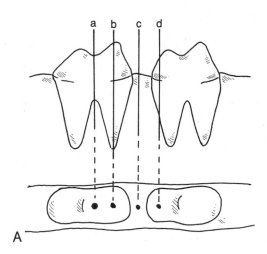

A

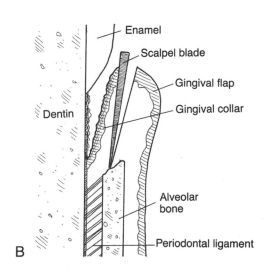

B

Enamel
Scalpel blade
Gingival flap
Gingival collar

Dentin

Alveolar bone

Periodontal ligament

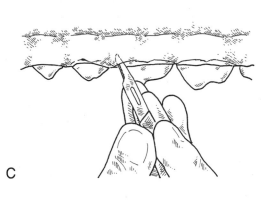

C

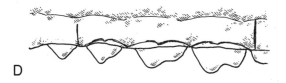

D

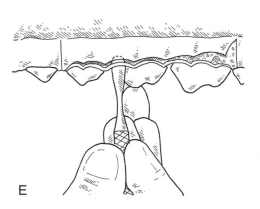

E

Step 4—The collar of marginal tissue is removed by incising the attachments, with the scalpel blade placed into the sulcus horizontally at the base of the pocket. Affected tissue is removed from the root surface with a sharp scaler or curette *(A) (B)*.

Step 5—The flap is retracted, and the root surfaces are planed smooth with sharp curettes *(C)*.

Step 6—Osseous defects and necrotic bone are removed with small round burs in a low- or high-speed handpiece accompanied by saline irrigation.

Step 7—The area is flushed with a 0.2% chlorhexidine solution.

Step 8—The flap is repositioned, being sure that the bone margin is covered, and sutured interdentally with 4-0 or 5-0 absorbable suture *(D)*. The releasing incisions are sutured with interrupted sutures.

Postsurgical Care

- Soft food is recommended for 1 week.
- Oral antibiotics, continued as necessary.
- Daily oral flushing with 0.2% chlorhexidine solution for 2 weeks.
- After healing, home oral hygiene to minimize further plaque accumulation.
- Frequent follow-up examinations and periodic periodontal therapy accompanied by radiographic examination to monitor healing progress.

Complications

- Infection.
- Dehiscence.
- Inadequate coverage of alveolar bone margin due to excessive cutting of tissue.
- Greater pocket formation if soft tissue sutured too high on the root surface.

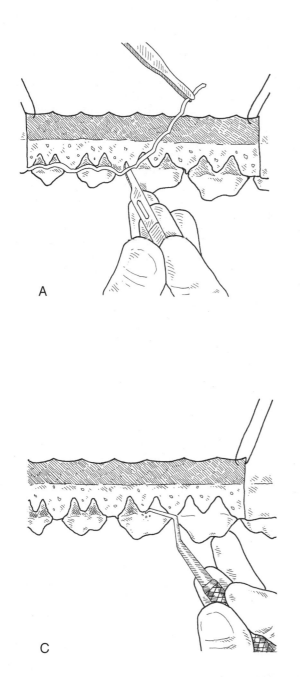

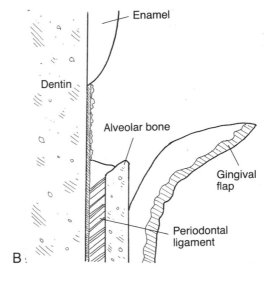

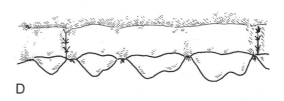

Apically Repositioned Flap Surgery

General Comments

- When performing apically repositioned flap surgery, the gingiva is removed, the periodontal pocket depth is reduced, and the soft tissue is reattached apical to its original location. Possibly, this exposes a furcation or dentin and permits better cleaning of the tooth and access for osteoplasty. The zone of attached gingiva may be increased.

Indication

- Areas with pocket depths greater than 5 mm where a reverse bevel flap is contraindicated; when there are pockets with minimal attached tissue so that the intent is to move the keratinized free gingival margin apically over bony surface.

Contraindications

- Loose teeth.
- Poor client compliance with home oral hygiene or with return for recall prophylaxis.
- Lack of keratinized free gingiva or attached gingiva to move apically.
- Poor health status of patient.

Objective

- To decrease pocket depth in areas with deep intrabony pockets bringing the free gingival margin just coronal to the level of the alveolar bone to allow for better self-cleaning of affected areas and to increase the zone of attached gingiva.

Equipment

- No. 11, 12, 15, or 15C scalpel blade with handle.
- Molt No. 9 periosteal elevator or number 7 wax spatula.
- 4-0 or 5-0 absorbable suture.
- Needle holders, thumb forceps, scissors.
- Burs, as necessary, for osteoplasty, ostectomy.
- Sharp curettes for root planing.

Technique

Step 1—The blade is used to create a reverse bevel incision around the involved teeth (A), and the epithelial attachments are cut buccally and palatally or lingually and interproximally (B).

Step 2—Vertical releasing incisions are made in the healthy gingiva mesial and distal to the involved teeth (C).

Step 3—A full-thickness flap is elevated apically with a periosteal elevator to expose the alveolar bone for about 3 to 4 mm; then a split-thickness flap is elevated apically, leaving periosteum to suture the apically repositioned flap (D).

Step 4—Sharp bony edges, irregular bone margins, or necrotic alveolar bone margins are removed with round burs and saline irrigation (E). (See the section on Osteoplasty.) Tooth-supporting bone is not removed.

Step 5—Granulation tissue and pocket lining are removed from the gingiva by curettage, and the root surfaces are planed (F).

Step 6—The surgical area is flushed to remove debris with sterile saline or 0.2% chlorhexidine solution.

Step 7—The gingiva is repositioned just coronal to the alveolar bone level and sutured (G) with vertical mattress sutures tacking down to the periosteum apically and securing the coronal full-thickness portion to the lingual tissue (H).

Step 8—The vertical releasing incisions are sutured with interrupted stitches. A fold of redundant tissue may be present and will reconform during healing.

Postsurgical Care

- Daily oral flushing with 0.2% chlorhexidine solution for 2 weeks.
- Return to routine home oral hygiene after 1st week.
- Follow-up periodic periodontal therapy as necessary to continue oral health.
- Soft food is recommended for 1 week.
- Oral antibiotics should be continued as necessary.

Complications

- Infection.
- Dehiscence.
- Inadequate coverage of alveolar bone due to excessive cutting of tissue.
- Greater pocket formation if soft tissue sutured too high coronally on tooth surface and not at bony crest.

Citric Acid

- Citric acid is applied to the root structure after any root planing procedure to enhance reattachment of gingival tissues.[7]
- Following root planing, a citric acid solution that has a pH of 1 is applied to the dentin for 3 minutes, then rinsed.
- Citric acid may be purchased at a pharmacy or through dental supply houses. It is

mixed with sterile water to form a super-concentrated solution.
- There is debate as to the effectiveness of citric acid treatment.

Periodontal Dressings

- Periodontal dressings are applied after periodontal surgery to protect gingival tissues.

- Lack of patient acceptance and lack of adequate adhesive areas limits their use.
- One product that does seem to stay in place fairly well is the light-cured paint on dam.*

*Paint on Dam: Den-Mat Corporation, 2727 Skyway Drive, Santa Maria, CA 93456

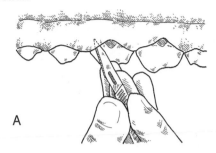

A

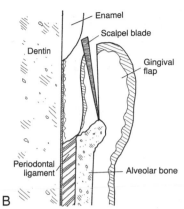

B

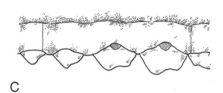

C

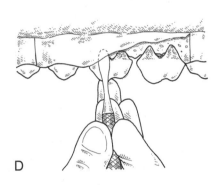

D

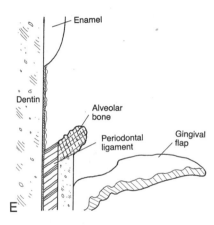

E

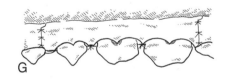

G

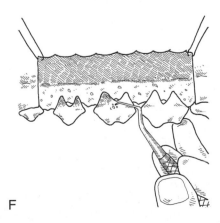

F

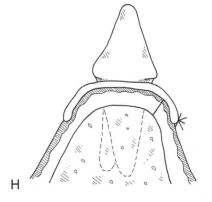

H

SOFT-TISSUE GRAFTING TECHNIQUES

Pedicle Graft

General Comments

- The pedicle graft uses adjacent attached gingival tissue to reestablish gingiva that has been lost.
- An area of exposed tissue from the donor site will heal by second intention.

Indication

- For use in an area with gingival cleft formation that has an adjacent edentulous area (A).

Contraindications

- Loose tooth.
- Unrealistic client expectations.

Objective

- To establish a functional margin of attached gingiva in areas of cleft formation associated with periodontal disease, combined periodontal/endodontic lesions, and frenula pull.

Equipment

- No. 11, 15, or 15C scalpel blade and handle.
- Molt No. 9 periosteal elevator or number 7 wax spatula.
- 4-0 or 5-0 absorbable suture.
- Needle holders, thumb forceps, scissors.
- Sharp curettes.

Technique

Step 1—The teeth are scaled and polished.
Step 2—A beveled incision is made along the gingival margin of the defect to remove diseased epithelial lining (B). The side adjacent to the graft is beveled externally, with the side away from the graft beveled internally. When treating a mandibular canine tooth, the graft should be taken mesial (anterior) to the canine tooth to avoid the mandibular frenulum.

Step 3—The exposed root surface is planed smooth with a curette, and the area is flushed with dilute chlorhexidine.
Step 4—A vertical incision is made at approximately two and one-half times the cleft width from the midline of the gingival border apically to match the length of the cleft (C). The object is to create the donor graft one and one-half times the size of the recipient width. A horizontal releasing incision is made along the midline of the gingiva to the depth of the periosteum.
Step 5—The portion of the graft adjacent to the cleft is elevated to the depth of the bone for the width of the cleft with a periosteal elevator, and the portion of the graft away from the cleft is elevated only to the level of the periosteum. This increases the blood supply and leaves periosteum over the exposed bone for granulation tissue formation.
Step 6—The graft is rotated over the cleft and sutured to the free gingival margin with interrupted sutures (D). The sutures are placed approximately 1.5 mm apart and are tied so that the margins are overlapped.
Step 7—The gingival edge away from the cleft is sutured to adjacent gingiva and periosteum. A cruciate (figure X) mattress-type suture may be placed to add additional support (E). Care should be taken not to create much pressure with the suture material.
Step 8—A periodontal dressing can be applied to protect the area for a few days.

Postsurgical Care

- Antibiotics as necessary.
- Remove periodontal dressing if the dressing is still present in 2 to 3 days.
- Twice daily oral rinsing with 0.2% chlorhexidine solution for 2 weeks.
- Continued daily home oral hygiene.
- Follow-up and periodic periodontal therapy as necessary to maintain oral health.

Complications

- Strangulation of gingival tissue by placing sutures too closely or tightly.
- Dehiscence, with failure to reform margin of attached gingiva.
- Exposure of bone with necrosis by elevating flap full thickness in area away from cleft.

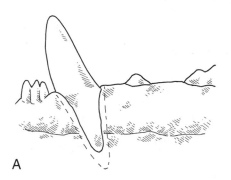

A

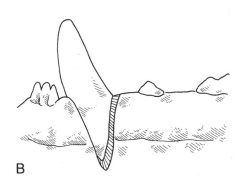

B

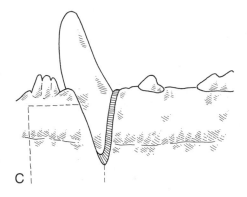

C

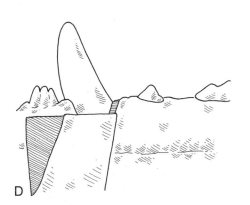

D

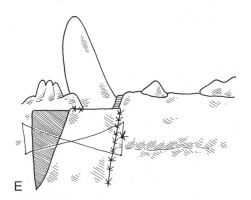

E

Free Gingival Graft

General Comment

* If gingival defect is related to endodontic disease, endodontic disease must be treated first.

Indications

* Individual teeth with deep gingival cleft formation close to or beyond the mucogingival junction that are otherwise healthy teeth *(A)*.
* Where adjacent gingival tissue that could be used to cover the defect is insufficient.

Contraindications

* Poor client compliance with aftercare or unrealistic client expectations.
* Systemic disease.
* Untreated and uncontrolled periodontal disease.
* Other dental disease; some gingival defects are caused by endodontic disease.

Objective

* To reestablish a border of keratinized attached gingiva around a tooth that has a deep gingival cleft, to retain the tooth, and to create 2 mm of attached gingiva, which means that approximately 4 to 5 mm of keratinized tissue will be needed to make up the free gingiva and attached gingiva.

Equipment

* No. 11, 15 or 15C scalpel blade.
* Template made from a small piece of paper or metal foil.
* 5-0 absorbable polyglycolic suture with swaged-on taper-point needle.
* Small periosteal elevator.
* Needle holder, thumb forceps.
* Periodontal dressing.

Technique

Step 1—The recipient site is treated by scaling and planing the exposed root surface. A reverse bevel incision is made around the gingival margin to remove pocket epithelium *(B)*.

Step 2—A 3 to 4 mm recipient bed for the graft is created by removing all the soft tissue down to the level of the periosteum in a rectangular pattern around the defect *(C)*. The bed should extend beyond the root surface sufficiently to allow for shrinkage during healing. Hemorrhage is controlled with a wet gauze and pressure.

Step 3—A donor area is selected where attached gingiva is sufficient, such as the area above the maxillary canine tooth or bucally by the mandibular first molar. The size of the recipient site can be measured, or a template can be made by using a small piece of aluminum foil.

Step 4—The template is placed on the donor area, and the outline is traced with a no. 15C blade *(D)*. Care should be taken to leave the periosteum intact and not expose root or bone.

Step 5—The donor incisions are deepened with the blade to the level of the periosteum.

Step 6—A corner of the donor tissue is elevated with the blade, leaving periosteum (split thickness) *(E)*, and tagged with a 5-0 suture with a swaged-on taper-point needle as a holder and marker.

Step 7—The remainder of the graft is elevated with the blade while tension is gently placed on the suture until the graft is free *(F)*.

Step 8—The graft is placed over the recipient bed (gingival side up), and pressure is applied for several minutes to help create a seal and force out air and blood between the donor and recipient site.

Step 9—The edges of the graft are sutured to the surrounding gingiva with interrupted sutures, spaced 2 mm apart *(G)*, using 5-0 absorbable suture with a swaged-on taper-point needle.

Step 10—Sling sutures are placed across the donor tissue and anchored on either side in solid tissue. Alternatively, or additionally, a periodontal dressing is placed over the graft site to protect it for the first few days.

Postsurgical Care

* Removal of the periodontal dressing in 2 to 3 days if the dressing is still present.
* Appropriate antibiotic therapy.
* Suture removal in 10 days if using nonabsorbable suture.
* Soft food for 10 to 14 days.
* Twice daily oral flushing with 0.2% chlorhexidine solution for 2 weeks.
* Home oral hygiene after healing to minimize progression of periodontal disease.

Complications

- Sloughing of the graft from rough handling, poor adaptation of tissues, or patient abuse.

- Sutures placed too tightly or closely, creating loss of blood supply.
- Bone necrosis at donor site if insufficient periosteum left for healing.
- Inadequate home care.

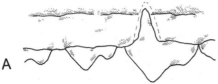

A

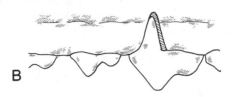

B

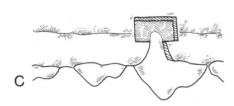

C

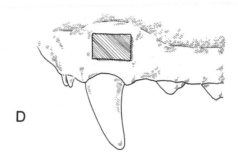

D

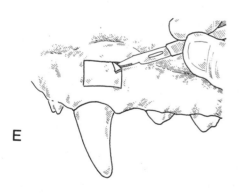

E

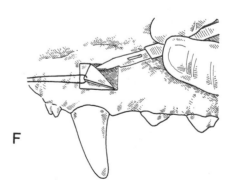

F

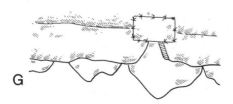

G

MANAGEMENT OF DEFECTS IN BONE

General Comments

- Osseous surgery techniques are performed according to the type of lesion present and the wishes and compliance of the client.
- Management of bony defects by elimination of bony pockets provides an environment for better gingival healing around periodontally affected teeth that have supporting-bone loss.
- Bony defects are further classified ac-cording to the number of remaining bony walls.
- Three-wall defect most commonly occurs in the interdental area, also called an intra-bony defect *(A)*. This condition has the best prognosis for treatment.
- Two-wall defect is the most common defect and occurs in the interdental area *(B)*.
- One-wall defect occurs interdentally *(C)*. This defect has the worst prognosis for treatment.
- Osteoplasty is the technique that removes or recontours nonsupporting bone.
- Ostectomy is the technique that removes tooth-supporting bone.

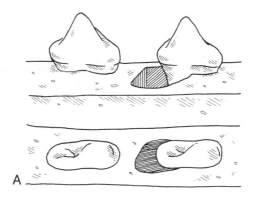

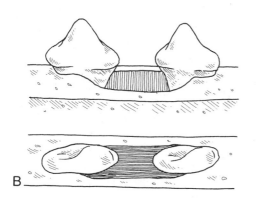

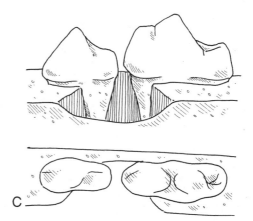

Management Techniques

- Induce regrowth of bone by grafting.
- Hemisect a multiroot tooth and extract one severely affected root while preserving the remaining root with appropriate endodontic procedure.
- Attempt to maintain pocket by frequent scaling, root planing, and plaque control. In pockets greater than 4 mm and in furcation areas, all of the subgingival plaque cannot be removed, and the disease process will progress.
- Attempt to maintain pocket by use of ultrasonic débridement combined with chemotherapeutic agents such as chlorhexidine. This may arrest the disease process; however, a refractory pocket may remain.
- Extract the tooth.

Osteoplasty

Indications

- Infrabony defect where the base of the periodontal pocket is apical to the level of the crest of the alveolar bone and resulting in sharp irregular bone contours.
- Need for thinning of bony ledges and establishing a scalloped contour to allow for periodontal flap closure.
- Irregular alveolar margins after extracting teeth.
- Leveling indicated for interdental crater formation.
- Ramping (smoothing) furcation ledges where periodontitis has caused bone loss in the furcation.

Contraindications

- Poor health status of patient.
- Lack of client commitment with aftercare.

Objectives

- To remove ragged alveolar bone, to improve bony contour in periodontally diseased areas so as to allow adaptation of the surgical flap, to improve healing, and to improve ability to maintain oral hygiene.
- In periodontally created one- or two-walled bony defects: to allow adaptation of a surgical flap with a parabolic flow with the highest point in the interproximal area.

Equipment

- Materials for flap surgery.
- No. 1, 2, or 4 bur in a handpiece.
- Sterile saline.
- Small (3 mm) bone rongeurs (postextraction).

Technique for Osteoplasty or Ostectomy

Step 1—A full-thickness flap is prepared as described on pages 188 to 191 with a reverse bevel incision (A).

Step 2—Granulation tissue is removed, and the roots are thoroughly planed and smoothed with curettes.

Step 3—Sharp edges and ledges of alveolar bone are removed and contoured as needed with a round bur in a handpiece, accompanied with saline irrigation (B). Minimal bone removal is desired, trying to make the parabolic architecture with the highest point interproximally (C).

Step 4—Irregular alveolar margins are recontoured in areas of tooth extractions.

Step 5—Surgical area is lavaged with sterile saline.

Step 6—The gingiva is replaced over bone margin and sutured interdentally (D) (E).

Postsurgical Care

- Periodontal dressing if desired.
- Antibiotics as indicated.
- Twice daily oral flushing with 0.2% chlorhexidine solution for 2 weeks.
- Home oral hygiene.
- Follow-up management/recall for periodic periodontal therapy.

Complications

- Excessive bone removal with loss of attachment. Supporting bone should not be removed (ostectomy).
- Excessive heat produced if inadequate irrigation or too high an rpm with bone necrosis.
- Inadequate bony contour or furcation ramping with poor gingival adaptation and poor healing or dehiscence.

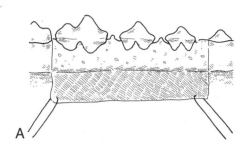

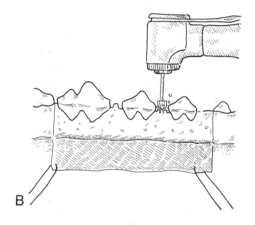

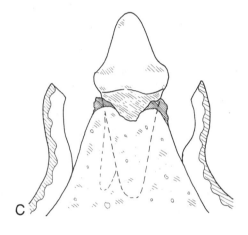

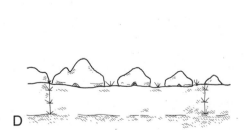

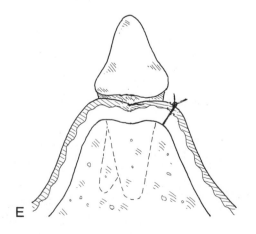

Guided Tissue Regeneration and Bone Grafting

Bone Grafting

General Comments

- The value of veterinary bone grafting in the treatment of periodontally diseased teeth varies. Occasional bone reformation has been reported following thorough root planing and curettage after flap surgery in humans without the use of a filling material in bony defects, but it is not predictable.[4] If these procedures are to be successful, client compliance is extremely important in follow-up of controlling plaque and monitoring the area.
- Bone grafting can be done in conjunction with osteoplasty to enhance new bone formation.

Indication

- Two- or three-wall defects where bone regeneration is desirable to maintain periodontal health of a tooth.

Contraindications

- Severely loose teeth.
- Poor health status of patient.
- Lack of client compliance with or patient acceptance of aftercare.
- Furcation invasion.
- Poor crown-to-root ratio.

Objective

- Regeneration of bone around periodontally affected teeth with bone loss, using autologous bone graft or synthetic implant material.

Equipment

- Autogenous cancellous bone taken from edentulous area.
- Hydroxyapatite.*
- Polylactic granules.†
- HTR.‡

- Consil.*
- Gore-Tex.†
- Calcium carbonate.
- Materials for periodontal flap surgery.
- Number ½ round or number 330 pear bur in handpiece.

Technique

Step 1—A full-thickness periodontal flap is created with a reverse bevel incision to expose the defect *(A)*.

Step 2—The bony pocket is débrided, and the root surface is planed smooth *(B)*.

Step 3—Lateral bony projections or irregularities can be smoothed with an appropriate-size round bur in a handpiece with saline irrigation *(C)*.

Step 4—The bony pocket walls are fenestrated with no. ½ or no. 330 bur in a slow-speed handpiece to a depth of 1 to 2 mm in several places to ensure release of bone-forming elements.

Step 5—Bone grafting material is mixed with saline or blood to form a paste and is packed into the defect to the height of the remaining bone *(D)*.

Step 6—The gingival flap is replaced immediately and sutured interdentally *(E)* *(F)*.

Step 7—Optionally, periodontal dressing is placed over the graft site.

Postsurgical Care

- Appropriate antibiotics.
- Periodontal dressing removed in 7 days if still present.
- Twice daily oral flushing with 0.2% chlorhexidine for 2 weeks.
- Follow-up plaque control; radiographs at 3 to 6 month intervals.

Complications

- Infection.
- Dehiscence.
- Progression of periodontal defect and bone loss.

---

*Interpore 200, 181 Technology Dr., Irvine, CA 92718

†Polylactic Granules: THM Biomedical, Inc., 325 South Lake Ave., Duluth, MN 55804

‡Bioplant, Inc., 20 North Main Street, South Norwalk, CT 68541

---

*Nutramax Laboratories, Inc., 5024 Campbell Blvd., Suite B, Baltimore, MD 21236

†W. L. Gore and Associates, Inc., 1500 North Fourth St., Flagstaff, AZ 86004

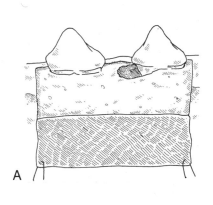

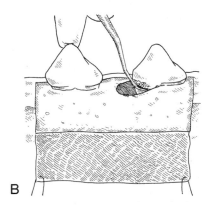

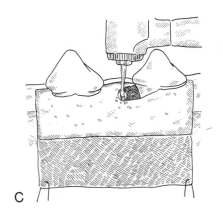

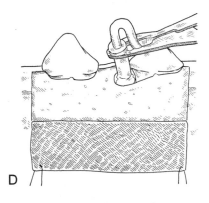

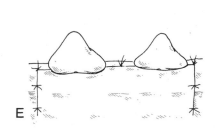

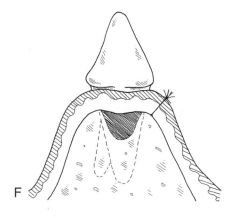

Guided Tissue Regeneration

Indications

- Three-wall defects, two- to three-wall defects, funnel-shaped defects greater than 5 mm deep, and class II furcation with or without a vertical component.

Contraindications

- Client's inability to perform home care.
- Loose teeth.
- Oral or systemic disease considerations.

Objective

- Exclusion of gingival epithelium and connective tissue from the root surface to allow formation of a periodontal ligament.

Equipment

- Periodontal surgical instruments.
- Gore-Tex*
- Shield†

---

*W. L. Gore & Associates, 1500 North Fourth St., Flagstaff, AZ 86003

†THM Biomedical, Inc., 325 South Lake Ave., Duluth, MN 55804

Technique

Step 1—Periodontal flap surgery is initiated; root planing and curettage are performed.

Step 2—An appropriate size membrane to extend a minimum of 4 mm apical to defect is selected. The membrane should overlap the lateral borders 2 to 3 mm over the entire defect. The collar should be at or below the cementoenamel junction.

Step 3—The material is placed and tightly secured to the tooth by a sling suture.

Step 4—The flaps are adapted with simple interrupted interdental sutures. The flaps should be full thickness to avoid tissue necrosis.

Postsurgical Care

- Antibiotic therapy for 1 week postoperatively.
- Commercially available chlorhexidine rinses or gels.
- If a nonresorbable material is used, it must be removed in 4 to 6 weeks, without disturbing the lining material.
- Periodic periodontal therapy, as indicated, to maintain oral health.

PERIODONTAL SPLINTING

General Comments

- Periodontal splinting is only semipermanent, at best, to immobilize teeth and improve gingival health; it does not lead to any long-term stabilization.[4]
- These techniques can be used with a dental acrylic or with a composite resin.

Indications

- Mobile incisors with solid adjacent teeth.
- When all six incisors are slightly mobile and can be stabilized as a unit.

Contraindications

- Client is unwilling to follow-up with adequate home care or to return for frequent, periodic professional care.
- Teeth with inadequate (less than 20%) bone support remaining.
- Single incisor without adjacent teeth present.
- Periodontal and endodontic involvement of a nonstrategic tooth.
- Traumatized primary teeth, while the jaw is still growing.
- Small breeds with root proximity problems caused by thin interseptal bone.

Objectives

- To stabilize teeth (most commonly incisors) loosened, secondarily, from bone loss.
- To improve healing after periodontal treatment/surgery.
- To preserve cosmetic function.

Equipment

- A .010 ligature wire for figure-of-eight or Stout interdental wire support technique.
- Fine square orthodontic arch wire for lingual splint technique.
- Minikin pins for lingual splint technique.*
- Light-cure composite resin.
- Dental acrylic.
- Howe wire-bending pliers.

*Whaledent International, 236 5th Ave., New York, NY 10001

- Small wire-cutting pliers.
- Finishing burs.
- Optional: Ribbond.*
- ProTemp II or Protemp Garant.†[8] (These materials are a combination of a composite resin and dental acrylic. The Protemp Garant comes in a mixing syringe, and the Protemp II is in separate tubes that are hand-mixed. This material can be placed directly on the teeth or over spot etching, as an alternative to using composite resin or acrylic material.)

Techniques

- Several techniques can be used, depending on the materials available, time needed for stabilization, and cosmetic appearance desired.

Figure-of-Eight Wiring Technique

Step 1—A no. ½ or 1 round bur is used in a high-speed handpiece to create a shallow, enamel groove circumferentially around each tooth at the middle of the crown (A). Do not enter the pulp chamber. (This step is optional if cosmetic appearance is not critical or splinting is temporary.)

Step 2—A .010 ligature wire is placed in a figure-of-eight pattern around the teeth, stabilized in the grooves, and tightened (B).

Step 3—The teeth are prepared by acid-etch technique.

Step 4—A dental acrylic or a light-cure composite resin is layered over the wires and grooves and is shaped and cured (C). When using dental acrylic, a fine camel-hair or Getz brush‡ is dipped into the liquid (monomer) and then into a small amount of the powder (polymer). This small amount of mixed acrylic is placed over the ligature wire. This step is repeated until the acrylic covers all the wire and the interproximal areas. It will take several minutes to harden.

Step 5—The acrylic or composite resin can be smoothed and shaped with finishing burs or sandpaper discs (D).

Step 6—The occlusion should be checked and any areas of interference adjusted.

*Ribbond, Inc., 1326 5th Ave., Suite 640, Seattle, WA 98101

†ESPE America, 1710 Romano Dr., Norristown, PA 19404

‡Teledyne-Getz, 1550 Greenleaf Ave., Elk Grove Village, IL 60007

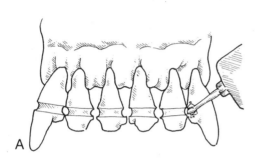

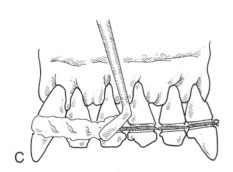

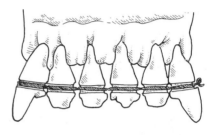

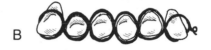

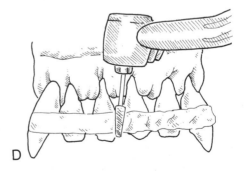

Lingual Wire or Pin Stabilization

- If cosmetics are important, this is the preferred technique.

Step 1—A number 33½ or 34 inverted cone bur is used to make a shallow groove across the lingual aspect of the incisors coronal to the cingulum *(A)*. Do not enter the pulp chamber.

Step 2—If an arch wire is to be used, it is shaped to conform to the lingual aspect of the incisors and fitted in the groove. The wire is cut and set aside.

Step 3—The teeth are prepared with acid-etch preparation. Do not etch exposed dentin.

Step 4—The wire is placed in the groove *(B)*.

Step 5—If Minikin pins are to be used, a small amount of composite resin or dental acrylic is placed in the groove first, and the pins are placed to overlap an interproximal space *(C)*.

Step 6—Composite resin material or dental acrylic is placed over the wire or pins and cured as necessary *(D)*. The material is shaped and smoothed *(E)*, and occlusion is checked and adjusted. The interdental spaces are left open.

Postsurgical Care

- Daily home oral hygiene.
- Frequent, periodic periodontal therapy as required to maintain oral health.
- Removal of the splint when the teeth have stabilized, if the splint is to be only temporary.

Complications

- Chipping of acrylic or composite and loosening of the teeth. If chipped or fractured, dental acrylic can be repaired by adding additional powder and liquid to the splint. Acrylic is less brittle than the composite resin.
- Exposure of wire, leading to uncosmetic appearance.
- Progression of periodontal disease, necessitating extraction.
- Endodontic involvement caused by entering pulp chamber or thermal injury.

Ribbond

- This is a bondable, reinforced ribbon material that can be used to splint periodontally involved incisors.
- It comes in 2 mm, 3 mm, 4 mm, and 9 mm widths. It requires special scissors to cut it, and cotton gloves to avoid oil contamination from the clinician's skin must be worn to manipulate it.
- A template of tin foil is used to measure the length of material needed to lay on the lingual aspect of the incisors.
- The Ribbond is cut to length with the special scissors and coated with filled bonding resin. It needs to be protected from ambient light.
- The teeth to be stabilized are prepared for bonding. Unfilled resin is placed on the teeth, and a thin layer of composite resin is placed with a Centrix syringe.
- Ribbond is placed on the resin material, compressed with a cotton-gloved finger, and adapted to the teeth.
- Excess composite material is removed, and each tooth is light-cured 30 to 40 seconds lingually/palatally and labially.
- Additional resin can be placed to create a smooth splint surface.
- The splint is smoothed and finished using conventional composite technique.

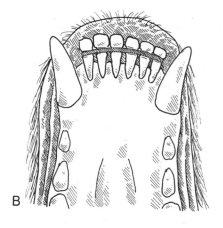

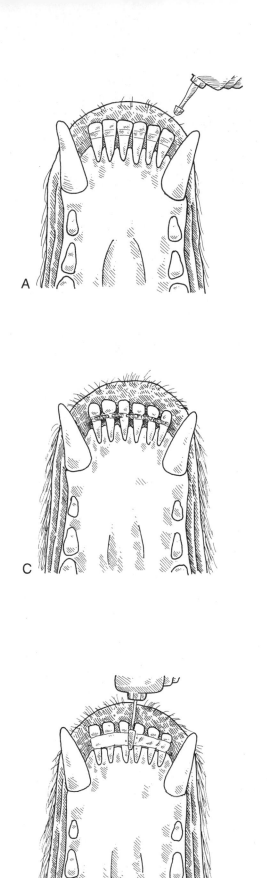

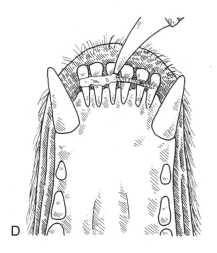

Maryland Bridge Splinting

- The Maryland Bridge is commonly used in restorative therapy. This technique can provide a long-term solution.
- The bridge must be manufactured by a dental lab.
- The bridge may allow retention of a pontic *(figure)*.

Technique

Step 1—Closed or open periodontal therapy is performed as necessary, in the first anesthetic procedure, when more than one is necessary to complete the treatment.

Step 2—An impression is taken. If the teeth are excessively mobile, the teeth may be temporarily bonded together for support.

Step 3—The bridge is manufactured by a dental lab.

Step 4—The bridge is cemented in place, in the second anesthetic procedure.

- The bridge should be at least 2 to 3 mm above the gingiva to reduce chance of irritation and to provide space for cleaning beneath.

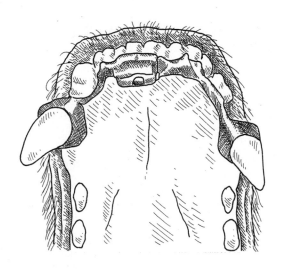

Tight Lip Surgery in the Shar Pei Dog

General Comments

- Tight lip in the Shar Pei dog is a condition in which the vestibule of the lower lip is excessively shallow.
- The lip is drawn against the mandibular incisor teeth.
- This may cause trauma to the lip and lingual displacement of the mandibular incisors.
- The client should be advised of possible genetic impact inherent in this problem. Appropriate consent, absolving the clinician of complicity to commit fraud, should be signed, and the client should be advised to remove the animal from the breeding line.

Indication

- Tight lip in the Shar Pei dog.

Contraindication

- Lack of client compliance or patient acceptance of aftercare.

Objective

- To relieve lip tension and draw the lip down.

Equipment

- Equipment for periodontal flap surgery.
- 2-0 PDS suture.

Technique

Step 1—An approximately 2 cm ventral incision in a craniocaudal direction is made over the mandibular symphysis (A).

Step 2—The skin is undermined in a craniodorsal direction (B).

Step 3—A suture is passed as far dorsally as possible toward the lip, taking an anchoring bite of tissue in order to pull the lip ventrally (C).

Step 4—The suture is tacked down to the periosteum as far caudally as possible on the mandibular symphysis (D).

Step 5—The suture is tightened. This should draw the lip ventrally. Additional sutures may be placed (E).

Step 6—The skin is sutured with fine nylon suture.

Postsurgical Care

- Broad spectrum antibiotics.
- Daily home oral hygiene.
- Skin suture removal in 10 to 14 days.

Complications

- Breakdown of suture if a sufficient anchor for the suture is not taken, or if the patient is not restricted from self-destructive oral behavior.
- Infection (sterile technique should be used).

REFERENCES

1. Grove K. Periodontal Therapy. Compend Contin Educ 1983; 5:660–664.
2. Grove TK. Periodontal Disease. Compend Contin Educ 1982; 4:564–570.
3. Zwemer TJ. Boucher's Clinical Dental Terminology, 3rd ed. St. Louis: C.V. Mosby, 1982:299.
4. Rateitschak KH, et al. Color Atlas of Periodontology. Stuttgart: Georg Thieme, 1986.
5. Woodall, IR. Comprehensive Dental Hygiene Care, 4th ed. St. Louis: C.V. Mosby, 1993:592.
6. Fedi PF Jr. The Periodontic Syllabus. Philadelphia: Lea & Febiger, 1985:115.
7. Linde J. Textbook of Clinical Periodontology. Munksgaard: Munksgaard/Saunders, 1985.
8. Emily P. Tenth Annual Veterinary Dentistry Forum, Houston, 1996.

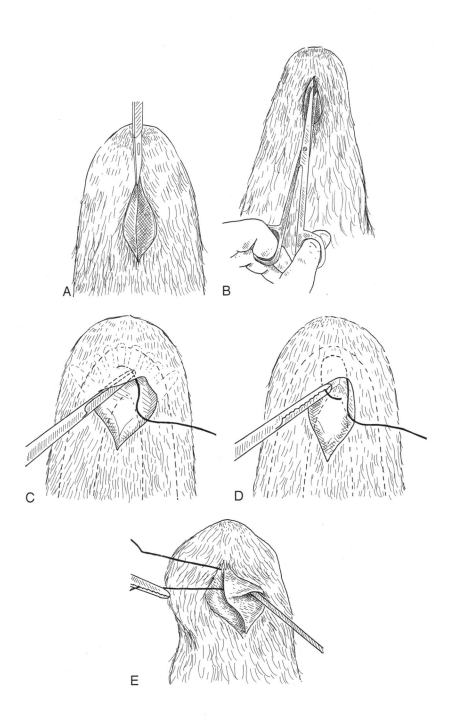

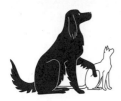

Chapter 6

EXODONTICS

GENERAL COMMENTS

- Teeth should not be sacrificed unnecessarily. In years past, when veterinary dentistry was taught in veterinary curricula, exodontics was one of the primary subjects. Students learned how and where to trephine and repel equine teeth. Entire books were devoted to equine dentistry (e.g., Merillat, LA. Animal Dentistry and Disease of the Mouth. Chicago: Alexander Eger, 1911). As the usefulness of the horse in industry declined, equine dentistry was not emphasized as much in the veterinary curriculum. As current practitioners endeavor to render good dental care to their clients, they should bear in mind that exodontics is the area of dentistry they should practice as infrequently as possible. Most veterinarians are sensitized to the term "euthanasia" and do not like to perform such a procedure wantonly. It may be helpful to use the term "euthanasia" interchangeably with the word "extraction." That way, every time a tooth euthanasia = "toothanasia" is performed, more sensitivity will be manifest, and the practitioner will look for other, more positive alternatives.

- When extractions are indicated, however, many animals will have greatly improved oral health and a better quality of life as a result of extractions being performed properly.
- Teeth are normally held in the alveolar bone by the periodontal ligament. When performing exodontics, the periodontal ligament must be stretched and then broken or torn. If this is accomplished properly, the rest of the extraction process is atraumatic.
- A radiograph is taken before most extractions to evaluate health of the alveolar bone; visibility of the periodontal ligament; variations in root anatomy; presence of ankylosis (decreased visibility of periodontal space, along with increased density of alveolar bone); or root resorption. This information helps determine the justification and logical approach for the intended extraction.
- Good accessibility and exposure to the surgical site may require changing the patient's position during the procedure.
- Good visibility must be maintained throughout the procedure. Bright lighting, magnification, suction, use of an air/water syringe, and relative position of the clini-

cian and patient are all factors affecting visibility.

- Buccal gingival flaps are used appropriately to improve visibility of and expedite access to and removal of solid teeth requiring extraction.
- The patient will generally be under a general anesthetic. A secured endotracheal tube with inflated cuff and gauze packed at the back of the pharynx will help prevent blood and debris from getting into the airways and esophagus. A pad or towel beneath the head will cushion the head from pressure during the procedure. Ophthalmic ointment in the eyes will protect them from drying, and a cloth covering the face will protect the face from soiling and the eyes from foreign objects and debris.
- Appropriate, sharp elevators of sizes and curvature should be used to match the tooth intended for extraction. The elevator is grasped with the butt of the handle seated in the palm and the index finger as close to the tip as possible to prevent slippage.
- The patient's head needs to be properly supported. During maxillary tooth extractions the patient's head is cradled over the bridge of the maxillary bone with the palm of the free hand. With small dogs and cats

the entire head may be cradled in the palm during caudal maxillary tooth extractions.

- During mandibular tooth extractions, the lower jaw can be cradled in the palm of the free hand, or the individual side can be grasped between the thumb and forefinger. These positions help prevent jaw fracture by neutralizing pressure applied during extraction. They also help prevent facial nerve damage due to pressure on the head if the head is resting on a hard table.
- Gentle tissue handling is important to minimize trauma and to allow rapid healing of both hard and soft tissues.
- After the extraction, the socket is thoroughly débrided, and rough alveolar bone edges are smoothed.
- Any exposed bone is covered by soft tissue and sutured.
- Preoperatively, the practitioner should consider the advisability of a preanesthetic hematologic database as well as other laboratory tests indicated by history or medical examination.
- The client's approval should be obtained for the extent of treatment, the cost anticipated by the clinician, and a plan of action in the event that an unanticipated disorder is discovered during the procedure.

Indications

- As a general principle, any tooth that is not contributing to function is a more likely candidate for extraction (with permission from the client).[1]
- Retained primary teeth *(A)*. Two homologous teeth should never be in the mouth at the same time. If a practitioner identifies an adult tooth erupting, and the primary tooth is not exfoliating naturally, it is time to extract the primary tooth.
- Interceptive orthodontics. Primary teeth are extracted when the mandible or the faciomaxillary structures are not developing appropriately and a malevolent interlock exists, interfering with normal jaw development.
- Supernumerary teeth *(B)*, when they cause crowding or interfere with occlusion and periodontal health.
- Malocclusion or malpositioned teeth, if orthodontics, occlusal equilibration, or other corrective techniques are declined by the client.
- Periodontal disease, if the periodontium cannot be restored, or if the client does not commit to a combination of the necessary home and periodic professional care *(C)*.
- Nonvital teeth, or fractured crowns with pulp exposure when root canal therapy will be unsuccessful due to extensive periapical abscessation *(D)*, or if the client declines endodontic treatment.
- Teeth that have structural damage, for which restoration is not feasible because of the extent or type of destruction or for economic factors.
- Retained roots or sequestered bone at fistulated, former extraction sites.
- Teeth experiencing internal or external resorption, if treatment is not possible *(E)*.
- Teeth in a fracture line that interferes with bone fracture repair or healing. Teeth in a fracture line may or may not require extraction.[2]
- Teeth involved with or surrounded by oral neoplasia.
- Any dental or oral disease, when the client desires less expensive but definitive treatment. NOTE: Extraction is not necessarily the easiest method of treatment, such as a request to extract an otherwise healthy, recently fractured canine tooth or carnassial tooth. It also may not be the least painful for the patient, postoperatively.
- Impacted or embedded teeth or ones involved with developmental root end cysts or tumors.

Contraindications

- Patients that are in poor health and may not tolerate the procedure or general anesthesia.
- Malignant conditions when the patient is undergoing radiation or chemotherapy that would inhibit healing.
- Bleeding disorders that cannot be controlled.
- Patients on medications that may cause prolonged bleeding times (e.g., aspirin, anticoagulants, and anticancer drugs).

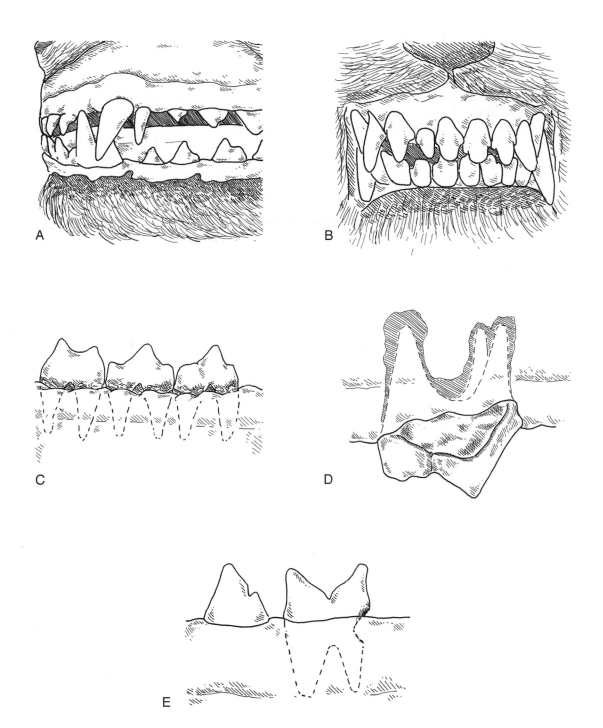

Objectives

- Controlled force should be used when extracting teeth. Patience is prudent for successful extractions.
- Adequate access to a smooth, unimpeded pathway of removal should be obtained.
- A tooth should be extracted completely with as little trauma to the oral tissues and bone as possible.
- All the tooth's roots should be extracted.

- Surgical elevators are used as levers to break down the periodontal ligament. Three basic types of lever are involved:[3]
- A first-class lever, with a fulcrum between the resistance and the force *(A) (B)*.
- A lever that is a wedge *(C) (D)*.
- A lever that is a wheel and axle *(E) (F)*.
- If the tooth root has not been displaced by the surgical elevator, extraction forceps are used to lift the tooth out of the socket after the periodontal ligament has been torn free.

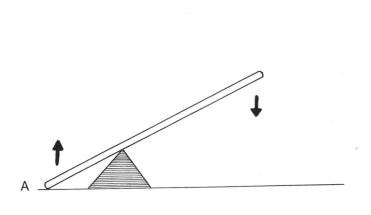

A

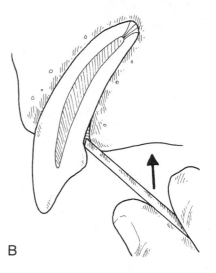

B

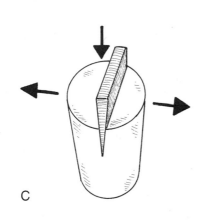

C

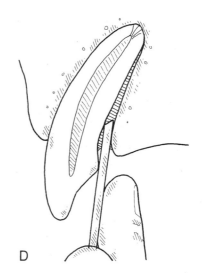

D

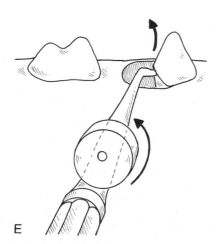

E

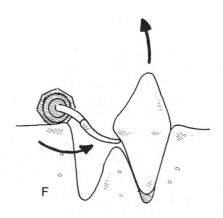

F

Materials

- See Chapter 2, Dental Equipment and Care, for details of specific instruments.

Nonsurgical Extraction Pack

- Scalpel handle and no. 11, 15, or 15C blades.
- No. 4 or 6 round bur; 701L, 557L, 1557, or 1558 crosscut cutting burs in a low- or high-speed handpiece.
- Surgical elevators (301S, 34, 304) or luxators.
- Periosteal elevators (Molt No. 2, 4 or 9, no. 7 wax spatula, ST 7* or Pritchard).
- Extraction forceps (small breed and large).
- Bone or spoon curette (5-0).
- 3 mm bone rongeur or bone rasp.
- Tissue forceps.
- Needle holders.
- Scissors.
- Gauze pads.
- Suture material: 3-0 or 4-0 resorbable suture, reverse-cutting needle or taper swaged-on needle.
- Surgical extraction pack.
- Root-tip picks.
- Apical elevator.
- Root-tip forceps.
- La Grange surgical scissors.
- Bone wax.
- Consil† or Collaplug.‡

Feline Extraction Pack

- Scalpel handle with no. 11, 15 or 15C blade.
- Small excavator.
- No. 7 wax spatula or Molt No. 2 periosteal elevator.
- Root elevators (301S or other feline elevators, 3 mm curved luxator).
- Apical elevator.
- Nos. 330, 2, 4, and 701 cutting burs with low- or high-speed handpiece.
- Small-breed extraction forceps.
- 5½ inch needle holders.
- Iris scissors.
- Adson-Brown or fine tissue forceps.
- 4-0 or 5-0 chromic catgut suture on reverse-cutting or taper swaged-on needle.

---

*Henry Schein, 135 Duryea Rd., Melville, NY 11747
†Nutramax, 5024 Campbell Blvd., Suite B, Baltimore, MD 21236
‡American Biomedicals Corp

SIMPLE EXTRACTION OF SINGLE-ROOTED TEETH

Incisors, First Premolars, and Mandibular Third Molars

Technique

Step 1—A radiograph is taken, and the tooth is evaluated for root structure, periodontal ligament health, and surrounding bone (A).

Step 2—The gingival attachment is incised by inserting a no. 11 scalpel blade into the sulcus and severing the gingival attachment around the tooth (B).

Step 3—A surgical elevator, or Molt No. 9 periosteal elevator, is used to break down the periodontal ligament by alternately stretching and compressing it. The tip of the elevator is inserted between the tooth and the alveolar crest at a slight angle to the tooth, with the concave side facing the tooth. This utilizes the elevator as a wedge lever. The instrument is forced apically, then rotated slightly until tension is exerted on the periodontal ligament. This position is held for 5 to 10 seconds. The elevator is gently moved around the circumference of the tooth in this fashion and gradually advanced apically (C). Movement of the tooth will be noticed as the periodontal ligament is stretched and torn. Hemorrhage from the torn periodontal ligament will assist in elevating the root.

- Alternately placing the elevator mesially and then distally while maintaining rotation as well as apical pressure on the tooth will result in further stretching and tearing of the remaining periodontal attachments. At this time the elevator can often be used as a first-class lever to elevate the tooth out of the socket (D). To gain additional purchase when using the elevator as a first-class lever, a notch can be made with a bur at the neck of the tooth (E).

Step 4—The loosened tooth is grasped with extraction forceps as close to the gum line as possible. The tooth can be rotated slightly on its long axis with a steady pull to remove the tooth from its socket. NOTE: Do not use force. If the tooth is not easily displaced, continue elevating it with either the wedge or first-class lever technique, intermittently using the extraction forceps, if necessary.

Step 5—The extracted tooth should be examined to ensure that the entire root has been extracted. If the root has broken into pieces, a radiograph may be needed to make this determination.

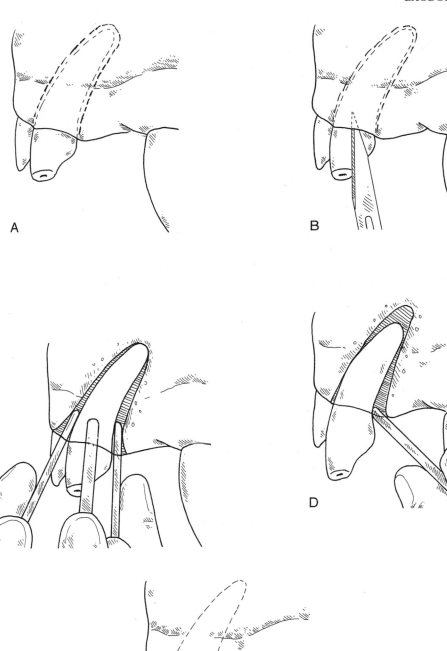

A

B

C

D

E

Step 6—The alveolus is débrided with a spoon *(A)* or bone curette *(B)* to remove any infected granulation tissue, debris, pus, and necrotic bone. The curette is placed at the apex and a scraping, pulling motion is used from the apex toward the rim of the socket.

Step 7—The crest of the alveolar bone may need to be reduced to facilitate suturing. This can be done by using a rongeur *(C)*, a bone rasp, or a large round bur with water spray. This step is performed to increase chances of primary tissue apposition, prevent fenestrations of soft tissue by sharp bony edges, and hasten the auto-osseous remodeling period.[4]

Step 8—The extraction site is gently lavaged with saline or dilute chlorhexidine or Betadine solution. Leave a blood clot. Use of a 35 ml syringe with an 18 gauge needle creates adequate pressure.

Step 9 (Optional)—If enhanced healing is desired, various products may be used. The alveolus can be packed with loose tetracycline powder, synthetic bone graft material,* or autogenous bone, as indicated. (Caution must be used when using tetracycline powder due to possible staining of adjacent structures.)

Step 10—Digitally compress the extraction area with gauze. This helps compress the alveolar plates, reduce hemorrhage, and oppose gingival tissues. Suturing may not be necessary after this step when extracting very small teeth and if minimal damage has occurred to the periodontal tissues.

Step 11—The gingiva is best sutured using a reverse-cutting or a taper needle and 3-0 or 4-0 absorbable suture material *(D)*.

---

*Consil, Nutramax Laboratories, Baltimore, MD 21236

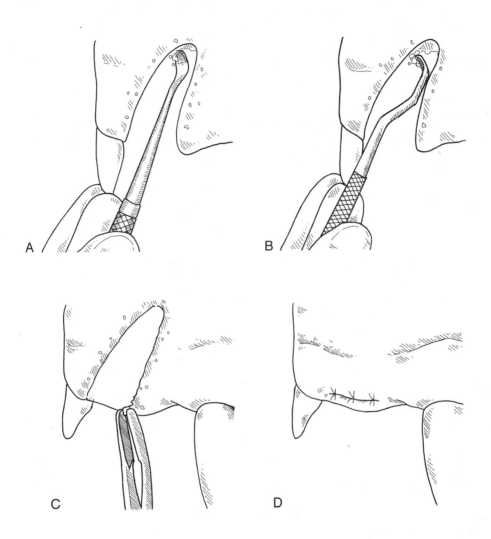

NONSURGICAL EXTRACTION OF TEETH WITH MULTIPLE ROOTS

- In the dog: maxillary second, third, and fourth premolars; mandibular second, third, and fourth premolars; and mandibular first and second molars. In the cat: the multirooted teeth in need of sectioning are usually the maxillary second, third, and fourth premolars; mandibular third and fourth premolars; and first molar.

General Comments

- If the multirooted tooth is first sectioned to provide "multiple" single roots, its extraction is no more difficult than that of multiple single-rooted teeth. A simple envelope flap may be used to separate the gingiva from the tooth for sectioning.

Indications

- Premolars and molars that are partially mobile secondary to periodontal disease or advanced periapical abscessation (A). These may include the maxillary fourth premolar and the upper and lower first and second molars.
- Retained primary premolars.
- Extraction of crowded or rotated premolars in a brachycephalic dog to preserve the periodontal health of adjacent teeth.
- Advanced root resorption.

Contraindications

- Solid teeth with abnormal root anatomy, ankylosis, or resorption that may lead to retained root fragments, excessive tissue damage, jaw fracture, or other complications (see the later section titled Surgical Extraction Technique).

Objective

- To extract a multirooted tooth completely and cover the resultant socket, causing minimal tissue.

Materials

- Nonsurgical extraction pack.
- High- or low-speed handpiece.

Technique

Step 1—The gingival attachment is incised around the tooth with an elevator or scalpel blade (B).

Step 2—A radiograph is taken and evaluated to determine whether the tooth can be extracted easily. If it can, it is extracted using those techniques and principles in the simple single-root extraction, with elevation proceeding around each root until the remaining periodontal attachments are loosened.

- If the tooth is mobile, the elevator can be placed in the furcation perpendicular to the long axis of the tooth to gain good purchase, and coronal pressure is applied to remove the tooth, providing the roots are not divergent or hooked. Care must be taken that all gingiva has been cut away from the tooth. If extraction forceps are used, each root must be completely loosened before extraction. Minimal twisting is used to remove the tooth. This reduces the risk of root fracture. If elevation cannot be easily performed, the tooth should be sectioned, separating each root.

Step 3—Using a periosteal elevator, the gingiva is elevated from the tooth and retracted, unless gingival recession is significant (C).

Step 4—A cross-cut fissure bur is used in either a high- or low-speed handpiece to section the tooth. Sectioning is performed taking the shortest, straightest pathway, starting from the furcation (D). This leaves each root separate. A water spray is used during sectioning to avoid heat necrosis of adjacent teeth and bone.

Step 5—Each root is elevated as in a simple single-root extraction (E). The elevator can also be placed perpendicular to the long axis of the tooth at the furcation between the roots and rotated slightly and held for 5 to 10 seconds to loosen the roots (F). Each root is loosened progressively, using adjacent roots for leverage when possible. If one root is more solid, the other root(s) can be removed first to allow easier elevation along the inter-radicular surface of the solid root.

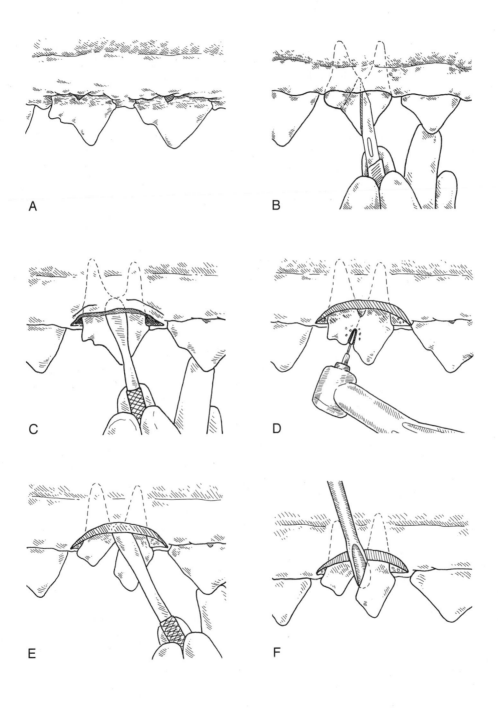

A

B

C

D

E

F

Step 6—Once all roots are mobile in the sockets, each is extracted using extraction forceps *(A) (B)*.

Step 7—The alveolus is curetted and débrided of necrotic and/or infected tissues.

Step 8—Irregular edges of the alveolar crest are smoothed using a rongeur, bone rasp, or bur in a handpiece *(C)*.

Step 9—The extraction site is lavaged with saline or a chlorhexidine or Betadine solution.

Step 10 (Optional)—The socket can be packed with tetracycline powder, synthetic bone, or polylactic acid granules or cube as discussed in the single root technique.

Step 11—The extraction site is digitally compressed with gauze to promote coagulation.

Step 12—The gingiva is sutured, tension-free, over the extraction site with 3-0 or 4-0 resorbable suture *(D)*.

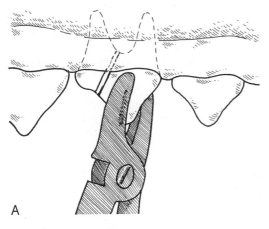

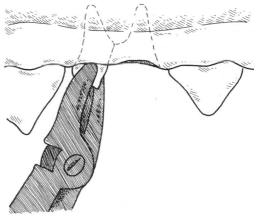

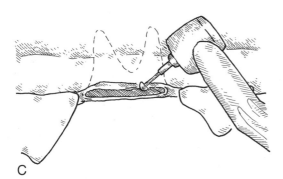

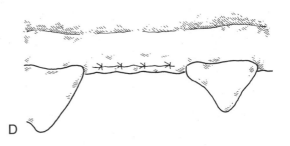

Maxillary Fourth Premolar

Additional Considerations

- Each root is separated using a cross-cut fissure bur in a handpiece *(A)*.
- The palatine root is separated by cutting in the fissure created by the base of the large mesial cusp and the palatine cusp.
- The mesial and distal roots are separated by cutting between the two large cusps in a straight line to the furcation *(B)*.

Maxillary First and Second Molar in the Dog

Additional Comments

- Each root is separated, using a cross-cut fissure bur in a handpiece *(C)*.

- The palatine root is separated from the rest of the tooth by cutting with a cross-cut fissure bur in the distomesial fissure created by the mesial-distal cusps and the palatine cusp.
- The mesial and distal roots are separated by cutting apically through the fissure formed by the large cusps in an apical direction to the furcation *(D)*.

Complications

- Root-tip fracture is more likely if the periodontal ligament is strongly attached and the roots are not extracted individually.
- Fracture of a root if the division is not made completely.
- Misdirecting and inappropriately separating one of the roots or damaging adjacent structures.

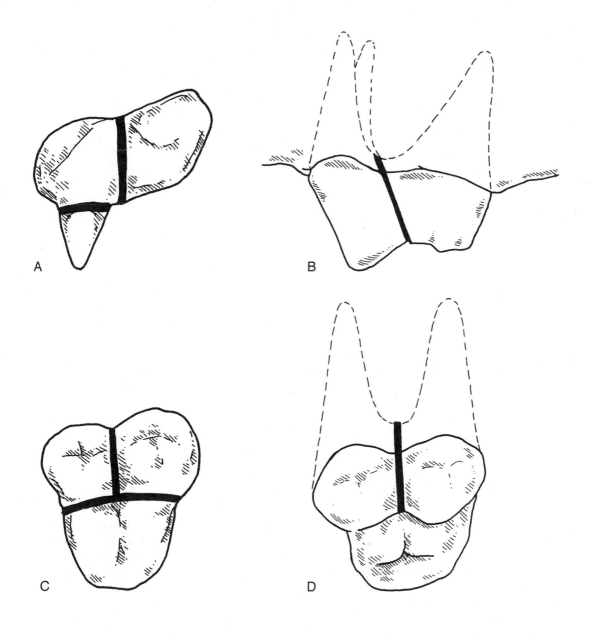

A

B

C

D

Surgical Extraction Technique

General Comments

- This technique is used for difficult extractions in which tooth size, number of roots, root anatomy, or pathologic problems on preoperative radiographs indicate potential for complications or increased difficulty in extraction.
- The process is more involved and should not be used if simple elevation will suffice. Surgical extraction techniques, however, can expedite difficult extractions and will save time by allowing better exposure, better access for root elevation, and improved postoperative healing.

Indications

- Larger, solid single or multirooted teeth that require extraction, when simple elevation techniques are insufficient for adequate removal.
- Generally, the canine teeth and carnassial teeth in the dog affected by endodontic or early periodontal disease, where other treatment options are not feasible or declined by the client.
- Maxillary canine tooth extraction due to periodontal disease extending into the nasal cavity.
- Solid teeth with divergent roots or curved root ends.
- Teeth with ankylosed roots.
- Root fracture.
- Abnormal root anatomy.
- Feline or canine teeth undergoing external odontoclastic resorption.

Objective

- To create a buccal gingival flap and remove alveolar bone, as necessary, to facilitate complete extraction of the tooth with minimal trauma.

Materials

- Surgical extraction pack.
- High- or low-speed handpiece.
- Irrigation capabilities.
- Magnification and bright lighting beneficial.

Technique

Step 1—A radiograph is taken and evaluated prior to extraction.

Step 2—The gingival attachment around the tooth is incised with a scalpel blade or surgical knife *(A)*. (A small excavator can be used in cats.)

Step 3—A buccal mucoperiosteal flap is created over the tooth with one or more vertical releasing incisions. Cuts making the releasing incisions should be made with a single motion, down to the bone. Apically diverging releasing incisions are made over healthy tissue one tooth mesial and distal to the tooth to be extracted *(B)*. This permits adequate circulation to the flap. (In cats with multiple extractions, the entire quadrant can be flapped.)

Step 4—It may be necessary to elevate the flap apical to the end of the juga (bony prominence covering the root). The flap should be carefully elevated from the buccal bone, mesial to distal, with a periosteal elevator. The lingual or palatal gingival tissue should be elevated as an envelope flap to expose the alveolar crest *(C)*.

Step 5—A cutting bur with water cooling is used to reduce the level of the alveolar bone buccally, mesially, and distally as necessary as much as 1 to 2 mm in a cat or 3 to 5 mm in a dog *(D)*. The bone height in the coronal furcation area can also be reduced. With canine teeth, the outline of the juga is cut through the bone with the bur. (The entire buccal apical surface of the root does not always have to be exposed.) This frees the buccal plate from the rest of the facial bone. An elevator can be used to remove the detached bony plate (see p. 238).

Step 6 (Optional)—If desired, a ledge can be drilled at the rostral and caudal aspect of the tooth at the junction of the alveolar crest and the root. This allows for elevator purchase.

Step 7—If the tooth is multirooted, it should be sectioned as described on page 226.

Step 8—An elevator can now be used as a wedge around the mesial, lingual, or palatal and distal surfaces, as in a simple extraction, to break the periodontal ligament or ankylosis of the root structure. Remember to hold the elevator with a slight rotating force for 10 to 30 seconds wherever it is placed. NOTE: Do not use the elevator vertically between crown pieces. This may lead to root fracture.

Step 9—The elevator can be placed perpendicular to the long axis of the tooth at the furcation area between roots and between the mesial or distal root and the adjacent tooth as a wheel-and-axle lever or as a first-class lever to gradually stretch the periodontal ligament. Finesse and patience while instrumenting each root will help achieve a successful extraction *(E)*.

Step 10—As the tooth is loosened, the elevator is moved apically until the roots are sufficiently freed so that they are either displaced by the elevator or are easy to grasp and extract with an extraction forceps.

- CAUTION: With maxillary canine teeth, care is taken not to lever the crown of the tooth too far buccally. This leverage could cause an implosion fracture to an unhealthy nasal bone plate at the apical end of the palatal alveolar wall. If this bone is damaged, an oronasal fistula may result.

Step 11—If the loosened root is not displaced coronally by the elevator, an extraction forceps is used to grasp the crown piece as far apically as possible. Traction is applied while the tooth/root is simultaneously rocked in an intermittent twisting motion on its long axis, with a prolonged torque pressure at the end of each twisting action, until it is extracted. If this action does not readily extract the tooth, further use of the elevator is required as in steps 8 and 9.

Step 12—The alveolus is gently débrided with a spoon curette or similar instrument to remove granulomatous tissue, pus, and debris as in a simple single-tooth extraction.

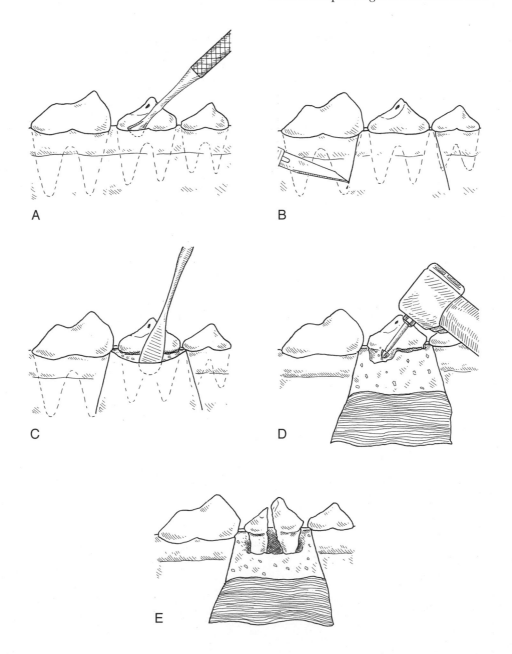

Step 13—Any sharp bony projections are smoothed using a bur *(A)*, rongeur, or bone rasp. The alveolar crest also may be further reduced, if needed, to facilitate suturing.

Step 14—The surgical area is lavaged with sterile saline or a dilute chlorhexidine or Betadine solution.

Step 15—Tetracycline powder[5] or Consil can be placed in the sockets, as appropriate. If the extraction site is free from infection, it can be packed with a carved polylactic acid cube or granules to increase bone fill, support the flap when an oronasal fistula is present, and reduce hemorrhage. The cube should be carved with a new scalpel blade in order to match the shape of the void.

Step 16—The elasticity of the flap is increased by making an incision in the periosteum of the flap. The flap is raised and held with a tissue forceps while a no. 15C scalpel blade, or smaller, is used on the exposed underside of the flap to incise the periosteal layer across the entire base of the flap. The tissue will expand as the inelastic layer of periosteum is cut *(B)*.

Step 17—Gingival margins are appropriately shaped with a fine scissors, and the flap is placed in position. The corners of the flap are sutured first *(C)*, placing additional sutures 2 to 3 mm apart and 2 to 3 mm from the gingival edges *(D)*. Absorbable 3-0 or 4-0 suture is adequate. Sometimes, 5-0 suture is preferable in the cat.

Complications

- Fracturing the root(s) due to too much force or improper leverage of the elevator.
- Fracturing the buccal bone if the overlying bone was not adequately removed.
- Creating an oronasal fistula as the maxillary canine tooth is extracted by creating an implosion fracture between the alveolus and the nasal cavity as the crown is elevated buccally during the extraction process.
- Fracturing the mandible by using improper elevation technique, such as by removing too little bone or by supplying too little digital support beneath the operative site.
- Alveolitis.

Aftercare: Follow-Up

- Pain should be considered and controlled with drugs and by offering softened food if warranted (see Chapter 11, Anesthesia/ Pain Control). Frequently, veterinarians are unable to recognize or diagnose pain in patients. It may be better to err on the cautious side and administer pain-relieving drugs if they are not contraindicated. Softened food additionally is less traumatic to the freshly sutured gingiva. The newly sutured tissue should also be spared by instructing the client to withhold hard treats and chew toys while the tissue heals.
- The client should be instructed to rinse the extraction site at least once daily.
- Antibiotics should be administered.
- The patient should be examined by the doctor in 10 to 14 days to evaluate healing.
- Periodontal dressings may be applied to protect the healing soft tissue.

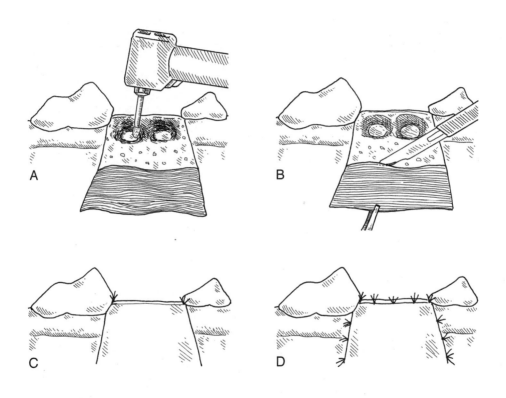

Canine Tooth Extraction

General Comments

- Extraction takes one of two forms, depending on how well the tooth is attached. If the attachment has been weakened sufficiently to allow some mobility, the tooth can be extracted in a manner similar to that of any single-rooted tooth. If the attachment is solid, as with normal periodontium, it is less traumatic and requires less procedure time to lay a gingival flap and remove the buccal plate of bone.

Indications

- Same general indications as on page 232.
- Disarming a vicious or biting dog or cat if coronal reduction and pulp capping are not permitted.

Contraindications

- With a fractured mandible or faciomaxillary complex, extraction may need to be postponed.

- In small-breed dogs with periodontal disease involving the mandibular canine teeth, it may be preferable to maintain these teeth with periodontal therapy, if there is still solid bone supporting the tooth (see Chapter 5, Periodontal Therapy).

Technique

- See the section on nonsurgical extraction technique for an easily extracted tooth, pages 222 to 224.
- See the section on surgical extraction technique for a tooth firmly in bone requiring extraction, pages 232 to 235.

Step 1—The gingival attachment is incised *(A)*.

Step 2—One or more releasing incisions are made *(B)*.

Step 3—The flap is elevated with a periosteal elevator *(C)*.

Step 4—The juga is outlined with a cutting bur *(D)*.

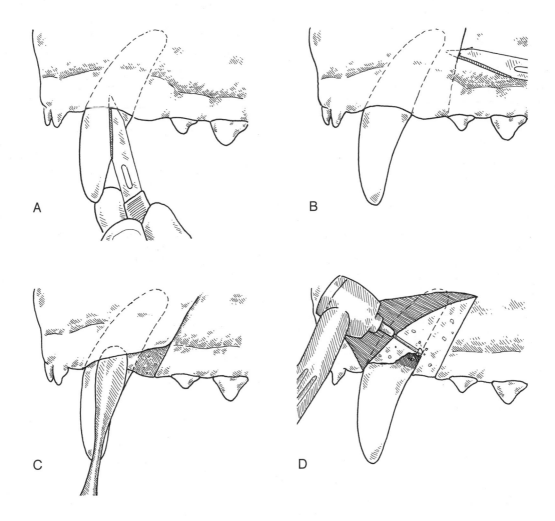

A

B

C

D

Step 5—The buccal plate is elevated with a periosteal elevator or root elevator *(A)*.

Step 6—Root elevators are used as a wedge lever around the mesial, palatal, lingual, and distal surfaces to stretch and tear the remaining periodontal ligament, loosening the tooth *(B)*.

Step 7—Once the tooth is loosened, extraction forceps are placed as far apically as possible; using gentle rotation clockwise and counterclockwise, the tooth is removed *(C)*.

Step 8—A spoon curette is used to remove granulomatous tissue and debris *(D)*.

Step 9—Any rough alveolar edges are smoothed with a cutting bur, and the extraction site is lavaged *(E)*.

Step 10—The buccal gingival flap is sutured in place *(F)*.

Complications of Canine Tooth Extraction

Tongue Hanging Out of the Mouth

Description
- The mandibular rostral teeth serve, among other functions, as a basket to contain the tongue when it is at rest. When lower canines are extracted, the tongue may not be held in the mouth all the time.

Treatment
- Discuss this possibility with client before extraction; this may give an added reason to perform alternative treatment.

- Osseous integrated implant will provide the patient with a new tooth.
- Cheiloplasty may be attempted, but success and healing are difficult to obtain.

Trapping Lip Between Gum and Mandibular Canine Tooth

Description
- After extraction of the maxillary canine tooth, the maxillary lip may be caught and pinched between the mandibular canine and gingiva of the maxilla, which may be very uncomfortable for the patient.

Treatment
- Coronal reduction and pulp capping of offending mandibular canine tooth.
- Extraction of the mandibular canine tooth.

General Extraction Complications
- Complications include fractured socket, fractured or broken root tips, hemorrhage, endocarditis, secondary infections, mandibular fracture, oronasal fistula, soft tissue trauma by the remaining opposing tooth, alveolitis, laceration of gingival tissue, retained root fragment, sequestered fractured bone plate, and inability to extract.[6]

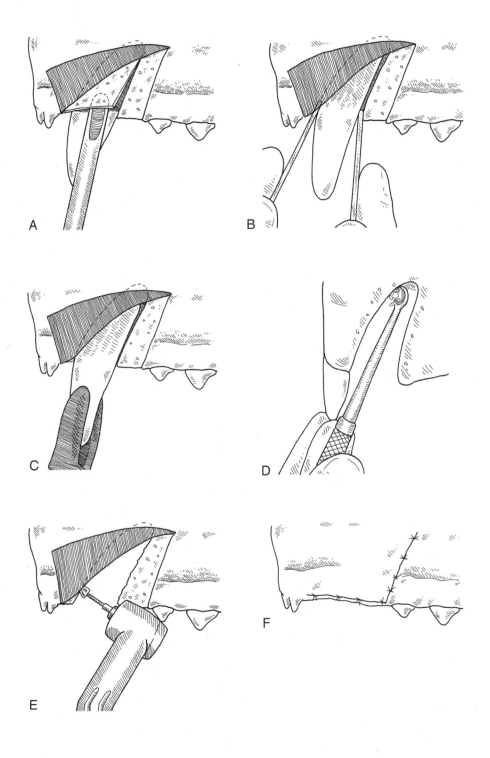

Fractured Socket

Description

- The alveolar bone is fractured in the process of extracting the tooth[4] *(A)*.

Treatment

- Fragments that are unstable or exposed should be dissected and removed before the gingiva is closed.
- Lightly pack synthetic bone grafting or scaffolding implant material in the socket, shaped to the size of the extracted tooth, and suture the gingiva.

Fractured or Broken Root Tips

Description

- A portion of the root is fractured and not extracted with the rest of the tooth.
- Can be a result of improper extraction technique, ankylosis, or resorbing roots.

Treatment

- See pages 232 to 234.

Hemorrhage

Description

- Bleeding from the extraction site.
- May be caused by careless technique, over-instrumentation, or handpiece bur perforation into the maxillary sinus or mandibular canal.

Treatments

Soft Tissue Hemorrhage

Pressure

- Pressure applied with gauze sponge, swab, or dental cotton roll directly to the extraction site to allow a clot to form *(B)*.

Cold Pack

- Application of cold compresses made from ice wrapped in a gauze sponge can reduce blood flow sufficiently to allow a clot to form and, at the same time, retard postoperative swelling *(C)*.

Ligation

- Ligation of bleeding vessels.

Electrocautery

- Most effective in controlling hemorrhage from small vessels. Caution must be exercised not to burn tissues.

Primary Closure of Site

- Suturing soft tissues over the extraction site with fine suture. NOTE: Controls only minor seepage. Do not use for extensive hemorrhage; see other techniques.

Aids for Coagulation

- Gelfoam*—packed into extraction site to serve as matrix for clot formation.
- Surgicel.†
- Collaplug.‡
- Synthetic bone§—packed into extraction site to serve as matrix for clot formation and then aid in formation of new bone; cube form carved by clinician and placed into socket *(D)*; granular form inserted into socket by syringe *(E)* or mixed to a paste with sterile saline and delivered on the blade of an excavator or placement instrument.

Hemorrhage of Bone

Crushing Bone

- Rongeurs may be used to crush bone.

Packing with Gauze

- The socket may be packed with gauze, a coagulation-enhancing material such as Gelfoam or Surgicel, or a biodegradable orthopedic implant.

Sterile Bone Wax

- Sterile bone wax may be placed into the alveolus onto bleeding bone.

Endocarditis

Description

- If the tooth being extracted is abscessed or severely affected by periodontal disease, a transient bacteremia should be expected. It will tend to localize in a distant area of inflammation.

Treatment

- If anticipated, pretreatment with an appropriate antibiotic is warranted.

Secondary Infections

Description

- Secondary infections create osteomyelitis or suppurative arthritis.
- Although infrequently diagnosed as direct sequelae of extractions, secondary infections, of which the practitioner should be aware, can occur.
- Signs include fever, reluctance or inability to eat, resistance to examination, depression, lack of healing, and foul oral odor.

---

*Pharmacia and Upjohn, 124 Campdell Dr., Canyon Lake, TX 78133

†Johnson & Johnson Medical, Inc., 2500 Arbrook Blvd., P.O. Box 9013, Arlington, TX 76014

‡Sutzer CAPeitek, 2320 Fariday Ave., Carlsbad, CA 92008

§Bioplant HTR-24 [Septodont] or biodegradable orthopedic implant (ADD): Consil, Interpore 200, Interpore International, 181 Technology Dr., Irvine, CA 92718

Treatment
- Radiographs, antibiotics, and surgical intervention may be necessary to assess and to treat cases of osteomyelitis, to débride diseased bone, and to cover exposed bone with soft tissue.

Mandibular Fracture

Description
- The severity of bone damage can be evaluated with a preoperative radiograph *(F)*. If severely infected or thin bone is found, advise the client of an increased possibility of fracture. The amount of force used in extractions must be controlled. Sectioning teeth is essential, and surgical extraction may be indicated in these situations to minimize torquing of weakened bone.
- A diseased mandible, once fractured, is often difficult to repair. It may never heal.

Small dogs with caudal mandibular fractures can often function with a fibrous union of the jaw.

Treatment
- Best to prevent.
- Perform complete extraction(s), including débridement of extraction site and suturing of gingiva to cover bone. Postoperatively, put patient on antibiotics.
- If only one side is affected, the contralateral side will give stability to allow fibrous union. If the fracture is bilateral, a tape muzzle can be used to support the jaw while the bone infection heals and a fibrous union is formed. Greater stabilization can often be achieved with interdental wiring alone or in conjunction with ex-

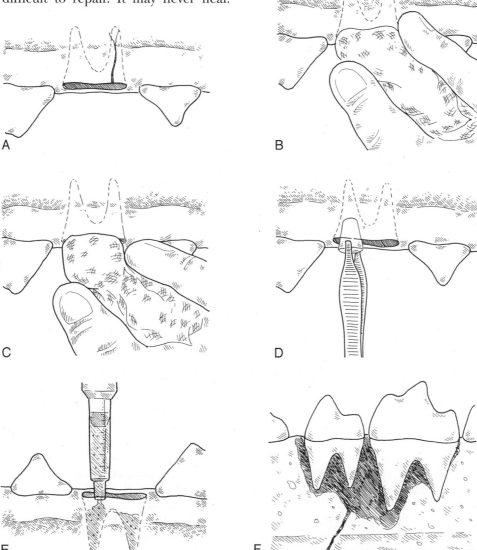

A

B

C

D

E

F

traoral splinting techniques (see Chapter 10, Dental Orthodontics). Bone plating often works well, but it is more invasive. Partial mandibulectomy is a last resort if other methods are unsuccessful or not possible.

Oronasal Fistula

Description

- A hole between the oral and nasal cavity may be present and not detected, or it may be created in the process of extraction.

Treatment

- Important to explain possibility of such occurrence to client before extracting tooth.
- See page 246.

Opposing Tooth Traumatizing Extraction Site or Lip

Description

- This most often occurs when a canine tooth is extracted. The lip or cheek is not held away from the gingiva, as it was formerly, by the maxillary canine, and the opposing tooth strikes it. The opposing tooth may only pinch the lip or may puncture or lacerate the lip.

Treatment

- The occlusion of the opposing tooth must be changed. This can be done by:
- Reducing the offending tooth coronally to a level that does not trap the lip. This will also require pulp capping if the pulp chamber is exposed.
- Orthodontically moving the offending tooth to a position that does not impinge on the soft tissue.
- Extracting the offending tooth.

Alveolitis: Painful Socket

Description

- This is due to inflammation or infection of the empty socket after extraction.

Treatment

- Best to prevent at time of extraction by débriding necrotic and infected tissues and suturing the socket closed.
- Antibiotic therapy after extraction.
- Irrigation.

Laceration of Gingival Tissue

Description

- Laceration occurs as the tooth is extracted if the gingival attachment is not incised completely or as a result of excessive elevation technique.

Treatment

- Suturing gingiva.
- Preventing by completely severing the gingival attachment and gentle elevation technique.

Ankylosis

Description

- Periodontal ligament space is not visible on radiograph.
- There is no tooth movement with the elevator because of ankylosis.

Treatment

- See page 243.
- Using bur and high-speed handpiece to pulverize root.

Large Tooth Surface

Description

- There may be tooth root surface so large that the practitioner is unable to exert enough force with the elevator to stretch/ break down the periodontal ligament.

Treatment

- See Surgical Extraction, pages 232 to 235.

Aftercare: Follow-Up

- The client should be instructed to rinse the area of extraction daily with a water-based commercial mouthwash such as Maxiguard, CET Spray, Listerine, chlorhexidine, or an iodine solution.
- Appropriate oral antibiotics are dispensed.
- The patient should be examined 10 to 14 days postoperatively by the doctor to determine whether healing has been normal and is complete or if further treatment is indicated.
- Softened diet and elimination of hard chew toys during the healing period are recommended.

Dental Radiology

- Any time it is suspected that a fragment of root has been left behind, a radiograph should be taken. It is better to find a piece of root at the time of extraction than to have to reoperate.
- The practitioner should always weigh the risk of leaving a portion of the root against the damage that may occur to tissue in extracting the root. If there is no infection at the site and circulation to the root tip is

undamaged, the root tip may be left in place without complication.[7] However, if the clinician's assessment of this is incorrect, a complication will occur.
- If the bone around the fractured root appears healthy on a radiograph and considerable tissue damage would be created by extracting the fractured root, then a decision may be made to leave it.
- A fractured root should be noted on the dental record/chart; possible complications and need for follow-up should be discussed with the client.

DENTAL PULVERIZATION

General Comments

- Occasionally, cases present with dilacerated roots or root tips or feline teeth that have resorptive lesions and are ankylosed such that they cannot be extracted with elevators and extraction forceps.
- In these cases, a high-speed handpiece and a pear-shaped, round, or cross-cut fissure bur in standard length or surgical length can be used to pulverize the remaining root fragment.
- This is a particularly effective technique in the cat, because of the cat's relatively short roots.
- The root tip is much harder than bone, and the bur tends to slip off and has a different feel and drilling sound than when pulverizing bone.
- The root tip does not bleed; adjacent bone does.
- The root tip is white; adjacent bone is a darker shade.

Indication

- Pulverization is done when there is difficulty extracting with elevators due to resorbing or ankylosed root ends. (If a root has undergone replacement resorption as evidenced radiographically, and there is no evidence of infection, only the coronal portion of the crown/root may need to be removed.[7])

Contraindication

- Pulverization has the potential for serious complications, including air embolism, and thus is not recommended if simple elevation or surgical extraction is feasible.

Objective

- Remove all the retained or ankylosed root fragment.

Materials

- Instruments to separate gingival attachment.
- High-speed handpiece with water cooling.
- No. 330, 2, or 4 FG burs.
- Magnification, additional light, forced air/water spray, or suction may improve visualization.

Technique

Step 1—A radiograph is made to evaluate the size and length of the root.

Step 2—The gingival attachment is cut with a blade, creating an envelope flap, and the crown of the tooth is cut off at the gingival line.

Step 3—The bur is used to remove the root structure carefully. Short periods of drilling should be used to prevent overheating of tissues and allow for visualization of progress. (Some practitioners consider only removing the pulp tissue until bleeding is no longer visible.)

Step 4—A radiograph is taken to show that the entire root has been removed. (Several radiographs may need to be taken intraoperatively until removal is complete.)

Complications

- Penetrating into adjacent structures such as nasal passages, sinus, or mandibular canal.
- Imploding a root fragment into nasal passages, sinus, or mandibular canal.
- Overheating tissue. Irrigate copiously to keep the tissues cool. The smell of burning bone can signal future problems of bone necrosis and delayed healing of extraction sites.
- Air embolism.
- Subcutaneous emphysema of the head, neck, and chest.

Aftercare: Follow-Up

- Reexamine in 7 to 10 days to evaluate healing.
- Antibiotics may be prescribed.

EXTRACTION OF RETAINED ROOT-TIP FRAGMENTS

General Comment

- Root-tip fragments may occur due to trauma, cavities, or resorption of the crown or as a complication of extraction *(A)*.

Indication

- If the root-tip fragment can be visualized, it should be extracted.

Contraindication

- If the risk of tissue damage is greater than the advantage gained by extraction, then the root fragment may be left and closely monitored. (When bone is healthy around a root tip, there is less chance of complications if only a small piece of root is left than if there is disorder involved, such as periapical disease or fistulation.)

Objective

- Removing the entire root tip without excessive damage to adjacent tissues.

Materials

- Same as for single-root and multiroot extractions.
- The fine root-tip picks are particularly effective (apical elevator, Heidbrink No. 1).
- Root-tip forceps.
- Magnification, additional light, forced air/water spray, and suction for improved visualization.

Techniques

- Of the several techniques for removing root tips, pulverization *(B)* (p. 243) and surgical extraction (pp. 232 to 235) have been described.
- Root-tip picks can be used as a wedge to expand bone and tease the root fragment out of the socket *(C)*.
- In a multirooted tooth, the inter-radicular septum can be opened with a bur on a high-speed handpiece to break down one wall of the alveolus. The root fragment may then be avulsed into the created space and grasped with a root-tip forceps.
- A trough can be cut adjacent to the retained root tip with a cutting bur to allow insertion of a root-tip pick or apical elevator.
- An oversized endodontic file can be used to retrieve the root fragment by inserting the file into the root canal and twisting to lock the file in place. With the aid of a root-tip pick, the root tip may then be retrieved by pulling on the endodontic file.
- A postextraction radiograph is taken to verify complete removal of the root fragment.

Complications

- Repelling the tooth fragment into the nasal cavity, sinus, or mandibular canal.
- Creating tissue damage (nerve, bone, or vascular).
- Additional hemorrhaging.

Aftercare: Follow-Up

- Monitor the healing process.
- Same as for other extractions.

EXTRACTION OF PRIMARY TEETH

General Comment

- The roots of primary teeth are longer, thinner, and more delicate than those of permanent teeth; therefore, they are more easily fractured.

Indications

- When the adult tooth is erupting and the primary tooth has not been lost.
- As soon as the adult tooth is noticeable, whether it has erupted through the gingiva or is pre-emergent.
- If mandible and facial maxillary complex is not developing properly, primary teeth may be extracted to allow independent growth of the two jaws. See Chapter 9, Interceptive Orthodontics.

Objective

- Remove the primary tooth and root without damaging the adult tooth or other oral structures.

Materials

- No. 11 scalpel blade.
- No. 301s root elevator or 3 mm luxator.
- 18 gauge needle.
- Small-breed extraction forceps.
- No. 15C scalpel blade.
- Needle holder.
- 3-0 or 4-0 absorbable suture.
- Gauze pads.

Technique

Step 1—Take a radiograph of the tooth to be extracted to identify the shape and length of the root(s).

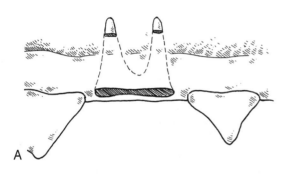

A

Step 2—Using a fine, sharp elevator or an 18 gauge needle as a wedge lever, elevate around the tooth. With primary teeth, it is important to elevate to the point that the periodontal ligament is broken and the tooth is free in the alveolus. Keep the elevator on the surfaces away from the permanent tooth as much as possible. In young puppies, when performing interceptive extractions of primary teeth, avoid deep apical elevation of the primary tooth, or damage to the permanent tooth bud may occur. Allow hemorrhage from the torn ligaments to create hydraulic pressure to help lift the tooth out of the socket.

Step 2a—For solid, retained primary canine teeth, it may be beneficial to make a small incision in the attached gingiva on the buccal aspect to reduce risk of fracturing the root. One or two stitches of resorbable suture are placed for closure.

Step 3—Extraction forceps are used to lift the tooth out of the socket. Rotational forces should not be used, because they often result in root fracture.

Step 4—A radiograph is taken if any doubt exists that the entire root was extracted.

Complication

- Fracture of the root.

Aftercare: Follow-Up

- Monitor healing.
- Monitor eruption of the adult tooth.

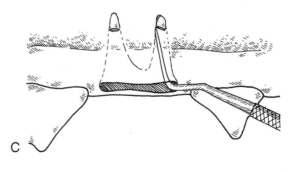

C

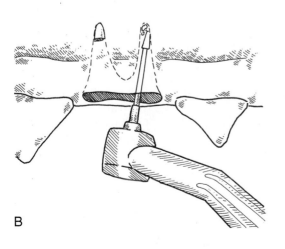

B

ORONASAL FISTULA REPAIR

General Comments

- Oronasal fistulae can occur associated with any of the maxillary teeth.
- Severe periodontal disease creating a palatal pocket and loss of the bone on the palatal side of the root may be noted when a probe is inserted deeply into an infrabony pocket radiographically or by irrigation of the pocket, resulting in irrigant dripping out of the nose. Clients may report chronic sneezing or snuffling with serous nasal discharge in patients. Dachshunds, poodles, and other small-breed dogs are often affected with oronasal fistulae secondary to periodontal disease.
- If an oronasal fistula is created by an extraction, it should be repaired.
- Traumatic avulsion of a canine tooth can create an oronasal fistula.
- Ideally, the repair should place an epithelial layer in the oral and nasal cavities.
- The flap must not have any tension on it after it is sutured in place.
- The suture line should not be over a void.
- Frequent irrigation of the surgery site and pressure with moistened gauze provides visibility and controls hemorrhage.

Indication

- A communication between the oral and nasal cavities.

Contraindication

- Severely infected tissue; best to wait to perform reparative surgery until after a course of antibiotics or until 7 to 10 days after an initial extraction stage.

Materials

- Surgical extraction pack.

Techniques

Single-Flap Technique: Buccal Mucoperiosteal Sliding Flap

- Used for fistulae where attached gingiva remains, providing a strong suture base. If the fistula is large or chronic, with no remaining attached gingiva, then the double-flap technique is recommended.

Step 1—The margins of the fistula are débrided of necrotic and epithelialized tissue (A).

Step 2—Releasing incisions are made with a no. 11 or 15C scalpel blade (B). The mesial incision is started at the gingival ridge, mesial to the fistula, and continued apically into the elastic buccal mucosa. The distal incision is started at the gingival ridge, in the area of the mesial line-angle of the first premolar, and continued apically into the buccal mucosa. The incisions should be diverging apically to ensure adequate circulation postoperatively. The cuts are made in one pass, to the bone, and include the periosteum in the flap.

Step 3—A reverse bevel incision is made at the buccal edge of the fistula connecting the releasing incisions. The palatal margin may be elevated slightly with a blade to facilitate suturing (C).

Step 4—The gingival flap, with its periosteum, is elevated apically with a broad periosteal elevator (D). Enough tissue should be elevated for the flap to be placed over the fistula without spontaneous retraction. This ensures that there will be no tension when the sutures are placed.

Step 5—The periosteum is incised mesiodistally on the underside of the flap at its base with a no. 15 or 15C blade (E).

Step 6—The alveolar crest may need to be reduced for better positioning of the flap. This can be done with a small rongeur, rasp, curette, or high-speed cutting bur.

Step 7—As conditions indicate, synthetic bone, a synthetic scaffold, or bone graft or tetracycline powder may be packed into the oronasal fistula before suturing.[5] This is contraindicated if there is no backing on the nasal wall.

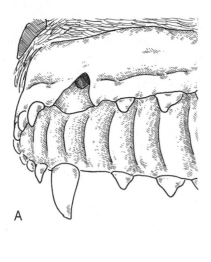

A

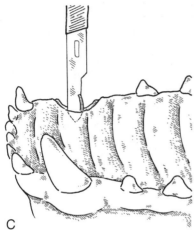

C

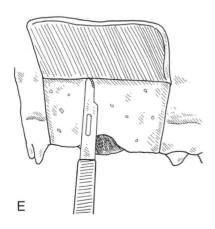

E

Step 8—The flap edge is trimmed, placed over the defect, and sutured with 3-0 or 4-0 resorbable suture on a reverse-cutting or taper swaged-on needle *(F)*. The corners of the flap are secured, and additional sutures are placed 2 to 3 mm apart and 2 to 3 mm from the gingival edge. Do not crush the tissue with sutures tied too tightly. Sutures are passed from unattached to attached tissue.

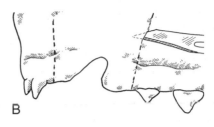

B

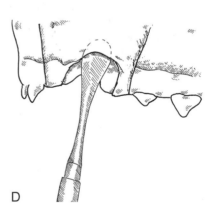

D

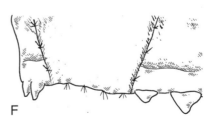

F

Double-Flap Techniques

- Double-flap surgery is more complicated and is usually used for large defects where no attached gingiva remains or when the single-flap technique has failed.[8]
- This procedure provides an epithelial surface toward the nasal cavity and provides greater support for the buccal flap.
- The mesial, distal, and buccal epithelial margins of the fistula are débrided and scarified with a no. 15C blade. The palatal margin is not débrided.
- Frequent irrigation of the surgery site and pressure with moistened gauze provide visibility and control hemorrhaging.

Double-Flap: Palatal Inverted and Buccal Sliding Flaps

Step 1—A full-thickness palatal flap is created by making parallel incisions from mesial and distal borders of the fistula to or past the midline on the palate, where they are convered and connected *(A)*. This must create a flap large enough, when inverted (folded over its base), to fit over the fistula and, after suturing, to have no tension on the suture lines.

This will create significant hemorrhage as the rostral palatine artery is transected. With careful dissection it may be possible to ligate the artery. Direct pressure with a moistened gauze will also control hemorrhaging.

Step 2—The palatal flap is based at the medial edge of the fistula and is elevated with a sharp periosteal elevator to the margin of the fistula *(B)*. It is inverted to cover the fistula. This inversion places the epithelium of the flap in contact with the nasal passage *(C)*.

Step 3—Using 3-0 or 4-0 absorbable suture, the palatal flap is sutured to the mucosa at the edges of the fistula. Simple interrupted or cruciate stitches are customarily employed *(D)*.

Step 4—A buccal mucoperiosteal sliding flap is created, placed over the sutured palatal flap, and sutured *(E)*, as described on pages 246 to 247, or, if more tissue is needed, a labial buccal pedicle flap may be created. Stitches are placed between the buccal flap and the underside of the palatal flap.

- The palatal defect will heal by second intention, if not covered by mucosa.
- Any epithelialized tissue that is covered by the flap should be scarified with a blade or bur to allow first intention healing.

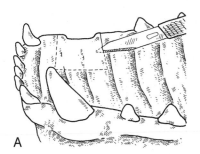

A

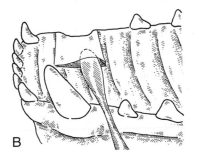

B

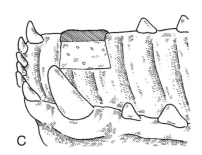

C

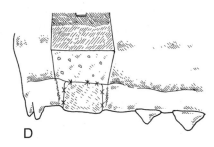

D

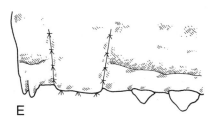

E

Double Flap: Palatal and Labial Buccal Pedicle Flap

Step 1—A palatal flap is created using the preceding steps 1 to 3.

Step 2—A partial-thickness pedicle flap is created by making an incision along the mucogingival junction from the area of the distal edge of the juga, extending mesially to create a flap long enough to completely cover the donor site of the palatal flap *(A)*. This may be past the midline in dolichocephalic and toy breeds. A second incision is made, and a pedicle flap with its width 1½ times the diameter of the fistula is created. This incision is made parallel to the initial releasing incision on the mucogingival junction. A third incision is made perpendicularly, connecting the two releasing incisions.

Step 3—Starting at the rostral end *(B)*, the flap is elevated *(C)*. Any epithelialized tissue that may be covered eventually by the flap should be scarified with a blade or bur to allow healing.

Step 4—The pedicle flap is sutured over the palatal flap and palatal defect using simple interrupted sutures of absorbable 3-0 or 4-0 suture on a reverse-cutting or taper swaged-on needle *(D)*. When fixing the buccal pedicle flap to the palate, the sutures will strengthen the repair if they include both flaps.

Step 5—The edges from the two releasing incisions are sutured together *(E)*.

Complications

- It is important to tell the client before extracting teeth that poor healing and/or dehiscence are a possibility.
- With any gingival flap technique, infection is a possibility.

Aftercare: Follow-Up

- Maintain the patient on a broad-spectrum antibiotic for 10 days.
- Area may need cleansing, but this can disturb the healing process. Using a water irrigation device or water spray bottle may be beneficial.
- The doctor should recheck the patient at 2- to 3-day intervals if quiet convalescence, client compliance, or technique is in question. It is better to troubleshoot complications early than to reoperate when the surgery has failed completely.
- The client should be advised against putting tension on the graft site by pulling on the patient's lip while cleansing the area or while examining the surgical site.
- A soft food diet should be provided and access to chew toys and hard treats withheld for 2 weeks.
- An Elizabethan collar may be necessary initially to keep the dog from pawing or rubbing the surgery area.

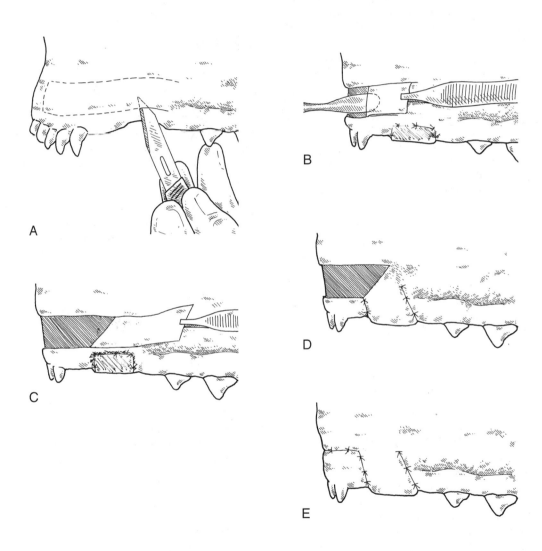

A

B

C

D

E

IMPACTED, UNERUPTED, OR EMBEDDED TEETH

General Comments

- An impacted tooth is one whose path of eruption is blocked or impaired.
- If the opposing tooth is erupted, then impaction should be suspected, and if the contralateral tooth is erupted, then impaction is almost certain.
- If a tooth is expected to erupt, it is called an unerupted tooth. Frequently, this is determined by clinically noting progress in the eruption process. If the eruption process has ended and the tooth is located beneath the mucosa, it is called an embedded tooth. This term is usually applied to teeth associated with some abnormality, e.g., gingival fibromatosis, supernumerary teeth, mesiodens, or pathologic states.

Indications

- Generally, most impacted teeth should be removed.
- To prevent infection (pericoronitis), pressure necrosis, and follicular pathologic processes such as odontogenic cysts and neoplasms.
- The presence of infection or disease due to impaction.
- To assist in maintaining occlusion.

Contraindications for Extraction

- Before the root has developed sufficiently to ensure that there is a problem.
- If there is an increased risk of injuring an adjacent significant structure (nerve tissue, vascular tissue, other teeth).
- When the patient's general health is not sufficient to tolerate the procedure.

Objective

- Extraction with minimal damage to other oral structures.

Materials

- Surgical extraction pack.

Technique

Step 1—A radiograph is taken to identify the location of the impacted tooth (A).

Step 2—A mucoperiosteal buccal flap is raised over the tooth as described on pages 232 to 233 (B).

Step 3—The bone covering the tooth is removed with a bur and high-speed handpiece (C). This creates access to the crown and root surfaces.

Step 4—The tooth may be sectioned for a stepwise removal of the tooth and to create space for elevation and instrumentation (D).[9]

Step 5—Once visualization is obtained, the remaining tooth structures can be displaced, elevated, and extracted (E).

Step 6—The site is closed using simple interrupted suture as described on pages 234 to 235.

Complications

- Delayed healing due to improper closure or poor flap design.
- Damage to adjacent structures or fracture of the mandible when too much bone is removed or improper extraction technique is employed.
- Infection of soft tissue or bone.

Aftercare: Follow-Up

- Standard postsurgical follow-up.

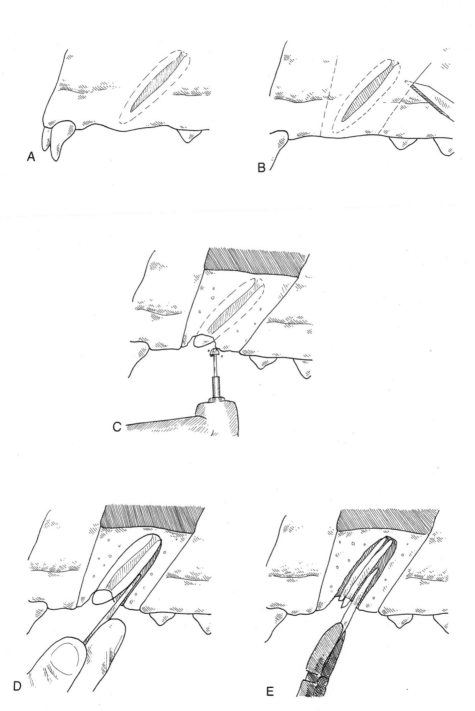

REFERENCES

1. Waite DE. Principles of Exodontia. In: Waite DE, ed. Textbook of Practical Oral and Maxillofacial Surgery. Philadelphia: Lea & Febiger, 1987:81–91.
2. Schloss AJ, Manfra Marretta S: Prognostic factors affecting teeth in the line of mandibular fractures. J Vet Dent 1990; 7:7–9.
3. Peterson LJ, et al. Contemporary Oral and Maxillofacial Surgery. St Louis: C.V. Mosby Co., 1988.
4. Maretta SM, Tholen M. Extraction Techniques and Management of Associated Complications. In: Bojrab MJ, Tholen M, eds. Small Animal Oral Medicine and Surgery. Philadelphia: Lea & Febiger, 1989:75–95.
5. Mulligan TW. Oral/Nasal Fistula Repair. New Orleans: Nabisco, 1988.
6. Dorn AS. Complications of Dental Extractions. Chicago: Surgical Forum, 1989.
7. DuPont G. Crown amputation with intentional root retention for advanced feline resorptive lesions—a clinical study. J Vet Dent 1995; 12:9–13.
8. Eisner ER. Nonsurgical and surgical tooth extraction and oronasal fistula repair. Part I. Canine Pract 1996; 21:12–15; Part II. Canine Pract 1997; 22:5–9.
9. Pedersen GW. Oral Surgery. Philadelphia: W.B. Saunders Co., 1988:69–71.

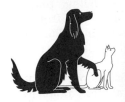

Chapter 7

ENDODONTICS

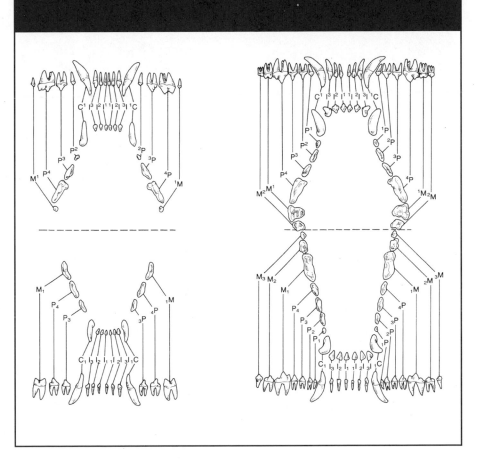

GENERAL COMMENTS

- The pulp is the innermost part of the tooth. The functional cells of the pulp are the odontoblasts, which produce dentin throughout the life of the tooth, creating a progressively thickened dentinal wall. Dental pulp consists of blood vessels, nerves, and connective tissue that support the odontoblasts and provide internal sensory and metabolic function to the interior of the teeth.[1, 2]

- The objective of endodontic therapy is to maintain a vital tooth or, failing that, to alleviate discomfort and infection from the tooth and periapical tissues by obliteration of the root canals.[3] It may also be considered preventive treatment in a patient without symptoms when a dead tooth is treated to prevent subsequent abscess, bone lysis, and possible infections and invasion into other areas.

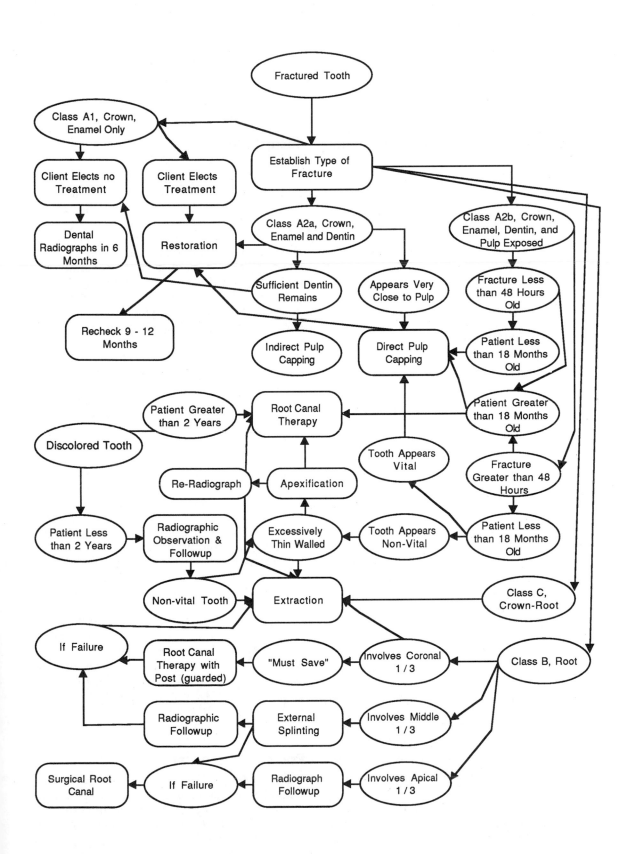

INDIRECT PULP CAPPING

General Comments

- Indirect pulp capping is indicated when a cavity or restorative preparation occurs within 1 to 2 mm of the pulp.
- During deep-decay cavity preparation, a layer of carious dentin can be left over the pulp. This layer will be sterilized with the application of calcium hydroxide.[4]

Indications

- Deep-cavity preparations where the pink hue of pulp is seen shining through the dentin.
- Extensive crown restorations on vital teeth.

Contraindications

- Direct pulp exposure.
- Nonvital tooth restorations.
- Radiographic evidence of periapical or apical disorder.
- Radiographic evidence of a root fracture.
- Radiographic evidence of a tooth with periodontal disease that is not salvageable.

Objective

- A protective layer of calcium hydroxide or glass ionomer is placed, in a vital tooth as a covering, on the floor of a restorative preparation or cavity preparation close to the pulp tissue to protect the pulp from thermal or chemical insult and to prevent sensitivity.

Materials

- Base material to cover the nearly exposed pulp. For many years, a fast-setting calcium hydroxide such as Life* or Dycal† has been recommended. Recently, glass ionomers have been used and may be the preferred material to use as a base.

*Kerr Corporation, 28,200 Wick Rd., Romulus, MI 48174

†Dentsply International, 570 West College Ave., P.O. Box 872, York, PA 17405

- Injection syringe or plastic working instrument.
- Materials, instruments, and equipment needed to prepare and complete a cavity preparation or restoration (see Chapter 8, Restorative Dentistry).

Technique

Step 1—The mechanically prepared cavity preparation or restoration site is irrigated with sterile saline to remove dentinal debris and is air-dried (A).

Substep 1—A dentin tooth conditioner is applied to the dentinal surface with a Getz brush for the manufacturer's recommended time, rinsed with water, and air-dried (B).

Substep 2—For deep-cavity preparations, it is desirable to use a calcium hydroxide and glass ionomer cavity liner. A minimum layer of 1 mm deep should be placed. The calcium hydroxide should be placed first. The tooth conditioner can be used over the calcium hydroxide product to prepare the dentinal walls for the glass ionomer. If possible, avoid getting the liner on the walls of the cavity coronally in the area of the final restoration.

Step 2—The cavity liner is applied over the base of the cavity or restorative preparation in a thin layer, using a Getz brush or plastic working instrument (C), and is allowed to dry. Bonding of the final restoration will be inhibited if the liner coats the walls of the cavity preparation (D). If the walls are coated inadvertently, they should be prepared again.

Substep 1—When using a light-cured glass ionomer liner, the material is cured with a visible-light gun for the prescribed length of time (E).

Step 3—In deep restorations, another layer of a glass ionomer can be placed to reduce the thickness of the final restoration (F). This reduces the polymerization shrinkage that occurs as the restoration material cures.

Step 4—The restorative procedure is continued (G), as described in Chapter 8.

Postoperative Care

- Follow-up radiographs at 6 and 12 months to evaluate pulp chamber size and evidence of apical abscess formation by comparison with other teeth.

Complications

- Entering pulp chamber during cavity preparation.
- Not allowing enough room for the final restorative material. The surface restorative needs to be thick enough for the patient to benefit from its abrasive and impact-absorbing attributes.
- Covering the walls of the preparation with the liner.
- Losing restorative material due to poor retention.
- Resulting imperfect margins in finished restoration.

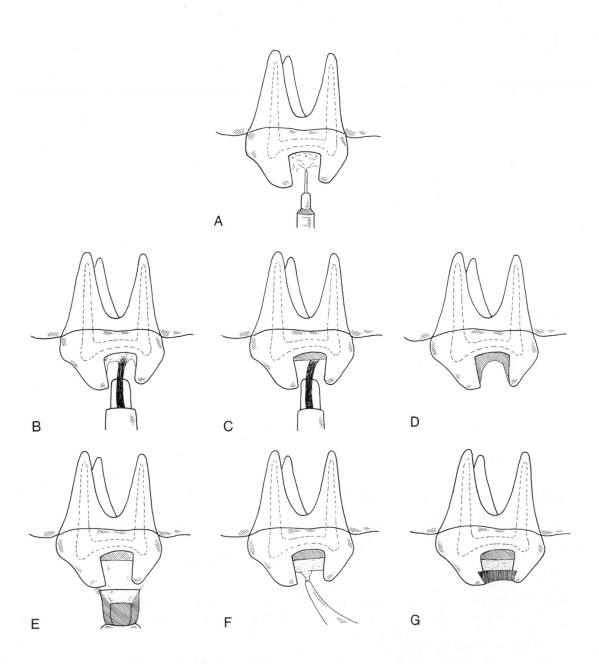

INDIRECT PULP CAPPING: CROWN THERAPY

General Comments

- Due to rules in most dog-show organizations, this treatment should not be performed on dogs intended to be entered in conformation-type dog shows.
- It is the best treatment to prevent further damage to the crown.
- A full-coverage crown *(A)* or half-coverage crown *(B)* may be placed to afford protection to the tooth to prevent chipping or further wear.

Indications

- Teeth that have fractures that have not exposed the pulp chamber.
- Teeth that have had excessive wear from such activities as carrying or chewing tennis balls or chewing on hard objects.

Contraindications

- Direct pulp exposure or radiographic evidence of apical disorder; endodontic therapy should be performed first.
- Animals intended for show. Although unfounded medically, animals may be disqualified from certain show events if they have crowns.

Objective

- To prevent further trauma and wear.

Materials and Technique

- See Chapter 8.

VITAL PULPOTOMY WITH DIRECT PULP CAPPING

General Comment

- In patients younger than 18 months of age, it is frequently desirable to achieve additional dentinal formation to increase the strength of a tooth that has been fractured. For recent fractures, vital pulpotomy with direct pulp capping is the treatment of choice. Patients that have received this treatment should be monitored closely with radiographs to observe changes in pulpal health. Root canal therapy is indicated if death of the pulp is evident on follow-up.

Indications

- Fractured tooth crowns with pulp exposure of less than 2 weeks' duration in patients younger than 18 months of age.
- Fractured tooth crowns with pulp exposure of less than 48 hours' duration in patients older than 18 months of age.
- Disarming animals by shortening the crowns of teeth used for biting.
- In patients with malocclusion to shorten any tooth crowns so as to eliminate interference with other teeth or soft tissues.
- Accidental exposure of pulp during deep-cavity or restorative preparation.
- Hemisection of vital multirooted teeth with extraction of one diseased or injured root when the remaining roots and crown are salvageable.

Contraindications

- Pulpal death.
- Pulp exposure longer than 2 weeks in patient of any age.
- Fractures of the primary teeth. This procedure can be performed on primary teeth but is usually not cost-effective when compared with extraction.
- Severely traumatized or grossly contaminated pulp when the pulp is unlikely to survive.

Objective

- Protect the pulp by stimulating dentinal repair with secondary dentin by using calcium hydroxide, as an irritant directly on the pulp tissue, and placing a restoration over the pulp access site.

Materials

- Diamond disc or no. 701 cross-cut, tapered-fissure bur for shortening the crown.
- No. 2 or 4 round bur in high-speed handpiece.
- Sterile saline.
- Sterile paper points.

- Dycal (Dentsply International).
- Calcium hydroxide paste (HypoCal,* Pulpdent paste†) or calcium hydroxide powder.
- Intermediate filling material (Life, Dycal, IRM2, [Dentsply] glass ionomer base materials).
- Injection syringe.
- Restorative material of choice is discussed in Chapter 8.

---

*Ellman, 1135 Railroad Ave. Hewlett, NY 11557
†Pulpdent Corporation, 80 Oakland St., Watertown, MA 02272

Technique

Step 1—The oral cavity, particularly the tooth to be treated, is disinfected with an antiseptic solution (0.2% chlorhexidine). Aseptic technique is used throughout the procedure.

Step 2—A no. 701 cross-cut, tapered-fissure bur in a high-speed or low-speed handpiece with water cooling can also be used to amputate a tooth crown *(C)* or hemisect a multirooted tooth *(D)*. (When disarming animals, the canine teeth are shortened to the level of the adjacent teeth) *(E)*.

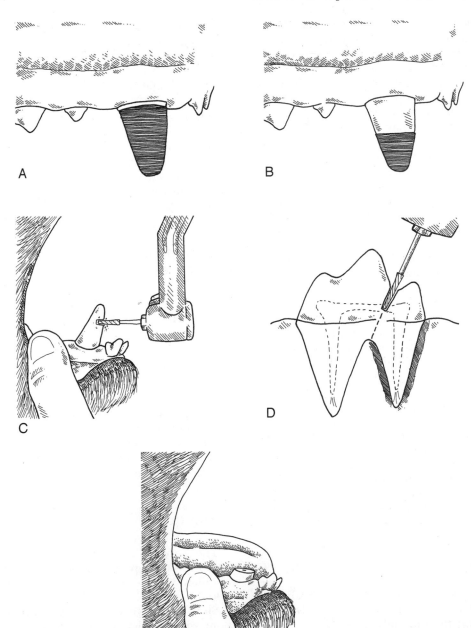

Step 3—A bur approximately equal in size to the diameter of the pulp chamber (round, pear, or tapered-fissure) is used in a high-speed handpiece to remove the coronal portion of the pulp from the amputated tooth, removing 5 mm of the pulp from the remaining endodontic system (A).

Step 4—Hemostasis is achieved using sterile saline lavage and the blunt end of multiple sterile, dry, paper points. Leaving a paper point in place for 2 to 3 minutes is often sufficient to control hemorrhaging. In cases with persistent hemorrhaging, lavage with a local anesthetic solution containing epinephrine can be used.[5] Caution should be used if employing a halothane (Fluothane) anesthetic agent. If hemorrhaging continues, the coronal portion of the canal should be inspected to be sure all pulp tissue coronal to the area cleaned out in step 3 has been removed. Any filaments of pulp left may cause continued hemorrhaging.[6] A coating of calcium hydroxide powder on the paper point may also help control hemorrhaging (B).

Step 5—When bleeding is controlled, calcium hydroxide paste is applied over the exposed pulp for a depth of 1 to 2 mm using the applicator syringe provided (C). The paste is tamped against the pulp stump with the blunt end of a sterile paper point. If using a calcium hydroxide powder, a sterile retrograde amalgam carrier can be used to gently place a layer of powder against the pulp.

Step 6—An intermediate filling material, such as glass ionomer, is placed over the calcium hydroxide paste with an injection syringe or jiffy tube and is allowed to cure (D).

Step 7—The pulpal access (cavity) opening is prepared (E) for the desired filling material, and the restoration is completed (F).

Postsurgical Care

- Postoperative antibiotics should be administered for 7 days.
- Radiographic follow-up at 6 months and 12 months, or at appropriate intervals, is necessary to detect pulp death and subsequent apical changes indicating the need for root canal therapy. (Compare with contralateral tooth.)

Complications

- Inaccurate history resulting, in reality, in an older injury and more extensive pulp infection than initially assessed.
- Loss of restorative material with possible contamination of pulp.
- Tooth discoloration due to hemorrhaging from pulp seeping into dentinal tubules coronal to pulp amputation. (Bleeding through intermediate filling material necessitates redoing the procedure.)
- Pulpal death, which may lead to apical abscessation.
- Pulpitis, which causes pain and may be difficult to detect.
- Internal resorption of the pulp chamber or root canal.

DIRECT PULP CAPPING WITH DENTAL ADHESIVES

General Comments

- Studies have shown that tissue responses after direct pulp capping may be caused by bacterial infiltration rather than directly by material toxicity.[7]
- The advantage of this technique is that it may provide a superior biologic seal due to the increased amount of resin contact.

Indications, Contraindications, Objectives

- Same as for calcium hydroxide technique in preceding section.

Materials

- In addition to those listed in calcium hydroxide technique in preceding section:
- Acid etch gel.
- Dentin adhesive.
- Unfilled and filled light-cured resin.
- Light-cure gun.

Technique

The coronal portion of the tooth is prepared as in the preceding section. Hemostasis is obtained, and this technique begins after step 5.

Step 6—Provisionally cover the exposed pulp with a calcium hydroxide paste with a sterile materials application syringe. This material is applied to protect the pulp during the next step and must not be skipped.

Step 7—A 37% phosphoric acid gel (contained in the composite resin kit) is applied for 20 seconds.

Step 8—After 20 seconds, the gel is wiped onto the enamel for a brief 10 seconds and then rinsed off.

Step 9—The area is blot-dried.

Step 10—The entire preparation, including enamel, dentin, and pulp tissue, is treated with the dentinal adhesive system for approximately 5 seconds, followed by 5 seconds of air drying.

Step 11—A light-cured unfilled resin is applied and activated.

Step 12—The filled resin is applied.

- See Chapter 8, pages 326 to 337, for further information on composite dental restoration.

Postsurgical Care

- Postoperative antibiotics for a minimum of 7 days.
- Radiographic follow-up at 6 months and 12 months, or at appropriate routine prophylactic recall–appointment intervals.

Complications

- A dead tooth may result from any vital pulp capping procedure.
- The risks should be explained to the client before treatment: (1) the tooth injury may be older or more severe than it was thought to be; (2) the undetectable overwhelming infectious organisms might have contaminated the pulp; (3) the patient may further insult and injure the tooth with inappropriate oral behavior.

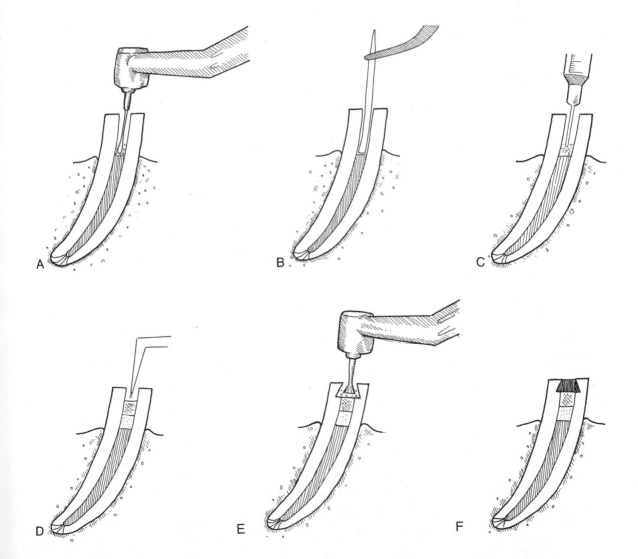

APEXIFICATION/APEXOGENESIS/ HARD TISSUE FORMATION

General Comments

- Apexification is the process of stimulating the formation of a closed apex when a necrotic pulp is present in an incompletely developed young permanent tooth.
- Apexogenesis is the stimulation of completion of normal developmental root lengthening in traumatized young permanent vital teeth.
- The injected calcium hydroxide paste can be intermittently removed and replaced during the healing period if there is no radiographic evidence of hard tissue formation.
- Hard tissue formation is usually seen in 3 to 6 months.
- Length of time to apexification has not been documented in dogs but can take up to 18 months in humans. [4]
- The prognosis is guarded in immature animals due to the fragility of the thin tooth wall that is subject to fracture upon minimal trauma.

Indications

- Fractured tooth crowns with severely traumatized or necrotic pulp in animals with a weak or absent apical seal (less than 18 months of age).
- Root perforations caused by overinstrumentation during endodontic therapy.

Contraindications

- Mature teeth with solid apex do not need apexogenesis or apexification; standard root canal therapy is treatment of choice and is usually successful.
- Inability of client to return for follow-up radiographs and completion of root canal therapy.

Objective

- To induce closure of the apical third of the root canal or formation of a calcified bar-

rier at the apex to allow for future obturation of the canal.

Materials

- Calcium hydroxide paste (Pulpdent Paste, HypoCal).
- Lentulo spiral paste filler.
- Endodontic files and stops.
- Sterile water or saline.
- Sterile paper points.
- Needle and endodontic syringe.
- Sterile cotton pellets.
- Fast-setting cement base (Dycal, Life, IRM2) or glass ionomer base material (see Chapter 8, pp. 338 to 347).
- Restorative material of choice.

Technique

Step 1—A radiograph is taken to examine development of root length and apical closure.

Step 2—Access to the pulp chamber is made per standard endodontic treatment (see the later section in this chapter, Coronal Access to the Pulp Chamber).

Step 3—A small file is placed into the canal to the approximate apical limit, and the tooth is radiographed again to determine a working length of the files, optimally to within 2 mm short of the apex, thus preventing injury to the periapical or apical tissues (A).

Step 4—The root canal is filed and shaped in a standard manner described in the later section in this chapter, Cleaning and Shaping the Canal, using only sterile water or saline for irrigation (B).

Step 5—The canal is dried, using the blunt end of sterile paper points (to avoid perforation into the apex) (C).

Step 6—The canal is filled with calcium hydroxide paste, using a spiral filler with a stop at the working length (D) or a sterile needle with an endodontic syringe.

Step 7—The calcium hydroxide paste is forced to the apex by placing a cotton pellet over the paste and using a blunt plugger to condense it apically (E). The cotton pellet is removed with an endodontic file or broach.

Step 8—The calcium hydroxide paste is removed 3 mm from the access area, and a fast-setting base is placed over the paste (F).

Step 9—A restoration is placed according to standard techniques.

Postoperative Care

- Follow-up radiographs are taken every 3 months to evaluate apical closure or root healing.
- When the desired hard tissue formation or apical closure is seen, the calcium hydroxide paste is removed, the canal is irrigated with sterile saline, and the canal is dried. Obturation can be completed using a tech-nique to fill a larger canal adequately (chloropercha, inverted cone, or thermoplasticized gutta-percha technique).

Complications

- Restoration may need to be replaced; use restorative material that can be removed with the least damage to the tooth.
- Chronic abscessation or drainage due to the thin wall of the tooth.
- Penetration of the apical seal obtained when refiling the canal.

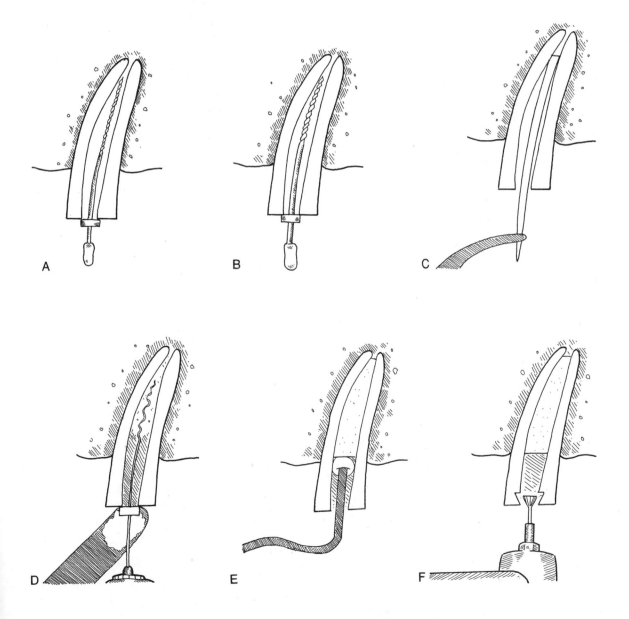

NONSURGICAL ROOT CANAL THERAPY (STANDARD ROOT CANAL THERAPY)

General Comments

- When the tooth pulp has been traumatized, the pathogenesis culminates in apical root-end resorption and abscess formation in the surrounding osseous tissue.[8, 9] The theory of standard root canal therapy is that if the source of the infection (the root canal) is cleaned, the body will successfully eliminate any residual escaped periapical infection.
- Bacterial pulpal infection can occur in an intact tooth. When a systemic infection occurs, microorganisms can ascend through the apical delta to contaminate the pulp canal (anachoresis).
- Patients requiring root canal therapy may present with a variety of signs.
- Patients may be asymptomatic.[10]
- Patients may show signs such as fever, localized facial edema, a draining tract out of the skin or orally, drooling, reduced biting pressure (some trainers report attack dogs bite and release as they bite—"typewriting"), or reluctance to eat (they may pick up food, start to chew, and then drop the food). Other clients report patients licking in the air, circling, or displaying other stress patterns. Trained tracking dogs or dogs used for their sense of smell may lose their ability to perform their tasks; other service dogs may lose their concentration.

Indications

- Fractured crown with pulpal exposure *(A)*.
- Worn tooth with pulp exposure *(B)*.
- Deep carious lesion with pulp exposure *(C)*.
- Discolored tooth with pulpal death *(D)*.

- Teeth that are opaque when transilluminated.
- Reimplantation of avulsed/luxated tooth.
- Radiographic evidence of periapical bone lysis.

Contraindications

- Fractured primary teeth.
- Teeth with an incomplete apex. Studies have shown, however, that the apex may close as early as 10 months of age.[11]
- In adult teeth of animals younger than 18 months of age, when the pulp chamber is large and dentinal layer is thin.
- Fractured crown with vertical root fracture.
- Tooth with internal resorption, creating a thin wall.
- Old animals with inaccessible or sclerosed root canals.
- Severe apical changes involving more than ⅓ of the root.
- Crown root fractures.
- Severe wear that has involved the periodontium and external resorption.
- Patients severely affected with systemic disease such as heart disease, diseases that slow healing such as diabetes, and terminal cancer.

Objective

- To remove diseased or necrotic pulp tissue and achieve a hermetic seal at the apex to preserve a tooth. Root canal therapy consists of three basic parts: (1) accessing the pulp canal, (2) cleaning and shaping the canal, and (3) obturating (filling) the canal. Each of these parts will be covered as a general procedure for restoring the tooth surface. Following are guidelines to adapt these general principles to individual tooth types.

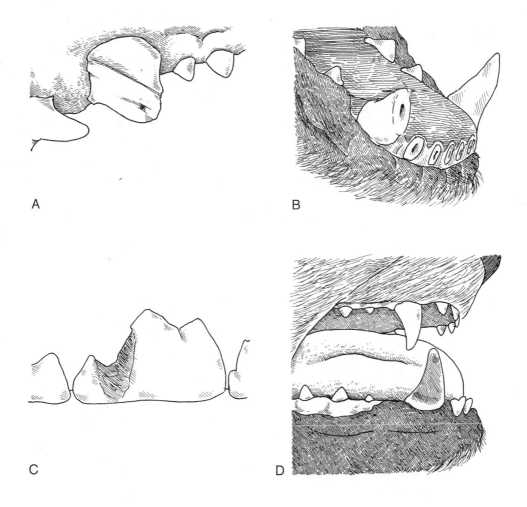

A

B

C

D

Coronal Access to the Pulp Chamber

General Comments

- The coronal access (perforation and entry to the pulp canal) is the first step in root canal therapy. The access may already be present, in the case of a fractured tooth, or may need to be created.

Objectives

- To obtain straight-line access to the apical (towards the apex) third of the root canal, which will permit free instrumentation of the canal and preservation of as much tooth structure as possible.
- To create a cornucopia-shaped convenience form that is widest at the access site and permits shaping the access to the width of the pulp chamber so that there are no overhangs of the root canal roof and the coronal walls to deflect the instruments during preparation.

Materials

- No. 2 or 4 round bur, no. 330 pear bur, or no. 701 or 701L cross-cut tapered-fissure bur for high-speed or low-speed handpiece.
- Intraoral x-ray film.

Technique

Step 1—A preoperative radiograph is taken to identify landmarks, to evaluate canal size and position, and to confirm the treatment plan.

Step 2—Evaluate the tooth clinically to determine root angulation, cusp position, and surface anatomy to guide position and angulation of the access site. (Access in specific teeth is outlined later in this chapter under specific tooth types.)

Step 3—The oral cavity is disinfected with 0.2% chlorhexidine solution.

Step 4—Using the desired bur, a hole is drilled through the enamel layer with the bur positioned perpendicular to the tooth surface. This step is eliminated if an open fracture site allows straight-line access to the apex (A).

Step 5—The bur is repositioned and aligned with the canal, and the access cavity continues to be cut (B).

Step 6—The access site is deepened until the pulp canal is entered. When using a high-speed handpiece, a reduced resistance and a higher pitched drilling noise are noted when the pulp canal is penetrated (C).

Step 7—The access can be enlarged, using a no. 701L bur or Gates Glidden reamer, and shaped to expose the entire width of the pulp chamber, removing ledges so as to appropriately accommodate the endodontic files (D).

Complications

- Removal of too much dentin at the cervical margin weakens tooth structure and may lead to postoperative fracture of the crown (E).
- Incorrect alignment of the bur with the root canal may lead to perforation of the root or cervical area (F).
- Inability to achieve pulp exposure (especially the palatal root of upper carnassial tooth).
- Ledge formation leading to excessive stress or bending of files during filing (G).
- A dull bur burning the enamel or dentin, causing heat and discoloration.
- A bur breaking and blocking the canal.

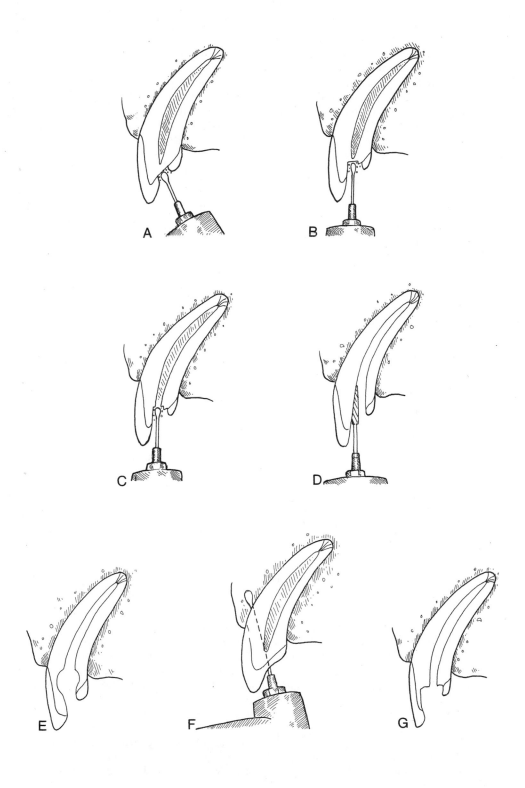

Cleaning and Shaping the Canal

Objective

- To débride the root canal, by removing all pulp tissue and necrotic or softened dentin, and to shape it in preparation for obturation. Endodontic files are used for this purpose, and the canal is disinfected by the use of disinfectant irrigating solutions.

Materials

- Endodontic files/reamers with rubber endodontic stops. (45 mm K-files* are minimum length for canine teeth in dogs. 60 mm Hedström files are available for larger patients.)
- Broaches.
- Intraoral x-ray film.
- Syringes with blunt-end 27 gauge irrigation needles.
- Sodium hypochlorite solution (dilutions vary with practitioner; preference: 1 part sodium hypochlorite, 3 parts water to full-strength sodium hypochlorite.)[5, 12]
- EDTA preparation (RC Prep,† REDTA Solution,‡ Endodialator§).
- Paper points.
- Ruler/measuring device/endodontic ring.
- Dressing forceps.
- Gates Glidden reamers.

Technique

Step 1—Length determination. A small-diameter endodontic file (usually size 10, but 06 and 08 sizes are available) with preplaced endodontic stop is inserted into the root canal 2 mm short of the estimated canal length as determined from a preoperative radiograph (A).

Step 2—Radiograph. A radiograph is taken to verify the file depth (how far the file has penetrated) and the working length (how far the file should penetrate.) This apical stop

*Brasseler USA, Inc., 800 King George Blvd., Savannah, GA 31419

†Premier Dental Products, 3600 Horizon Dr., King of Prussia, PA 19406

‡Roth International, 669 West Ohio St., Chicago, IL 60610

§Union Broach Dental Products, Division of Moyco Industries, 589 Davies Dr., York, PA 17402

indicates that the pulp canal does not extend beyond the file. The ideal working length is 1 mm short of the apex. The canal usually needs to be instrumented further, and the file may be inserted farther and additional radiographs taken until the working length is achieved. Once the working length is achieved, the endodontic stop is moved down the shaft of the file until it contacts the crown, with the file fully inserted. The length is noted (C) and recorded. To provide consistency as to the measurement, the stop should be perpendicular to the file.

- In small canals, the liberal use of a chelating agent (RC Prep) alternated with sodium hypochlorite may help open up the canals to allow access for smaller pathfinder files.
- Subsequent files are fitted with endodontic stops at the predetermined file length (B). If the file is not close to the desired depth, it is instrumented further, and a repeat radiograph is taken until the correct length is achieved.

Step 3—Filing. The canal is cleaned and shaped using the files in an appropriate manner:

- Hedström files: push-pull only (D).
- K-files: push-pull, or push-rotate clockwise 90 degrees and pull (E).
- Reamers: push-pull, or push-rotate past 90 degrees to carry debris to the access site with an auger action.
- The files are used in sequential order, with each file being inserted to the predetermined length and drawn against the sides of the canal in all directions until it moves freely.

Substep 1—An EDTA preparation can be used to help soften the dentin and to lubricate the files by placing a small amount in the canal with a curved tip syringe or, if using a bulk supply, by placing a small amount on an Endo-Ring and running the tips of the files through the ring before entering the canal. When using these products, make sure all of the chemical is removed from the canal in the filing/irrigating process.[13]

Step 4—Pulp tissue removal. Once the working length has been prepared with at least a size 25 file, any residual pulp tissue is removed from the canal by inserting the largest broach that will fit loosely in the apical third of the canal, twisting 90 degrees and pulling it out with attached pulp tissue.

- This step can be repeated several times with a clean broach.
- In large canals, two or three broaches can be placed and rotated simultaneously to ensnare the pulp tissue.

- While treating the same patient, pulp material may be removed from the broach by passing it through a rubber glove or rubber dam. Broaches are made of soft iron and fatigue and break easily if forced into a tight canal space. They are intended to be disposable and should be appropriately discarded as "sharps" after use.

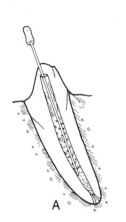

A

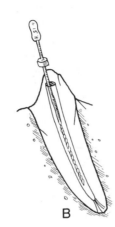

B

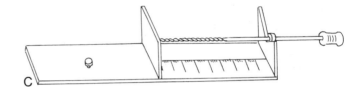

C

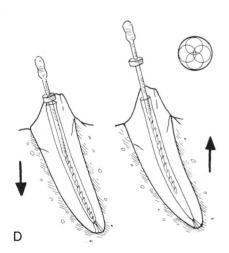

D

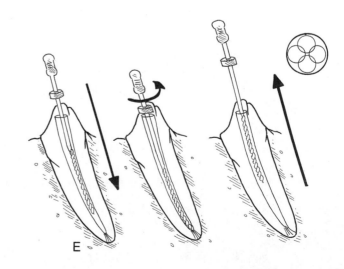

E

Step 5—Irrigation. The canal is irrigated and lubricated between file sizes, using a syringe with a blunt tipped needle. The needle is inserted into the canal so that it does not bind. Irrigating solutions used are sodium hypochlorite and EDTA preparations *(A)*.

Step 6—Recapitulation. Periodically, a smaller file should be inserted to remove any dentinal filings that may have been packed into the apical portion of the canal by previous larger files *(B)*.

Step 7—Shaping. By using standard (rigid core technique), step-back (which creates a tapered, flared, serial, telescoping, or funnel shape), or crown-down (which also creates a tapered, flared, serial, telescoping, or funnel shape) technique, the canal is shaped wider at the crown and tapered to a narrower diameter apically.

Substep 1—Standard Technique *(C)* (ideal for straight, narrow canals). This technique is used to prepare a canal that has the same size, shape, and taper as a standardized instrument. Each size file is placed to its working limit as the canal is cleaned and shaped *(D) (E) (F)*.

- Cleaning and shaping continue until clean, white dentinal filings are seen on two to three successive file sizes *(G)*, and the next-size file binds before reaching the working length *(H)*.

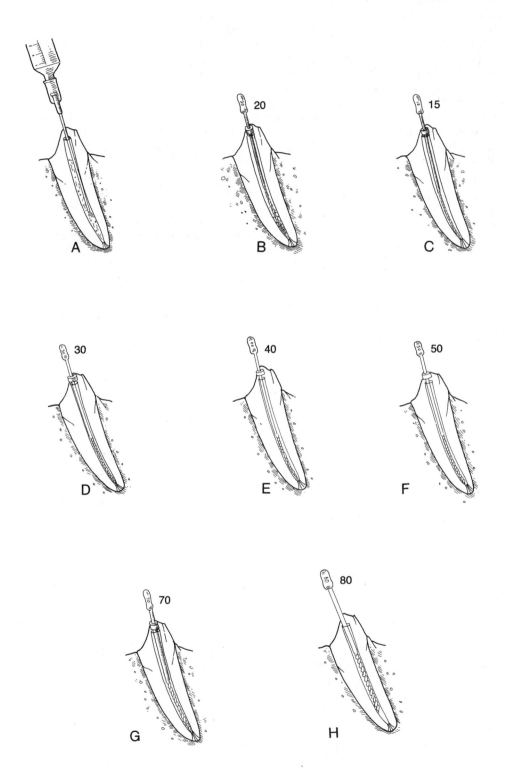

Substep 1—Step-Back Technique *(A) (B) (C) (D)*. Filing is started in the standard manner until the first file that binds at the apical limit is reached. Filing is continued in the standard sequential manner, increasing the file size one to two sizes larger. Next, the tapered or funnel shape is created by placing the stop on subsequently larger file sizes 1 to 1.5 mm closer to the file tip to create a working length for that file shorter than the previous file length. For curved canals or large-diameter canals, a sweeping motion is made with the file along one side of the canal at a time to create a smooth, tapered canal.

- A Gates Glidden reamer can be used to complete the taper in the coronal third of the root canal.

Substep 1—Crown-Down Technique. This technique is useful in narrow canals where difficulty, due to binding of the shaft of the file, is encountered attempting to penetrate with files to the apex. Filing is started, with a larger file first, to open the coronal end of the canal *(E)*. In addition, a Gates Glidden reamer may be used to open the coronal portion of the canal. Filing is continued, using progressively smaller size files *(F) (G)*. The result may be a ledged canal *(H)*, which may be smoothed by additional small files. Small Hedström files may be useful in this step.

Substep 2—Between each step-back file and the last full-length file, a smaller file is used to clean accumulated debris from the terminal portion of the canal. This is called recapitulating.

Substep 3—Between each file size, the root canal is irrigated with sodium hypochlorite.

Step 8—Disinfection. The canal is irrigated with sodium hypochlorite.

Step 9—Drying. The canal is dried by successively inserting absorbent points (paper points) into the canal with endodontic forceps *(I)*. The canal is dry when a paper point remains dry after insertion into the canal. When wet, the paper point has a grayish appearance, as compared with the whiteness of a dry paper point.

Postoperative Care

- The canal is now prepared to be obturated with a root canal sealer and a filling material of choice.

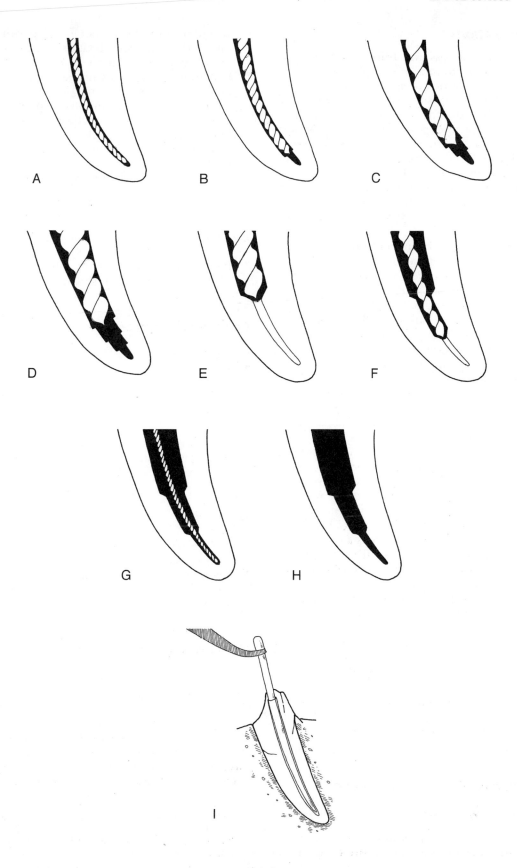

Complications

- Improper access and filing technique may result in a number of complications.
- The endodontic file may end up in a variety of incorrect positions. Transportation occurs when the file starts to widen the canal in the apical region (A). If filing in this direction continues, a ledge may be formed (B). Finally, a perforation may result when the file exits the wall of the canal (C). The file may perforate through an apical foramen. If filing continues, a larger apical opening is created; this is known as a zip (D).[14, 15]
- A root that has been perforated with a file and whose perforation has been treated should be observed radiographically because it may subsequently require retrograde filling (see p. 312).
- Separating (breaking) a file in the canal may occur. If the canal is clean, and the file seals the apex, one option is obturation with paste, leaving the broken file in place. If the file tip is lodged short of the apex but can be bypassed, the endodontic therapy can proceed as originally planned. If this is not possible, a retrograde filling is the best way to ensure success.
- To prevent breaking files in the pulp chamber, the safest practice would be to use a new set of files in every case. However, in veterinary practice, this is often not economically feasible. In every instance files should be discarded when acute bends, deformation, or reverse twists (unraveling) are noted. Endodontic files should be treated as sharps and disposed of according to local regulations.
- Incomplete filing may be performed. Leaving remnants of pulp tissue or contaminated dentin will lead to failure, with pain, persistent bleeding, and apical abscessation, and will require a repeat root canal procedure or a retrograde filling (see p. 312).
- Inadequate shaping leads to difficult or incomplete obturation. The canal should be reshaped with Gates Glidden reamers or larger files.

Persistent Pulp Hemorrhage

General Comments

- For a successful procedure, the root canal must be completely dry before obturation.

- When performing a root canal treatment on teeth with fresh fractures, persistent hemorrhaging may occur.
- If hemorrhaging does not stop with flushing, attempt dry blotting or use a hemostatic on a paper point inserted into the canal. An alternative method is to mummify the bleeding vessels with a formaldehyde preparation. A temporary surface restoration is installed, and the final filling is completed at a second visit, 1 to 2 weeks later.

Indication

- Persistent hemorrhaging after complete filing of a canal in a freshly fractured tooth.

Contraindications

- Open apex.
- Fractured root (class B fracture).

Objective

- To treat persistent apical hemorrhaging during root canal therapy by fixing residual apical vessels with the use of formocresol.

Materials

- Formocresol.*
- Cotton pellet.
- Temporary cavity material (Cavit G).†
- Sterile saline.
- Sterile paper points.

Technique

Step 1—The canal is irrigated with sterile saline and dried (E) with sterile paper points (F).

Step 2—A paper point or small cotton pellet is dipped in the formocresol solution, blotted dry, and placed into the canal with a dressing forceps (the paper point can be cut shorter, as necessary, to fit entirely into the canal) (G).

---

*Sultan Chemists, Inc., 85 West Forest Avenue, Englewood, NJ 07631
†Premier Dental Products, 3600 Horizon Dr., King of Prussia, PA 19406

Step 3—The access opening is sealed with a temporary cavity filling. *(H)*

Postoperative Care

- The patient is reanesthetized in 1 to 2 weeks. The temporary filling material is removed with a cutting bur, and the paper point or cotton pellet is removed with a broach or small file. The canal can now be obturated as desired.

Complications

- Failure of the client to return when requested with subsequent irritation of apical tissues by formocresol and eventual abscessation.

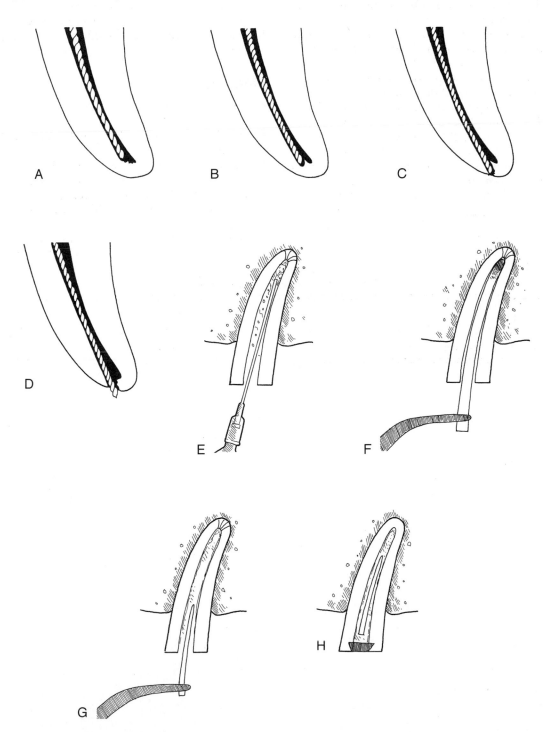

Rotary Filing Technique

General Comments

- The use of rotary instruments to open and file the canal has advantages versus the use of conventional hand files. This type of instrumentation allows for more complete cleaning of the canal, with less strain on the operator, and often results in a faster procedure.
- The major disadvantage of this technique is the expense of the instrumentation. Very low speed is required—no more than 350 rpm. Most low-speed handpieces turn at approximately 3,000 rpm. Therefore, a 10:1 or greater reduction gear is needed.
- The Taper Series 29.04 taper (ProFile .04 Taper Series 29*) provides a consistent 29% increase in file size as opposed to the International Standards Organization (ISO) files that increase at first as much as 50% (10 to 15) and later 10% (100 to 110).

---

*Tulsa Dental Products, 5001 E. 68th St., Suite 500, Tulsa, OK 74136

This series of files gives more sizes of files in the smaller range, where it is needed most, and fewer in the smaller range where it is not as important.
- The Taper Series 29 can be ordered for manual use as well as in rotary format.

Advantages

- There are fewer files in a Taper Series 29 set of files than in an ISO set of files.
- Using the Taper Series 29 is a more efficient use of time.

Materials

- Standard endodontic materials (Table 7–1).
- ProFile .04 Taper Series 29 Rotary Instruments.
- Contra-angle and low-speed handpiece (air or electric) capable of no more than 350 rpm; 150 to 300 rpm is preferred.
- RC Prep (essential for lubrication while using rotary files).
- Irrigation solution, syringe, and needles.

Table 7–1 • COMPARABLE FILE SIZES

.04 Taper Size	2	3	4	5	6	7	8	9	10
ISO Equivalent	.129	.167	.216	.279	.360	.465	.600	.775	1.00
Closest ISO File Size	10	15	20	30	40	50	60	80	100

Root Canal Preparation Technique (Premolar and Incisor Teeth)

Step 1—A size 08 or 10 manual K-file is used to open the canal to the apex, and radiographs are taken.

Step 2—Depending on the size of the canal, additional, sequentially larger, hand files are introduced, just to the point of the file actually working the canal. The last file size is noted.

Step 3—RC Prep is applied to a No. 5 Taper Series 29 rotary file, and the file is used to open the coronal half of the canal halfway down the canal.

Step 4—Continuing to use the RC Prep on the file and continuing to clean the file, sequentially larger Taper files are used to taper and shape the coronal half of the canal.

Step 5—Once the coronal half is opened, the equivalent file size three sizes larger than the last hand-file size is selected and used to shape approximately three quarters of the canal. Liberal use of RC Prep is encouraged to lubricate the file and soften the necrotic dentin in the canal. For example, if a No. 20 ISO file was the last hand file, a No. 7 Taper Series 29 rotary file is used. In no case should the file be forced into the canal.

Step 6—The next smaller taper file size is connected, and approximately seven eighths of the canal is opened. Using the above example, a no. 6 file is used.

Step 7—The next size smaller taper file is used to the apex. Using the above example, a no. 5 file is used.

Step 8—The next smaller taper file (approximately the same size as the hand file) is used to smooth and complete the shape of the canal. Hand files and irrigation are used as necessary to ensure complete removal of dentinal filings.

Complications

- Breakage of the file can occur. This can be caused by a variety of reasons: running a handpiece too fast or with too much pressure, lack of irrigation, lack of intraoperative cleaning of the file, or overuse of the file.
- To prevent breakage, the rotary file must be run slowly. The little dot on the shaft of the file should be visible as the file spins. If the dot is not visible, the speed is too fast.
- The file should not be in the canal for more than 5 seconds.
- Discard the file after using in not more than six canals.
- If binding occurs, an evaluation must be made as to the cause. In the initial opening of the coronal portion of the canal, it may be necessary to step back a size and reopen. In the crown-down phase, if binding occurs, opening the canal with hand instruments or further opening of the coronal portion of the canal may be necessary.

Obturation

General Comment

- Obturation is filling of the prepared root canal. The goal is to obtain an apical seal.

Contraindications

- Persistent hemorrhaging (see p. 276).
- Open apex (see p. 264).

Objective

- To fill the entire root canal system and any accessory canals completely and densely with nonirritating inert material, resulting in a fluid-tight seal.

Materials

- All materials may not be needed, depending on the method used.
- Root canal sealer. Many types are available. Traditionally, zinc oxide–eugenol (ZOE) has been used in veterinary dentistry. Other reduced-eugenol or non–eugenol-containing products are Thermaseal,* AH26,† Can-a-Seal,‡ NOgenol,§ Pulp Canal Sealer EW and Sealapex,‖ and KetacEndo.¶
- Gutta-percha points.
- Root canal pluggers or condenser.
- Root canal spreaders.
- Dressing forceps.
- Source of heat.
- Glass slab.
- Mixing spatula.
- Spiral fillers.
- Files.
- Chloroform.
- Eucalyptus.
- Alcohol in dappen dish.

---

*Tulsa Dental Products, 5001 E. 68th St., Suite 500, Tulsa, OK 74136

†L.D. Caulk/Dentsply, Lakeview and Clark Avenues, Milford, DE 19963

‡Henry Schein, 135 Duryea Rd., Melville, NY 11747

§G.C. America Inc–Fuji Products, 3737 W. 127th St., Alsip, IL 60803

‖Kerr Corporation, 28,200 Wick Rd., Romulus, MI 48174

¶ESPE America, 1710 Romano Dr., P.O. Box 111, Norristown, PA 19404

- Heated gutta-percha applicator.
- Electrically heated plugger.
- ZOE applicator.

Obturating Techniques

Application of Sealer

- In any filling technique, the root canal sealer is placed into the canal first. The choice of product is by individual preference. ZOE, either United States Pharmacopeia or incorporated into a product, is the traditional sealer. Concern has been expressed about eugenol slowing or inhibiting the ability of composite restorations to set up. Therefore, many reduced-eugenol or non-eugenol products have been developed.
- The root canal sealer is mixed according to directions to a thick consistency and placed into the canal, using one of the following methods:

1. A spiral paste filler with a reduction gear on a low-speed handpiece is loaded with the paste and inserted into the canal to depth, activated, and moved slowly in and out to distribute the paste along the canal walls.

2. Using a file two to three sizes smaller than the largest file to reach the apical limit, the file is placed into the sealer paste, inserted into the canal to the apical limit, rotated counterclockwise to coat the walls, and withdrawn. More paste is added, and the file is pumped in and out while being rotated until the walls and the apex are coated (A).

3. The sealer paste can be injected into the canal using pressure with a syringe and blunt-end needle that is small enough not to fit snugly into the canal (B).

4. The sealer paste can be placed on the master gutta-percha cone after sizing and inserted into the canal with the cone.

Advantages
- Improved apical seal.
- Bacteriostatic.
- Radiopaque.

Disadvantages
- Some toxicity to tissues if forced periapically.
- Soluble when exposed to oral or tissue fluids; therefore, if used as the only obturant, may wash out and fail.

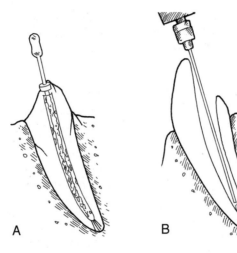

A   B

Spiral Filling or Injection

- A ZOE mixture is spatulated on a glass slab until smooth and the consistency is such that a thread of material is formed when the spatula is elevated off the slab 1 to 2 cm *(A)*.

Spiral Filling Technique

Step 1—A spiral filler is placed in a reduction gear contra-angle on the low-speed handpiece. Spiral fillers come in assorted sizes; one is chosen that can be inserted to the apical limit of the canal without binding.

Step 2—The tip of the spiral filler is loaded with the ZOE mixture *(B)*, and the spiral filler is placed into the canal to the apex.

Step 3—The rotary movement is activated, and the spiral filler is carefully moved back and forth in the canal without completely withdrawing it to fill the canal with paste. A spatula with additional paste on the tip is held near the access opening to continuously place paste into larger canals *(C)*.

Step 4—When the canal is full, paste will be extruded out of the access opening(s) as the filler is moved toward the apex *(D)*. The low-speed handpiece with reduction gear must be set to rotate in forward direction (clockwise) to get proper filling.

Complications

- Binding and breaking the spiral filler in the canal may occur if the spiral filler is too large in relation to the canal diameter.
- Abnormally shaped canals may be inadequately filled or contribute to instrument breakage.

Injection Technique

Step 1—A small syringe is loaded with the ZOE paste or other sealer, and a blunt-end or notched-end needle is placed into the canal to the apical limit. The needle is slowly withdrawn as the paste is injected into the canal *(E)*.

Step 2—Injection guns are available that have cannulas of premixed root canal sealer* for injecting the paste into the canal under pressure.

Advantages

- Faster fill technique.
- Fewer materials needed.

Disadvantages

- Potential for inadequate fill, air bubbles, accessory canals not filled.
- Without a denser filling material such as gutta-percha present, ZOE may be resorbed at the apex losing the fluid tight seal.
- Shrinkage of ZOE paste, after setting, leading to microleakage if the paste is used as the only obturator.

Application of Solid Filling Material

General Comments

- Many types of techniques have been devised to fill the root canal with solid filling material.
- Due to the variety of situations, each practitioner should have many techniques available.
- A three-dimensional fill is desired.[16]

---

*Pulp canal sealer: Kerr, Romulus, MI 48174; Endoseal System, Endoseal, Centrix, Inc., 770 River Rd., Shelton, CT 06484

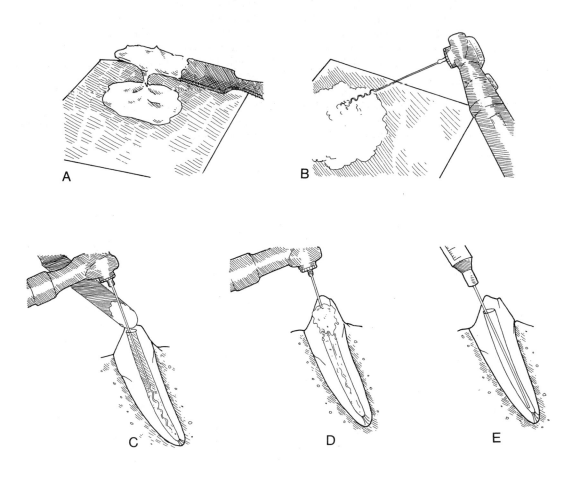

Obturation: Single-Cone Technique

- A dry gutta-percha or silver cone equal to the size of the last file used during instrumentation is selected. If the cone comes from a sterile container, it may be placed into the canal to the apex *(A)*. There should be a little resistance or tug-back felt when removing it. If nonsterile cones are used, the cone should be placed in sodium hypochlorite to disinfect it before inserting it into the canal.

- A radiograph is taken with the point in place to check for fit and fill. The entire canal should be filled. When the appropriate fit is achieved, the gutta-percha point can be marked at the coronal access by pinching with dressing forceps *(B)*. If a stiffer gutta-percha point is desired, the point may be soaked in alcohol before insertion.

- A root-canal sealer is placed in the canal as a liner using the method described in the section on Obturating Techniques.

- The point is cut off at the pinch mark, placed into the canal, and pushed in with a plugger or condenser until the pinch mark is at the desired level *(C)*.

Advantages

- Provides a dense filling material at the apex to provide a longer-term success rate.
- Can provide sufficient fill in smaller, shorter canals prepared with standard technique.

Disadvantages

- Inadequate procedure in larger, longer canals because only the apical 2 to 3 mm of canal is solidly filled.
- Single-cone technique has greater amount of leakage than techniques that condense gutta-percha.
- Difficult to force smaller gutta-percha point (less than 30) to the apical limit; alcohol helps stiffen gutta-percha.

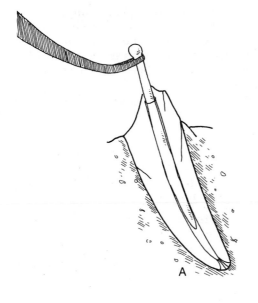

A

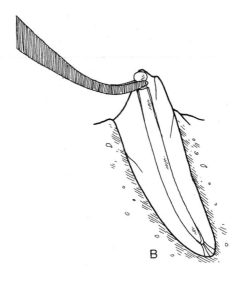

B

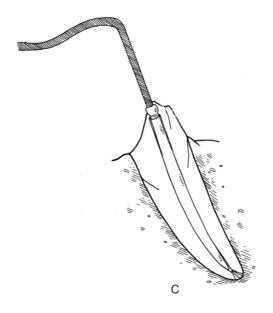

C

Cold Lateral Condensation

- The canal is shaped in either a step-back or a crown-down technique, creating a flare of the coronal limit of the canal.
- A root-canal spreader is chosen that can be inserted to within 1 to 2 mm of the working length of the canal alongside the master cone *(A)*. Larger files or reamers can be used as spreaders in longer canals. The spreader must not be wider than the canal because it may cause excessive lateral force and expansion fracture of the root.
- A standardized gutta-percha point (master cone) is placed in the canal and checked for a snug fit to the apical limit of the canal *(B)*. Use a point the same size as or one size smaller than the last file used. This will allow space for sealer. The length of the point is marked by pinching the cone with dressing forceps at the level of the access hole.
- Root-canal sealer is placed into the canal as previously described.
- The master cone is placed into the canal to the predetermined length.
- A root canal spreader is inserted along the master cone to within 1 to 2 mm of the working length with apical pressure only *(C)*. This seats the gutta-percha point to the apical stop.
- The spreader is rotated on its axis clockwise and counterclockwise several times and is removed.

- An accessory gutta-percha point slightly smaller than the spreader is immediately placed into the space created by the spreader.
- These two steps are repeated until it is impossible to insert an accessory cone farther than 2 to 3 mm into the canal *(D)*.
- The excess gutta-percha is removed with a heated instrument below the access opening *(E)*.
- A radiograph is taken to confirm a complete fill.

Advantages
- Provides more complete obturation of canal with inert filling material.
- Places gutta-percha into apical stop during condensation to prevent overfill.

Disadvantages
- More time is required.
- A variety of gutta-percha sizes and spreaders is needed. Additional veterinary-length spreaders must be added to the inventory to reach desired limit in longer canals.
- Vertical root fracture may occur if excessive lateral force is applied.

Complications
- Splitting of root by overinstrumentation.
- Inadequate filling of canal.
- Old gutta-percha becoming hard and brittle and no longer compressible and malleable.

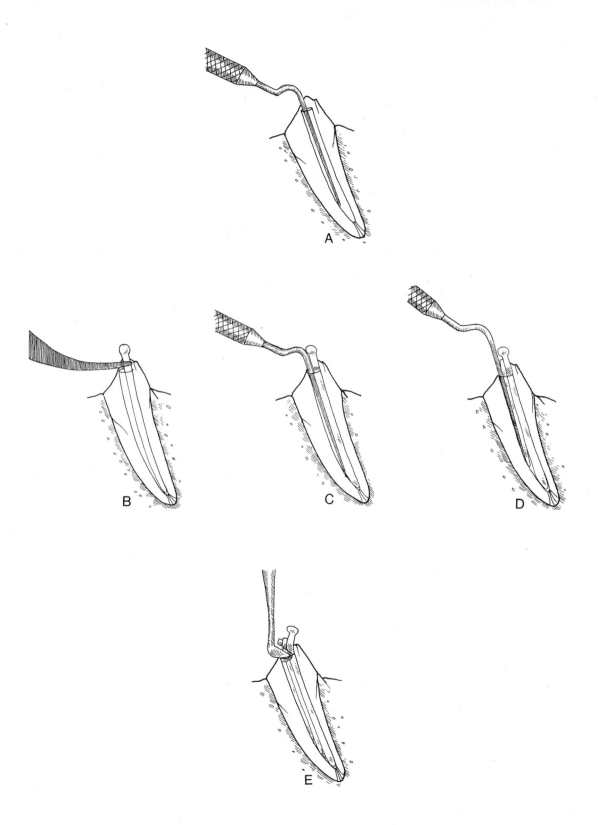

Warm Lateral Condensation

- This technique uses the same instruments as the cold lateral condensation. In addition, a heated carrier is used to soften the gutta-percha to allow further condensing of gutta-percha against the canal walls.
- The canal is prepared and shaped in either a step-back or a crown-down technique with coronal flare.
- A master cone is fitted, and sealer is applied to the canal, followed by the master cone *(A)*. Several accessory points are placed as in the cold lateral condensation technique.
- A carrier (spreader) is warmed in a flame *(B)* and is inserted into the gutta-percha in the canal *(C)*. It is rotated and moved up and down continuously to keep it from sticking to the gutta-percha and dislodging it as the spreader is removed (an electrically heated spreader* simplifies this technique).

---

*Touch and Heat, Analytic Technology Corporation, 15233 NE 90th St., Redman, WA 98052

- A cold lateral spreader is inserted into the space created and is removed.
- An accessory point is inserted *(D)*, and the process is repeated until the canal is full *(E)*.
- The excess gutta-percha is removed with a heated instrument below the coronal access opening *(F)*.
- A radiograph is taken to confirm the fill.

Advantages

- A denser fill and elimination of irregularities (caused by accessory canals, lateral canals, or filing procedure) are achieved.
- The microleakage potential is reduced.

Disadvantages

- Time-consuming.
- Accidental removal of gutta-percha from canal with heated carrier (avoided with proper technique and experience).
- Flame-heating of spreaders causing loss of temper and weakening instrument.

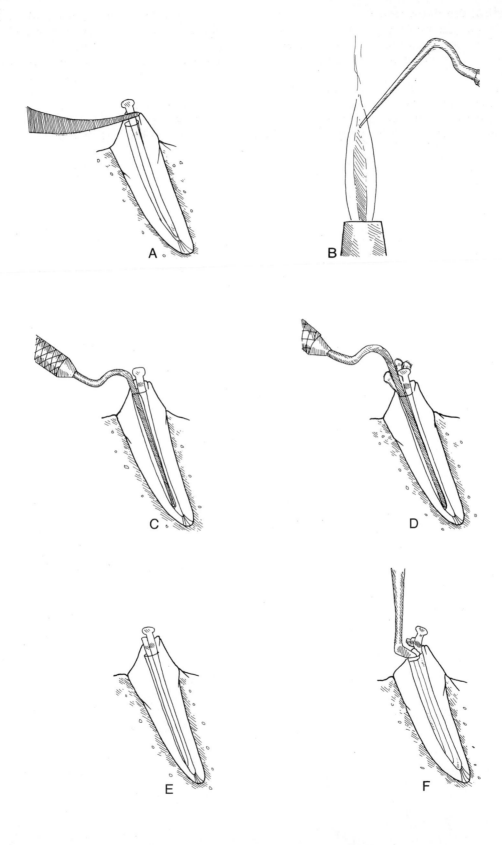

Vertical Condensation

- After placement of a single cone in the canal, a root canal plugger or condenser is used against the end of the point to push it apically.
- As a complete filling technique, a set of pluggers with depth markings is required, and the canal is prepared in step-back technique *(A) (B) (C)*. The pluggers should reach the desired length and be wide enough to cover as large an area of gutta-percha as possible at the desired depth.

Step 1—A master cone is fitted, the canal is lined with sealer, and the master cone is seated *(D)* as described in the earlier section on the single-cone technique.

Step 2—The coronal portion of the cone is removed with a hot instrument *(E)*.

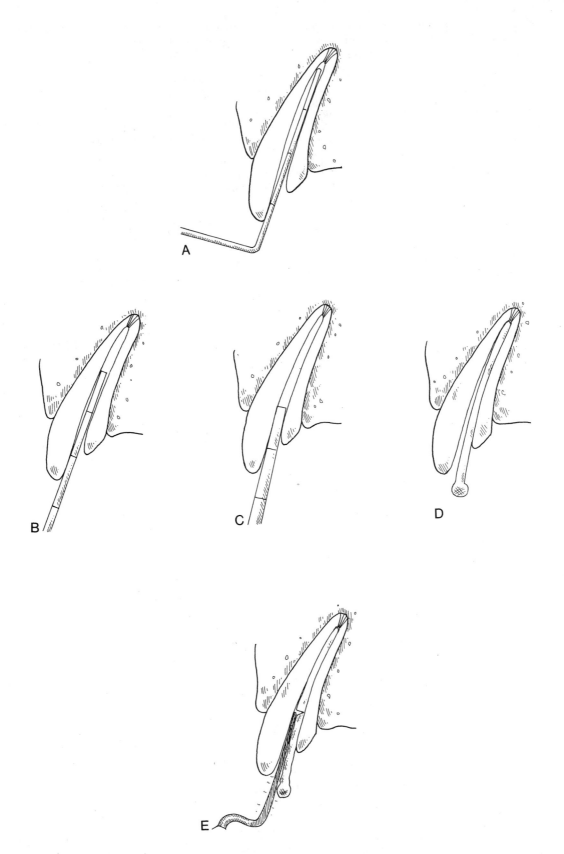

Step 3—A heat carrier (spreader or plugger) is warmed in a flame, inserted into the coronal third of the gutta-percha, and removed *(A)*. (Some gutta-percha will be removed with the instrument.)

Step 4—A cold vertical plugger of the appropriate length and width is inserted, and the gutta-percha is condensed apically *(B)*.

Step 5—An additional piece of gutta-percha 3 to 4 mm in length and matching the width of the canal is inserted into the canal *(C)*, and the process is repeated until the canal is full *(D)*.

- As an alternative to gutta-percha points, 4- to 5-millimeter increments of plasticized gutta-percha can be inserted into the canal with a special device (see p. 302) and condensed apically with an appropriate-size plugger for the entire fill or in addition to a master cone.

Advantages
- Complete obturation of canal apex and accessory and lateral canals.
- Available commercial spreaders that are sized for large canine teeth.*

Disadvantages
- Time-consuming.
- Requires variety of pluggers and spreaders and is more complicated technically.
- Greater chance of overfill.

---

*Cislak Manufacturing, Inc., 1866 Johns Dr., Glenview, IL 60025

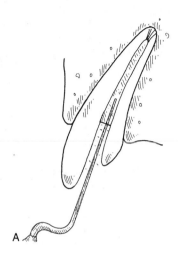

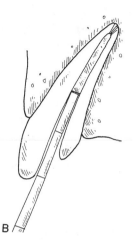

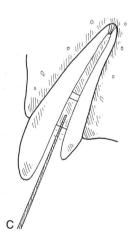

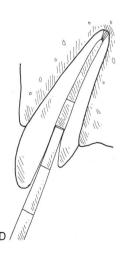

Lateral and Vertical Condensation

- The two previous techniques are used together to achieve complete fill of the canal.

Advantage

- Complete obturation of canal with gutta-percha.

Disadvantage

- Time-consuming.

Chloropercha/Eucapercha Technique

- This technique uses chloroform or warm oil of eucalyptus as a solvent to soften gutta-percha and allow its condensation into canal irregularities.
- Several large standardized gutta-percha points are placed in the solvent to produce a thick paste similar in consistency to that of ZOE. This paste is used as a sealer with a master cone and lateral condensation technique.

Advantage

- The softened gutta-percha can be forced into fine, tortuous canals.

Disadvantages

- Chloroform is a hazardous material and should be used with caution.
- Chloroform is a reported carcinogen; however, this does not appear to be a problem in the amounts used.
- Gutta-percha is less solvent in oil of eucalyptus.

Softened Gutta-Percha Condensation (Chloroform Dip Technique)

- This technique is useful when the apex is open or the apical portion of the canal is irregular *(A)*.
- A master cone is fitted that stops 2 to 4 mm short of the apex *(B)*. A pinch mark is made with dressing forceps at the desired working length as determined by previous radiographs.
- The apical 2 to 3 mm of the master cone is dipped in chloroform for 1 to 2 seconds *(C)*.
- Fluothane may be used to soften gutta-percha in place of chloroform.
- The canal is wetted with irrigant (sodium hypochlorite or saline) to prevent sticking to the walls. The cone is inserted into the canal and is tamped apically with a plugger until it reaches the working length *(D)*. (The cone can be removed, dipped in chloroform, and retamped until the working length is achieved; make sure it is reinserted in the same direction each time.) Confirm the fill with a radiograph. The cone can be 1 mm short of the working length.
- The shaped cone is removed and is allowed to dry for several minutes.
- The apical third of the cone is coated with sealer, and the cone is reinserted into the canal to the set length *(E)*.
- The canal is filled using lateral condensation; each accessory point is coated with sealer before insertion *(F)*.
- A radiograph is taken to confirm the fill.

Advantage

- Adequate apical seal obtainable in irregularly shaped canals.

Disadvantages

- Chloroform is a hazardous material and should be used with caution.
- Chloroform is a reported carcinogen; however, this does not appear to be a problem in the amounts used.
- Shrinkage of the gutta-percha as the chloroform evaporates may lead to microleakage.

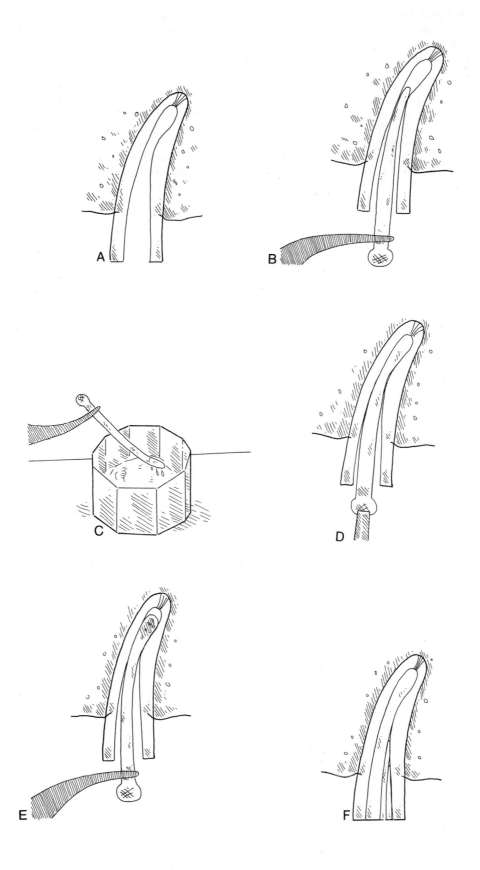

Custom-Point Fill

- A custom-point fill is used in canals that are larger than the largest standardized gutta-percha available.
- Several large cones are softened in a flame (A).
- The softened points are rolled into a cone shape between two glass slabs (B).
- When the point is the approximate size of the canal, it is cooled in water and trial-fitted (C) (D). The process is repeated until the cone fits 1 to 2 mm from the apex.
- The custom cone is used as the master cone, and either the warm or cold lateral condensation technique is used to fill the canal completely.

Advantage

- Allows obturation of large canals.

Disadvantages

- Time-consuming rolling gutta-percha to proper size.
- Gutta-percha must be softened sufficiently to minimize seams or apical voids—difficult to remove them all with this technique.

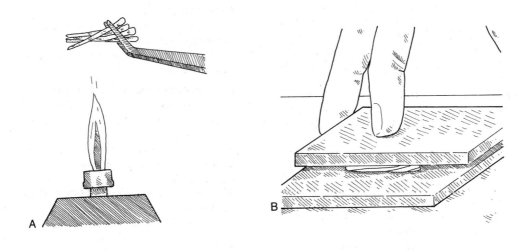

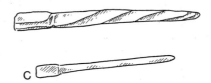

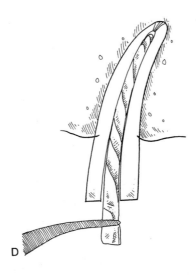

Thermomechanical Condensation (McSpadden Method)

- A McSpadden compactor, which looks like a Hedström file but with reverse flutes, is used in a low-speed handpiece and is inserted alongside a master gutta-percha cone placed 1 to 2 mm short of the apex. The compactor chops up the gutta-percha, thus plasticizing it and forcing it apically and laterally.
- A master cone is fitted in the canal, which has been prepared either in a step-back or crown-down technique, 1.5 mm short of the apex *(A)*.
- The McSpadden compactor selected is the same size as the last file that came 1 to 1.5 mm from the apex. The working length is marked on the compactor.
- The master cone is coated with sealer and is inserted into the canal.
- The compactor is inserted alongside the cone until resistance is felt and is rotated at maximum speed *(B)*.
- After 1 second, the compactor is advanced apically to the predetermined length and is slowly withdrawn while rotating.
- Accessory points can be dipped in sealer and placed alongside the master cone and a larger compactor used until the canal is full *(C)*.
- A radiograph is taken to confirm the fill.

Advantage
- Rapid condensation technique, forcing softened gutta-percha into canal irregularities.

Disadvantages
- Breakage of compactor tip in canal.
- Heat generation.
- Compactor not being long enough for use in canine teeth.

Broken-Instrument Technique

- If an instrument tip is broken inside the canal and cannot be retrieved, and an apical seal can be achieved, the tip can be left in place and a filling technique used to fill around it, if the canal has been completely cleaned *(D)*.
- The instrument breakage should be noted in the chart.
- The client should be informed, and follow-up radiographs should be taken at 6 months or earlier if complications are noted.

Advantage
- Do not have to remove a broken file tip.

Disadvantages
- If the canal is not adequately prepared, the procedure may fail.
- If a larger file tip is broken, it may not allow fill around it, necessitating an apicoectomy with retrograde filling.

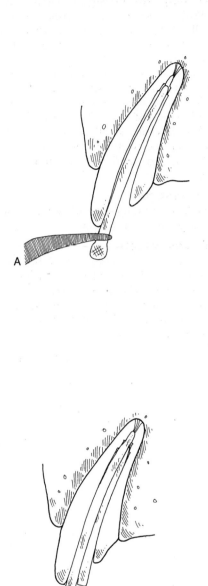

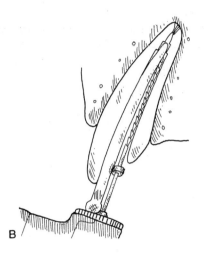

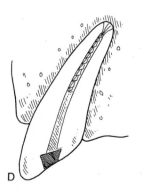

Inverted Cone Technique

- Some canals may have a wider apical portion that makes them difficult to fill with standard-size cones (feline canine teeth).
- Root canal sealer is placed as previously described.
- A gutta-percha cone is placed with the larger, rounded end toward the apex *(A)*.
- Using lateral and/or vertical condensation techniques, the remaining canal is filled with accessory gutta-percha points *(B)*.
- KetacEndo* used as a sealer in feline canine teeth can eliminate the need of accessory points in many canals.

Advantage

- Allows fill of atypical root canals, using standard gutta-percha and root canal sealer.

Disadvantage

- Time-consuming.

---

*ESPE America, 1710 Romano Dr., P.O. Box 111, Norristown, PA 19404

Orthograde Amalgam Technique

- This technique can be used when trying to fill a large open canal, as in an immature canine tooth, to provide greater strength for future restorations.[17]
- Amalgam is mixed and placed into the canal with an amalgam carrier *(C)*.
- The amalgam is condensed vertically with custom-made amalgam condensors *(D)*. (Condensors must be sized to reach the length and width of the canal.)
- These two steps are repeated until the canal is full.

Advantage

- Makes a stronger tooth when dentinal development is minimal.

Disadvantages

- Amalgam can be extended beyond apex if apical development is incomplete.
- Technique discolors tooth.
- Amalgam may expand and fracture tooth.
- Adequate-length condensing instruments needed for complete fill.

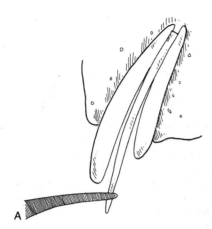

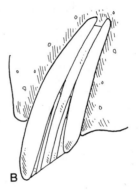

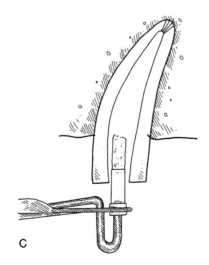

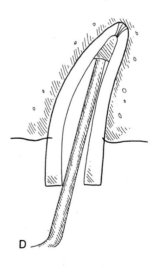

Thermoplasticized Gutta-Percha

Heated Gun Technique

- A special device (Ultra Fil System*, Obtura II†) is used to heat gutta-percha, which is injected into the canal with a pressurized syringe. The canal must be filed to a size 60 or 70 to allow the needle to be inserted near the apex. Cannules are supplied, loaded with gutta-percha of different levels of flowability. The more flowable gutta-percha is preferred.
- Root canal sealer is placed in the canal with a file or spiral filler.
- A cannule of gutta-percha is heated and loaded into the syringe.
- The needle (22 gauge) of the cannule is placed into the canal to within 1 mm of the apex.
- Melted gutta-percha is slowly injected into the canal as the needle is withdrawn *(A)*.

---

*Coltene/Whaledent, 750 Corporate Dr., Mahwah, NJ 07430

†Obtura Corporation, 1727 Larkin Williams Rd., Fenton, MO 63026

- In longer canals, a few millimeters of gutta-percha are placed in the canal *(B)*. After cooling for 20 to 30 seconds, a root canal plugger is used to push the gutta-percha apically *(C)*.
- This step is repeated until the canal is full *(D)*.
- Final condensation is performed with a root canal plugger to ensure an apical seal *(E)*.
- Excess gutta-percha is removed from the access opening with a heated instrument *(F)*.

Advantages

- Rapid filling method in larger canals.
- Can fill accessory or lateral canals.

Disadvantages

- Not applicable in small canals because the cannule needle is equivalent to a size-60 file.
- Needle of cannule not long enough for most canine teeth; must be combined with the vertical condensation technique to fill long teeth completely.

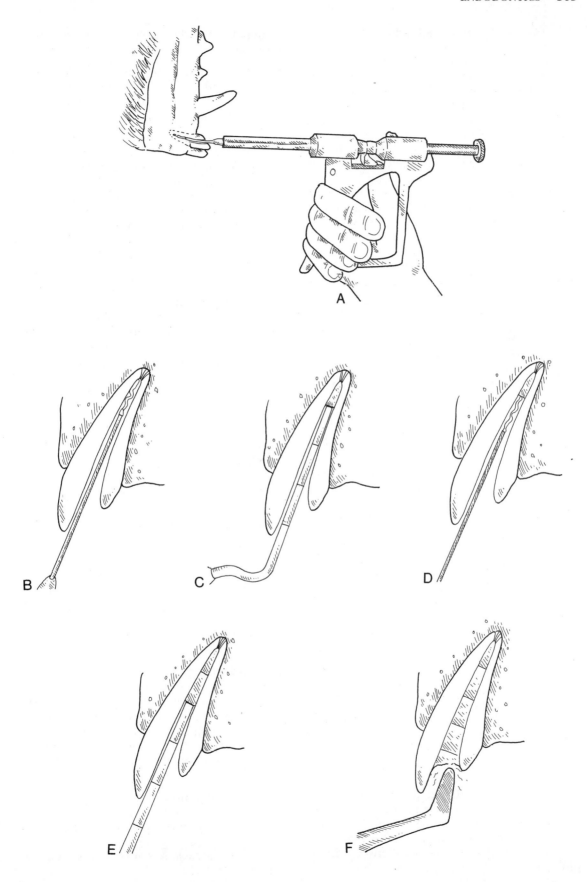

Heated Syringe Technique

General Comments
- This system employs a heater to heat gutta-percha in a syringe. The gutta-percha is then transferred to either a titanium core carrier or a sterile endodontic K-file with endodontic stop to be inserted into the canal. The SucessFil syringe may be reheated and used until empty.

Advantage
- A good, solid fill of the canal can be obtained.

Disadvantages
- Moderate expense for start-up and for materials.
- Learning curve to work with material.
- Can be time-consuming on larger canals.

Technique
- This technique has two options: leaving the file in the canal with the gutta-percha or removing the file after the gutta-percha is placed. The latter is the most commonly used.

Step 1—The syringe of gutta-percha is warmed in the heating unit *(A)*.

Step 2—A clean file two to three sizes smaller than the last file used to reach the apex is selected.

Step 3—Sealer is placed in the canal by one of the described methods.

Step 4—The selected file is inserted into the end of the syringe of warm gutta-percha and, while the plunger is simultaneously pressed, the file is withdrawn to create a thin, tapered coating of gutta-percha on the file *(B)*.

Step 5—The file is quickly inserted into the canal to the working length.

Substep 1—The file is held in place while the gutta-percha cools slightly; the file is then twisted counterclockwise and withdrawn, leaving the gutta-percha in place. A plugger is used to condense the softened gutta-percha apically. Additional gutta-percha can be placed and condensed until the canal is adequately filled.

Substep 1—An alternative method is to place a rubber stopper on the file before coating the file with gutta-percha. After the file is placed in the canal, the rubber stopper is placed against the tooth, and the file is withdrawn, keeping the gutta-percha in the canal. The gutta-percha is then condensed with a plugger.

Step 6—A radiograph is taken to confirm the desired fill.

- In large canals, this technique can be combined with using a cannule of warm gutta-percha injected to fill the coronal portion of the canal.

Complications
- May result in apical voids and coronal fill if too much material is placed on carrier.
- Gutta-percha may cool and not be taken to the working length if the insertion is too slow.
- Removing the gutta-percha with the file—wait a few seconds until gutta-percha has cooled; then twist the file out.

Obturation with Thermafil*

General Comments
- The Thermafil system uses a plastic carrier to which a rubber stopper and thermally plasticized gutta-percha have been applied.
- After standard endodontic preparation, the gutta-percha on the carrier is warmed, and the carrier is inserted into the treated canal.
- After taking a radiograph to evaluate proper fill, the carrier is cut off in the canal.
- Thermafil is available either in specific carrier sizes or in an assortment of sizes.
- The carrier sizes are from standard file size 20 to 140.

Advantages
- Thermafil allows filling of narrow, medium-length canals where using standard gutta-percha techniques may be difficult.
- Thermafil provides a good apical seal.
- Although relatively rare in the dog and cat, if lateral canal or apical canals are present, Thermafil provides introduction of gutta-percha into these secondary canals.

Disadvantages
- Currently, the carriers are manufactured only in 25 mm lengths; therefore, canals longer than 25 mm cannot be treated. Longer lengths may be manufactured.
- The carriers are expensive, and using the system is moderately technique-sensitive.

Technique
- Before beginning, the oven that will heat the plastic gutta-percha carrier must be turned on and allowed to warm up.

---

*Tulsa Dental Products, 5001 E. 68th St., Suite 500, Tulsa, OK 74136

Step 1—The endodontic obturator* is selected by using a size verification kit. From the kit, a carrier blank of the same size as the largest file used to the full working length is selected. The blank carrier is disinfected in a 5.25% sodium hypochlorite solution for 1 minute, followed by a rinse in 70% alcohol.

Step 2—The carrier blank is inserted to the working length. The carrier blank should fit without forcing. If it does not fit to the apex, either the canal must be reworked or a carrier blank the next size smaller must be selected and tried. A radiograph is taken to ensure proper fit to the apex.

Step 3—The same size plastic endodontic obturator as fits the canal properly is selected (C) and placed in the oven (D). The carrier should be warmed for 5 to 8 minutes before being inserted into the canal.

---

*Thermafil: Tulsa Dental Products, 5001 E. 68th St., Suite 500, Tulsa, OK 74136; Densfil: L.D. Caulk/Dentsply, Lakeview and Clark Avenues, Milford, DE 19963

Step 4—As the endodontic obturators are warming, Thermaseal* is spatulated. The material may be placed in the canal by coating gutta-percha points and swabbing the canal.

Step 5—Once heated, the endodontic obturators are inserted into the canals, being careful to make as direct an insertion as possible.

Step 6—Once inserted, radiographs are taken to confirm obturation to the apex of all canals.

Step 7—The endodontic obturators are cut with a heated instrument.

Complications

- There may be an inability to insert the endodontic obturator to the apex. In this case, the obturator should be reheated and reinserted; another obturator should be chosen and heated; or another method of filling the canal should be selected.

- In the maxillary fourth premolar, where the mesiobuccal and palatal roots come together, it is best to fill one canal, take radiographs, cut the obturator with a heated instrument, and then fill the other canal. Otherwise, the obturator from the first canal may prevent a direct insertion of the operator for the second canal.

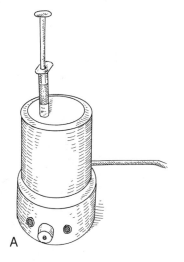

A

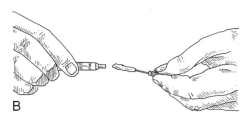

B

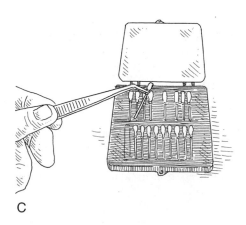

C

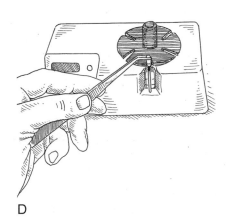

D

Additional Filling Techniques

Comments
Additional techniques are available, but they are not recommended by the authors. They are included to list their advantages and disadvantages.

- Paste injection system.
- Tubli-seal.*

Advantages
- Easy.
- Fast.

Disadvantages
- Overfill of canal possible.
- Sets up fast and may be difficult to remove if necessary, such as if post space or reinstrumentation is needed.
- May fill coronal end and leave an apex open.

Solid Fillers
- Silver points.

Advantages
- Do not shrink.
- Do not encourage bacterial growth.
- Nonirritating.
- Radiopaque.
- Easily introduced.

Disadvantages
- Difficult to remove.
- Rigid; often do not match canal shape.
- Not suited for curved canals.
- Corrosion may release cytotoxic silver and staining.

Removal of Gutta-Percha
- The following techniques may be used to remove gutta-percha:

1. An instrument may be used to heat the gutta-percha and remove it from the pulp chamber.
2. Endodontic files may be used to refile the canal.
3. Chloroform, Fluothane, or rectified turpentine oil may be introduced into the canal to soften it.

- Rectified turpentine oil has the advantage that it is not carcinogenic.

___
*Kerr Corporation, Romulus, MI

Restoration of Coronal Access

- A base of glass ionomer or other suitable material is placed over the gutta-percha ends.
- The access site is restored using a technique discussed in Chapter 8.

Postoperative Care
- Recommend soft food for 48 hours.
- Follow-up radiographs are recommended at 6 months, 1 year, 2 years, and 5 years.
- Oral antibiotics for a minimum of 1 week should be prescribed.
- Minimize aggressive chewing activity. Patients should be allowed to chew only items softer than the teeth.

Complications of Nonsurgical Endodontics
- The primary complication of a nonsurgical endodontic procedure is failure of the procedure related to improper operator technique.
- The patient may be asymptomatic; therefore, radiology is an important tool to enable diagnosis of a failed treatment. The radiograph may demonstrate that the lesion has remained the same, has enlarged, or has only slightly diminished in size, and total healing has not occurred.
- Common causes of procedure failure are incomplete obturation and inadequate apical seal, pathologic or iatrogenic root perforation, and broken instruments in the canal.
- Other causes of failure are root end resorption, coexistent periodontal-periapical lesions, and endodontic disease in adjacent teeth.

Variations with Individual Tooth Types

Incisors

Access Opening
- If the crown is fractured or worn (A), the opening to the pulp canal can be enlarged with an appropriate-size round or pear-shaped bur in a high- or low-speed handpiece.

- If the crown is intact, the access hole can be made on the lingual surface between the crown tip and the cingulum *(B)*. The bur is directed toward the center of the tooth along the long axis to avoid perforation of the root.

Filing and Irrigation of the Canal

- Smaller and shorter files are used to clean and prepare incisor canals. The root of the third maxillary incisor curves dramatically,

and it may be necessary to pre-bend files to reach the apex *(C) (D)*.

General Comment

- Incisor teeth can be treated relatively quickly. In small dogs it may be difficult to enter the canals of the central incisors and nos. 06 and 08 files may be necessary, initially, to start filing. Generally, the canal is filed to size 35 to 40 for the average-size dog.

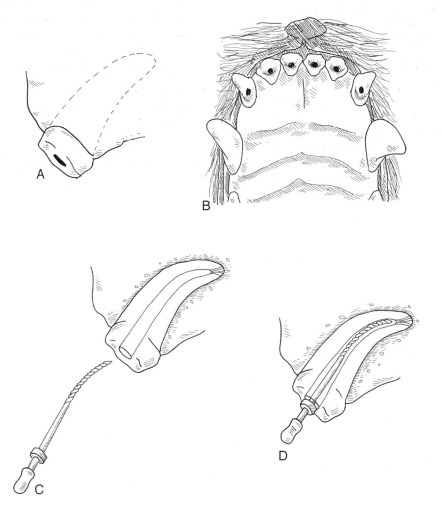

Canine Teeth

Access Opening

- An access hole can be made at the fracture site by enlarging the pulp canal opening with a no. 2, no. 4 round, or no. 330 pear-shaped bur in a high-speed or low-speed handpiece *(A)*. This access may be sufficient in fractured teeth with little remaining crown. An additional access hole is made on the mesial surface of the tooth 2 to 3 mm coronal to the gingival margin in a line with the root canal visualized on a preoperative radiograph in intact teeth or in teeth with incisal crown fractures to allow complete instrumentation of the entire canal length without undue bending of files. The access hole begins with an initial cut made through the enamel and perpendicular to it *(B)*. The bur is directed apically to penetrate the pulp chamber while being in a straight line with the apex *(C)*.
- Access holes must be just large enough to allow unimpeded instrumentation.

Filing and Irrigation

- Filing and irrigation are completed as described on page 270; files or reamers 40 to 60 mm long are necessary to reach the apex in large dogs. In dogs with smaller canals, it is beneficial to enlarge the coronal portion of the canal with a Gates Glidden reamer on a low-speed handpiece to eliminate binding the shaft of the larger files.
- Alternating between file types can be beneficial in completing the instrumentation and ensuring a clean canal. Reamers work well throughout the canal length, whereas K-files are best used in the apical third of the canal; Hedström files are preferably used to shape the coronal two thirds of the canal.
- Wide pulp canals in younger dogs necessitate circumferential filing to remove all pulp remnants and softened dentin.
- The average canal size ranges from no. 25 × 23 mm in small dogs to no. 50 × 36 mm in large dogs.[18]

Filling Techniques

- The techniques most commonly used are spiral filling, lateral condensation with multiple gutta-percha points, combinations of lateral and vertical condensation with standard gutta-percha, and thermoplasticized gutta-percha techniques.
- Large canals in young dogs can be filled with amalgam or Core Paste.*
- Longer plugger/spreader instruments designed for use in canine teeth are available (PLG/SP50, PLG/SP65, PLG/SP90).†

*Den-Mat, 2727 Skyway Dr., Santa Maria, CA 93456
†Cislak Manufacturing, Inc., 1866 Johns Dr., Glenview, IL 60025

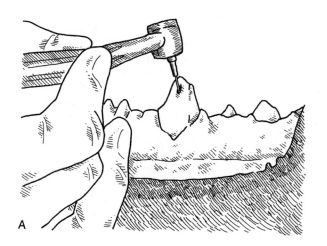

A

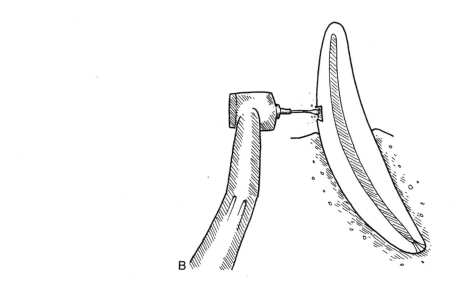

B

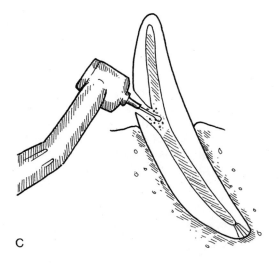

C

Teeth with Two Roots

Access Openings

- Openings need to be made into each root *(A)*. Premolars can be accessed from the fracture site, if large enough; otherwise, a separate hole is drilled into the crown over each root. The least amount of tooth structure as possible should be removed in making the access. Some authors advise opening the common pulp chamber liberally to allow removal of pulp tissue. The risks of using a single access site to instrument a two-rooted tooth are incomplete débridement and root-wall perforation when filing and creating voids when filling.
- In a mandibular molar, access is made into the mesial root by drilling a hole just lingual to the small fissure on the buccal surface of the tooth *(B)*. The distal root is accessed by a hole drilled in the center of the occlusal surface. Comparing the anatomic features with those in a radiograph helps determine the proper site and angle of the access hole.
- The roots may be filed sequentially or simultaneously *(C)*.

Teeth with Three Roots

Maxillary Fourth Premolar

Access to Mesiobuccal Root

- The mesiobuccal root can be accessed by drilling a hole at the point of intersection of a line approximately two thirds the distance between the developmental groove and buccomesial line angle at the waist of the tooth and one quarter the distance from the gingival margin to the full length of the normal cusp tip. If the cusp is missing, the distance is approximated by comparing the injured tooth with the contralateral one.

Palatal Root

Transcoronal Approach[19]

- The palatal root can be accessed through the hole discussed above by directing the file toward the palatine root *(D)*.
- The access to the palatine root can vary from a site in the chamber floor to a site in the chamber wall. It is helpful to externally visualize the palatal cusp and visible portion of the root. The access site may also be enlarged to provide better visualization of the chamber while locating the access to the palatine root.

Three Access-Hole Approaches

- The palatal root can also be accessed by drilling directly over the palatal cusp close to the notch created by the large cusp surface. This is more difficult, particularly in older dogs and in larger dogs.
- A third approach to the palatal root is to create a groove between the mesial root access hole and the palatal cusp across the surface of the tooth. In difficult cases, this will allow visualization of the common pulp chamber, and the files can then be directed into the palatal root, but it does require removal of an increased amount of tooth structure.
- Occasionally, in older or small dogs, the palatal root cannot be filed to the apex due to partial calcification of the canal. If there is no periapical disorder visible and further filing cannot be accomplished with additional use of chelating agents, a clinician may choose to file and fill the canal to the depth reached, after which the canal should be monitored closely. This may be preferable to root amputation.

Palatal Root Amputation

- If the palatal root cannot be accessed or if root perforation occurs in attempts to locate the canal, the palatal root can be sectioned and removed and the common pulp chamber filled with a restorative.
- One potential problem is that when the palatal root is amputated, its buttressing effect will be lost and the tooth will be weaker and more subject to fracture.[20, 21]

Access to Distal Root

- The distal root access hole is drilled two thirds of the distance between the distal surface of the tooth and the developmental groove and halfway from the gingival margin to the distal cusp.[19] These holes are made large enough to allow free instrumentation of all the canals in the maxillary fourth premolar.

Molar Teeth

- Access sites in the three-rooted molar teeth are best made on the occlusal surface after study of preoperative radiographs and study models.

Filing and Irrigation

- Filing and irrigation of all three roots are completed using 21 to 30 mm files, as described throughout this chapter. The distal root is generally larger and may often be filed to size 80. The mesiobuccal root averages size 30 to 35 and the palatal root size 25 to 30.[18]

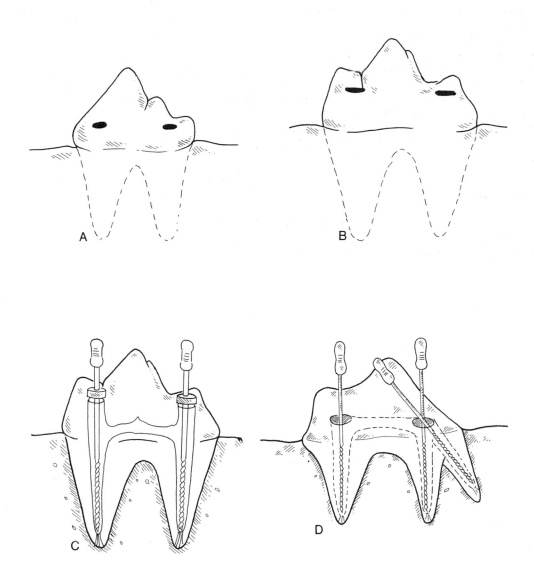

SURGICAL ENDODONTICS (APICOECTOMY WITH RETROGRADE FILLING)

General Comments

- The teeth most commonly requiring apicoectomy are the upper and lower carnassial teeth and upper and lower canines.
- A surgical root canal treatment can be successful only if the basic tenets of canal cleaning and shaping have been accomplished.
- All roots should be treated in multirooted teeth.
- It is very difficult to surgically access the palatal root of the upper fourth premolar. It can be resected and extracted, as necessary, to salvage the tooth. If it is adequately filled, and it is not the reason for the surgical decision, it may be left in place.
- Utilizing a study skull to reference anatomic features, with preoperative radiographs, is very often a helpful clinical aid.

Indications

- A tooth with an open apex and concomitant periapical infection that does not respond to standard endodontic treatment.

- Apical perforation during endodontic treatment that subsequently leads to clinical or radiographic failure.
- A separated endodontic file tip embedded in the root canal or wall, which interferes with complete preparation and filling of that canal and subsequently leads to clinical or radiographic failure.
- Failure of a standard root canal procedure resulting in clinical or radiographic failure (underfill, overfill, root perforation, etc.). May need to redo standard root canal treatment first, if canal is underfilled.
- Coronal approach impossible (narrow canals, aberrant canal formation, pulp stones, or calcified canal).
- Horizontal fracture of root tip.

Contraindications[22]

- Brittle health status of patient.
- Difficult access, the most common site being the palatal root of maxillary fourth premolar, resulting in poor technique.
- Complex root and crown structure.
- Excessively weak or damaged roots.
- Necessity to remove excess bone in the mandible, which may further weaken mandible.

Objective

- To ensure a seal of the root canal system at the apex by exposing the apical area and sealing the canal with a retrograde filling.

Materials

- Instruments and materials for standard root canal therapy.
- No. 10, 15, or 15c scalpel blade with handle.
- Periosteal elevator.
- Senn retractors.
- No. 701L, 2, 4, 33½, or 34 bur.
- Small-bone rongeurs.
- Dental excavator.
- Lucas 75 Curette.
- Bone curette.
- Dressing forceps.
- Cotton pellets, sterile gauze squares, hemostatic agent.
- Sterile saline.
- Retrograde amalgam or composite carrier.
- If amalgam technique is used: amalgam plugger and carver, non-zinc amalgam, amalgamator, amalgam well.
- If amalgam technique is not used: IRM or Super EBA Cement.*
- 4-0 absorbable suture material with swaged-on taper needle.
- Needle holders, scissors, thumb forceps.
- Cotton pellets.
- Hemostatic agent.
- Suction.

Technique

Step 1—Standard root canal therapy is performed first. (Retreatment and refilling of the canal may be first treatment option if failure is due to inadequate obturation, etc.)

Step 2—The mouth is disinfected with 0.2% chlorhexidine, and aseptic technique is employed.

Step 3—The tooth apex is located by feeling the bulge of the root (juga) beneath the alveolar mucosa and is exposed by incising the soft tissue superficial to the apex with a semilunar incision. The incision is made through the periosteum. (The area can be infiltrated with lidocaine with epinephrine to enhance hemostasis.)

Substep 1—A preoperative radiograph is taken to locate the apex.

---

*Bosworth, 7227 N. Hamlin Ave., Skokie, IL 60076

Access Sites

- Access to the maxillary canine tooth is made with a curved incision starting mesial to the root in the alveolar mucosa, extended distally to the level of the distal root of the second premolar, with the ventral depth of the curve at the coronal third of the root *(A)*.

- Access to the maxillary fourth premolar is made with a semilunar incision through the alveolar mucosa starting at the level of the third premolar and extending distally to the first molar, with the depth of the curve at the coronal third of the root. (Do not disturb the infraorbital nerve exiting above the mesiobuccal root or the distal root of the third premolar.) An approximation of the apical locations can be made when it is realized that the mesiodistal width of the tooth approximately equals the distance from the gingival margin to the apex. It can be visualized as a square. [21]

- Access is made to the first mandibular molar either intraorally, on the buccal mucosa, with a semilunar incision starting at the level of the fourth premolar and continuing distally to the second molar, with the depth of the curve at the coronal third of the root *(B)*, or through a ventral approach to the ramus of the mandible.

- Access to the mandibular canine teeth is made through a ventral approach to the mandible *(C)*.

The maxillary canine tooth is used as an example for a surgical root canal.

Substep 2—An incision is made through the alveolar mucosa and periosteum over the tooth to be treated *(D)*.

Step 4—The gingiva and periosteum are reflected *(E)*. The bulge (juga) over the root is palpated, and the apical area is determined by comparing with the file length used in preparation of the canal to locate the apex. Soft-tissue retractors are used to increase visualization. Avoid tearing the flap by using a sharp periosteal elevator and elevating a full-thickness flap including mucosa, fascia, and periosteum. Partial-thickness flaps are not recommended due to reduced healing capabilities caused by interrupted blood supply.

Step 5—The bone is drilled away, with a feather motion, using the side of the cutting bur, in a small circle encompassing the apex to expose the distal 4 mm of the root with a high-speed no. 2, no. 4 round, no. 701L cross-cut fissure, or no. 330 pear-shaped bur with accompanying sterile saline irrigation. If a draining fistula is present, the bone will be soft and can be removed with a rongeur or bone curette *(F)*. If difficulty is encountered in reaching the apex, a surgical length cross-cut fissure or tapered-fissure bur may help. The buccal bone plate is often very thin. A light touch and paintbrush feather-light strokes with the cutting bur are recommended.

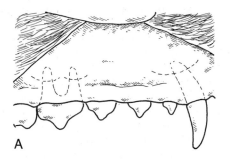

A

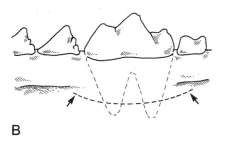

B

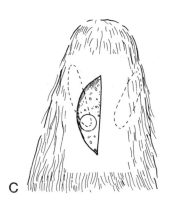

C

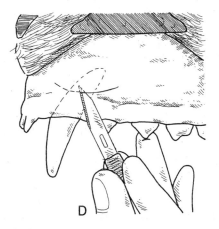

D

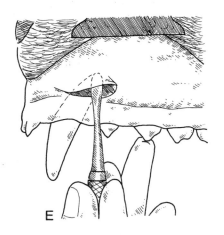

E

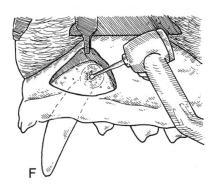

F

Step 6—The necrotic tissue in the apical area is curetted away from the bone with a surgical excavator or sharp curette *(A)*.

Step 7—The apex is resected at a 45 degree angle to the long axis of the tooth with a no. 701L tapered-fissure or no. 331L bur in a high-speed handpiece with sterile saline irrigation *(B)*. Necrotic apical material is removed so that solid hard root material is seen at the cut surface. More than 4 mm of root tip may need to be removed. This creates an oval opening of the pulp canal and exposes the canal filling material. The apex should always be removed because the terminal portion of a normal canine or feline root canal usually develops apically into the apical delta, where multiple fine vascular and neural elements enter and exit.

Step 8—The surgical site is flushed liberally with sterile saline to remove debris.

Step 9—Hemorrhaging is controlled by packing the area around the apex with sterile cotton pellets soaked in a hemostatic agent or by using bone wax, and visualization is enhanced by using suction equipment.

Step 10—The opening into the canal is undercut with a no. 33½ or no. 34 inverted cone bur to make adequate retention for the filling *(C)*. This preparation should extend 2 to 3 mm into the canal.

Step 11—The periapical area is flushed, dried, and repacked with cotton pellets or bone wax to keep the area dry and to allow entrapment of amalgam particles *(D)*. The cotton pellets or bone wax are removed before closure. Pellets should be counted before insertion and after removal.

- Many filling materials have been proposed to seal the apex. Amalgam has been used for years,[22-24] and zinc-free amalgam has been recommended because of the moist environment in which the restorative material is placed. Most recently, IRM2 or Super EBA Cement has been recommended.[25]

Step 12—If amalgam is used, the amalgam is mixed in an amalgamator, placed in the opening with the retrograde amalgam carrier *(E)*, and condensed in place with a small plugger. If IRM2 or Super EBA Cement is used, it is mixed and placed into the opening with a Centrix syringe.*

Step 13—The filling material is carved smooth with a carver and allowed to set.

Step 14—The hemostatic packing is removed, and the area is flushed with sterile saline or 0.2% chlorhexidine.

Step 15—The gingival flap is closed with interrupted sutures, using 3-0 or 4-0 absorbable suture material *(F)*.

Step 16—A postoperative radiograph is taken to verify the seal.

Postoperative Care

- Oral antibiotics for a minimum of 1 week; in some cases, 1 to 2 months.
- Follow-up radiographs at 6 months.
- Softened food and no hard treats or chew toys for 2 weeks to avoid tearing out sutures.

Complications

- Drilling into nasal cavity around maxillary canine. (This will generally heal with the closure of the flap.)
- Injury to infraorbital nerve during access to mesial root of upper carnassial tooth.
- Dislodging of retrograde filling due to inadequate preparation, placement, condensation, or finishing.
- Infection.

---

*Centrix, Inc., 770 River Rd., Shelton, CT 06484

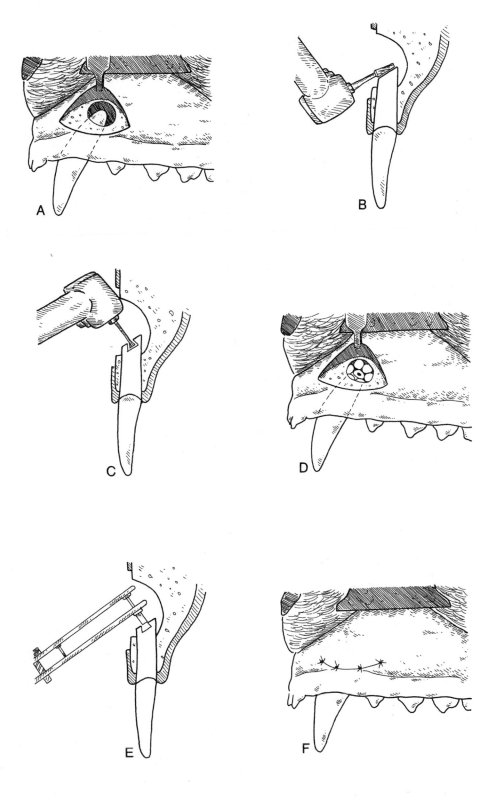

Table 7–2 • **PERIODONTAL/ENDODONTIC RELATIONSHIPS**

Condition	Signs	Treatment
Primary endodontic	Fistula Drainage into mucosa Normal crestal bone	Standard root canal therapy
Primary endodontics with secondary periodontal disease	Lysis of periodontal ligament Pocket formation J-shaped radiographic lesion	Standard root canal therapy Periodontal therapy
Primary periodontal	Lost crestal bone Normal apical region	Periodontal therapy
Primary periodontal with secondary endodontic disease	Mobility Loss of crestal bone Apical lysis Increased periodontal ligament loss	Periodontal flap Endodontic therapy
Combined endodontic and periodontal disease	Facial swelling Lateral swelling adjacent to apex	Endodontic treatment followed by periodontal treatment Poor prognosis

PERIODONTAL-ENDODONTIC RELATIONSHIPS

Comments

- The practitioner must consider the overall relationship and involvement of the periodontal and endodontic systems. Disease can originate inside the canal and spread to the periodontal tissues; conversely, disease can arise in periodontal structures and result in disease of the pulp.
- Table 7–2 may be helpful in defining the condition, signs, and treatment.

REFERENCES

1. Emily P, Tholen MA. Endodontic Therapy. In: Bojrab MJ, Tholen MA, eds. Small Animal Oral Medicine and Surgery. Philadelphia: Lea & Febiger, 1990:158–193.
2. Ross DL. The Oral Cavity. In: Kirk RW, ed. Current Veterinary Therapy VI. Philadelphia: W.B. Saunders Co., 1977:921–923.
3. Wiggs RB. Standard Endodontics. Las Vegas: Veterinary Dentistry, 1990:51.
4. Messing J, Stock C. Color Atlas of Endodontics. St. Louis: C.V. Mosby Co., 1988:170, 176.
5. Grossman LI, et al. Endodontic Practice, 11th ed. Philadelphia: Lea & Febiger, 1988.
6. Cohen S, Burns RC. Pathways of the Pulp, 5th ed. St. Louis: C.V. Mosby Co., 1994:643.
7. Heitmann T, Unterbrink G. Direct pulp capping with a dentinal adhesive resin system: A pilot study. Quintessence International 1995; 26:765–770.
8. Rubin LD, Maplesden DC, Singer RR. Root canal therapy in dogs. Vet Med Small Animal Clinician 1978; 73:593–589.
9. Ridgeway RL, Zielke DR. Nonsurgical endodontic technique for dogs. J Am Vet Med Assoc 1979; 174:82–85.
10. Goldstein GS, Anthony J. Basic Veterinary Endodontics. Compend Contin Educ 1990; 12:207–217.
11. Wilson GJ. Implications to the time of apical closure in relation to tooth fracture in dogs. Aust Vet Practitioner 1996; 26:65–75.
12. Visser CJ. The use of bleach and hydrogen peroxide in endodontics irrigation. J Vet Dent 1988; 5:3–4.
13. Products PD. Premier RC-Prep Instructions for Use. Norristown, PA: Premier.
14. West JD, Roane JB, Goering AC. Cleaning and shaping the root canal systems. In: Cohen S, Burns RC, eds. Pathways to the Pulp, 6th ed. Philadelphia: Mosby, 1994:179–219.
15. Grossman LI, Olivet S, Del Rio CE. Preparation of the root canal. In: Endodontic Practice, 11th ed. Philadelphia: Lea & Febiger, 1988:179–228.
16. Anthony JMG. Endodontic Filling Techniques. New Orleans: Veterinary Dentistry 1989:29.
17. Fahrenkrug P. Crowns: Indication, Preparation, Proceedings. New Orleans: Nabisco, 1988.
18. Eisner E. 353 Sequential Endodontic Cases: A Retrospective Study of Dogs and Cats in Veterinary Practice. New Orleans: Nabisco, 1989:33–37.
19. Eisner E. Transcoronal approach to the palatal root of the maxillary fourth premolar in the dog. J Vet Dent 1990;7.
20. Eisner ER. Performing surgical root canal therapy in dogs and cats. Vet Med 1995; 90:648–661.
21. Ross DL, Myers JW. Endodontic therapy for canine teeth in the dog. J Am Vet Med Assoc 1970; 157:1713–1718.
22. Wiggs RB, Lobprise HB. Veterinary Dentistry Principles and Practice. Philadelphia: Lippincott-Raven, 1997.
23. Taylor RA, Raymond P. Endodontia in the dog. Vet Med Small Animal Clinician 1972; 67:1197–1200.
24. Lawer DR. Root canal with retrograde amalgam filling. Cal Vet 1979; Mar:11–15.
25. Emily P. Surgical Endodontics. Las Vegas: unpublished, 1990.

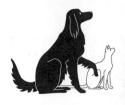

Chapter 8

RESTORATIVE DENTISTRY

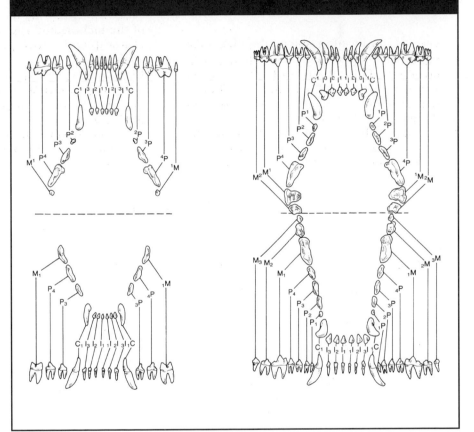

GENERAL COMMENTS

• Teeth are restored in an attempt to return the tooth to normal function and to normal appearance. In veterinary dentistry, this service is most commonly needed after endodontic therapy has been performed.

CLASSIFICATION OF LESIONS

• Various classification systems have been designed to communicate the extent of a dental lesion. One of the early classification systems was developed by G.V. Black. Black's system classifies cavities based on the location of the lesion.
• "Cavities," here, refers to defects in the tooth surface from any cause (such as a carious lesion, fracture, or abrasion).

Classification by Location of Lesion

• Class 1—Cavities beginning in structural defects in a tooth's pits and fissures (occlusal surface) *(A)*.
• Class 2—Cavities in the proximal surfaces of premolars and molars *(B)*.
• Class 3—Cavities in the proximal surfaces of the incisors and canines that do not involve damage to and restoration of the incisal angle *(C)*.
• Class 4—Cavities in the proximal surfaces of the incisors and canines that involve the removal and restoration of the incisal angle *(D)*.
• Class 5—Cavities that are not pit cavities in the gingival third of the crown of the labial, buccal, palatal, or lingual surfaces of the teeth *(E)*.
• Class 6—Defects on the incisal edges of anterior teeth or the cusp tips of posterior teeth *(F)*.

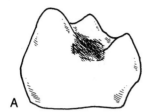

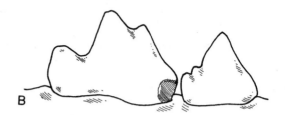

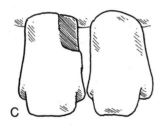

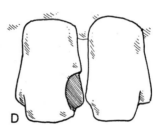

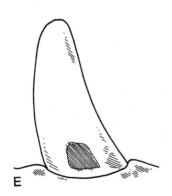

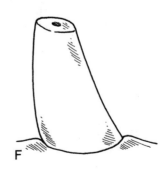

Classification by Extent of Fracture

- Although Black's system classifies cavities by location, the system does not classify the extent of the lesion. Basrani developed a classification system that accomplishes this goal.[1] This system is amenable to discussing treatment plans as well.

Class A1 Crown Fractures—Enamel

Description

- Fractures that involve chips of enamel only (A).

Treatment

- In the dog, observe radiographically every 6 months to 1 year; at the next periodic dental care appointment, smooth the damaged enamel margins to prevent enamel stripping. If injury is acute, a pit and fissure sealant or a fluoride containing varnish is appropriate to prevent progressive disease. Root canal therapy is indicated if there is any sign of pulpal death.
- In the cat, root canal therapy is recommended; most chip fractures are caused by enough trauma to these small teeth that trauma will lead to pulpal death and apical abscess formation.
- If on the cusp, crown therapy may prevent further damage.

Class A2a Crown Fractures— Enamel and Dentin

Description

- Fractures that have penetrated the enamel and include the dentin but have not exposed the pulp (B).

Treatment

Dog
- If enough dentin remains, indirect pulp capping and restoration with a glass ionomer, composite resin, or crown therapy.
- If very close to the pulp, direct pulp capping or root canal therapy followed by glass ionomer, composite resin, or crown therapy.

Cat
- Root canal therapy followed by glass ionomer, composite resin, or crown therapy.

Class A2b Crown Fractures— Enamel and Dentin

Description

- Fractures that involve enamel and dentin and have invaded the pulp.

Treatment

Young Animal (Younger than 1½ Years) (C)
- Vital pulpotomy, followed by glass ionomer, (composite resin), or crown restoration if the fracture is less than 2 weeks old.
- Extraction or root canal therapy and reinforced crown techniques if the fracture is open longer than 2 weeks (prognosis guarded; see Chapter 7, Endodontics, p. 260).

Older Animal (Older than 1½ Years) (D)
- Vital pulpotomy, if pulp exposed less than 48 hours.
- Root canal therapy followed by glass ionomer, composite resin, or crown restoration if pulp exposed longer than 48 hours.

Class B Crown Fractures— Root Fractures

Description

- Fractures involving the roots of teeth (E).

Treatment

- If the fracture is in the coronal third of the root, endodontic therapy followed by a post in the endodontic system of both pieces of the tooth may be attempted (prognosis guarded).
- If the fracture is in the middle third of the root, extraction is the best option in most cases.
- If the fracture is in the apical third of the root, a surgical root canal and extraction of the apical fragment can be performed.

Class C Crown-Root Fractures

Description

- Fractures involving the crown and root (F).

Treatment

- Most of the time, extraction is the best alternative.
- Root canal therapy followed by bonding of the split root may be attempted.

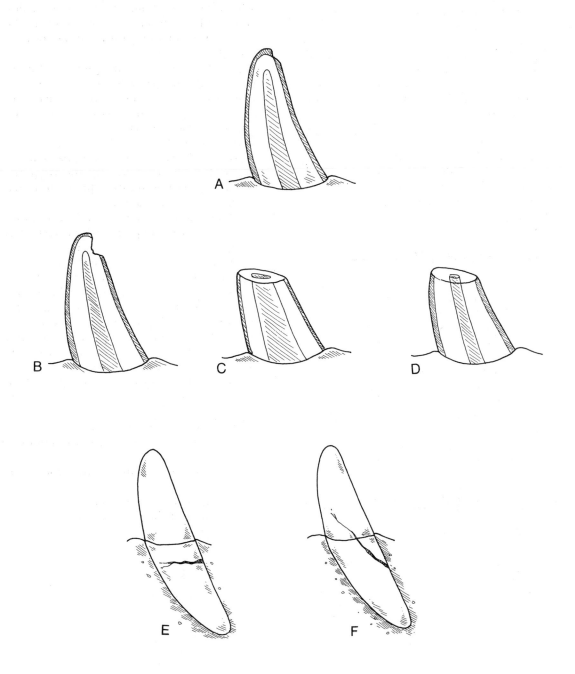

RESTORATIVE TECHNIQUES: GENERAL

Cutting Techniques

- Cut away from the enamel; i.e., when doing a crown preparation, cut with the bur approximately parallel to the long axis of the tooth; in a counterclockwise rotation around the circumference of the tooth (the bur is rotating clockwise) *(figure)*.
- When drilling into teeth, an intermittent pressure is applied. The period is two counts with pressure on to one count with pressure off to limit heat generation and maintain bur speed.
- The operator should be aware of the change in audible pitch in the handpiece as an indication of pressure placed on the tooth. A higher pitch indicates a higher speed, which is desirable.

Cavity Preparation Techniques

- The outline of the preparation is made using a round bur or a tapered-fissure bur to a depth of at least 1.5 mm.
- Macroretention is created using an inverted cone or pear-shaped bur.
- Additional retention can be created by making retention grooves in the base of cavity walls (intersection of wall and floors) with a round bur of appropriate size.
- The walls and floors may be smoothed with chisels or hatchets.
- Any carious dentin or poorly supported tooth structure should be removed.

RESTORATIVE MATERIALS

General Comments

- Many types of dental materials have evolved.

- The ideal material for restorative work would form a chemical bond to the enamel and dentin, would not distort after placement, would not break or fatigue, would have a high-impact strength, would have the same coefficient of expansion as dental structures, would match the tooth color, and would wear at the same rate as the teeth. Unfortunately, this material does not yet exist.[2]
- Given the different functions of different teeth and the areas to be restored, obtaining the best results from the materials available requires familiarity with the properties of each material.
- Restorative materials to be used should be picked according to the conditions to be restored so as to maximize the desirable properties and minimize the undesirable properties of the material.
- The restorative materials and techniques discussed in this chapter can be classified as plastics (restorative resins), glass ionomers, amalgams, and crown restoratives.
- It is important to store restorative materials correctly. An improper storage environment can rapidly destroy the material. The first thing one should do when receiving a material is to note the expiration date and read the package insert, paying particular attention to use and storage.
- Simplified, restorative dentistry can be broken down into five steps:

  1. Preparation of the surface.
  2. Placement and curing of the bonding agent.
  3. Placement and curing of the restorative agent.
  4. Shaping of the restoration.
  5. Smoothing of the restoration.

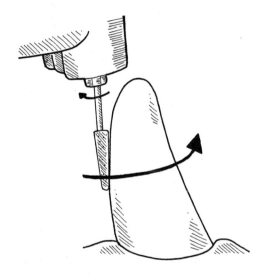

Plastics

General Comments

- As in many industries, dentistry has been dramatically changed by the development of synthetic plastics.
- Dental plastics are polymers created by a series of chemical reactions combining large numbers of similar smaller molecules (monomers) into a compound of high molecular weight.[3]
- Throughout the "life" of the material, polymerization continues. It is a continuous reaction that is never entirely complete.
- The polymerization reaction is activated either chemically or by light.
- Chemical-cure plastics usually come in two parts that, after mixing, cause molecules to join and the material to harden.
- Acrylic (composite) resins can be generally classified as filled or unfilled.
- Unfilled resins do not have fillers; they flow readily, are translucent, and are used to coat "cavity" preparations before application of the filled resins.
- The unfilled resins are applied to prevent microleakage and to promote the attachment of the restorative material to the tooth.
- Applying an unfilled resin to an acid-etched surface creates effective microprojections and therefore microretention of resin into the tooth's crystalline structure.
- The filled resins contain fillers and are more viscous, opaque, harder, and have better wearability than unfilled resins.
- The filled resin is bonded onto the unfilled resin.
- Fillers added to the filled resins give them hardness, strength, color, resistance to temperature change, wearability, and control of polymerization shrinkage.[4]
- Composite resins contain at least 60% (usually 70 to 80%) inorganic filler (quartz, lithium, or silica) by weight.
- The filler particles are described according to size: conventional (20 to 35 μm), intermediate or macrofilled (1 to 5 μm), microfilled (equal to or less than 0.04 μm), and hybrid (containing either a conventional or intermediate particle in addition to a microfilled particle).[4]
- The conventional and macrofilled compounds are more resistant to fracture and can be safely exposed to more abrasive and concussive "wear and tear" than can microfilled restoratives.
- Two disadvantages of the macrofilled compounds are a decreased ability to be finely polished because of larger particle size and becoming pitted with wear.
- Microfilled compounds polish to a very smooth surface; however, their disadvantage is that they tend to fracture more easily. They are best used in areas with less exposure to wear.
- In an attempt to reach a compromise between the microfilled and macrofilled qualities, hybrid compounds were developed to combine smoothness with durability.
- Both filled and unfilled resins cure by either chemical reaction or light exposure.
- Some products require use of a "bonding agent" before application of the unfilled resin so as to improve bonding to the tooth structure. Many types of systems are used for bonding agents, and the practitioner should refer to the instructions on the restorative kit for specific instructions.
- Care should be used with unfilled resins or bonding agents to apply only a thin film to the tooth.

Indications

- Restoration of a damaged tooth crown.
- Restoration of access holes after endodontic therapy.
- Bonding wires used for fracture repair and splinting teeth.

Contraindication

- Patients who chew rocks, bones, etc. Their surface defects should be restored with a stronger material.

Materials

- Flour pumice.
- Prophy cup.
- Dental handpieces.
- Mixing pad.
- Mixing spatula.
- Centrix syringe.
- Brushes/sponges.
- Acid-etch materials.
- Bonding agent.
- Composite resin restorative material.
- Plastic working instrument.
- Light-curing gun (light cure).
- Smoothing/polishing materials.

Technique

- Although many different applications and variations of chemical and light-cure restorations exist, the following example is a step-by-step method for placement using a two-rooted tooth that has undergone endodontic therapy.

Step 1—Preparation of the Surface

- Preparation of the surface is identical in chemical-cure and light-cure restorations.

Substep 1—Prepare the filling site, considering the following:

- All unsupported enamel should be removed using a handpiece and bur, chisel, or sharp curette *(A) (B)*.
- Margins should be made at sites least susceptible to caries.
- The preparation may include deep grooves on the side or base for retention.
- The border of the preparation should not terminate on cusps.[5]

Substep 2—Clean the surface using a prophy cup and flour pumice (not prophy paste, which may contain fluoride and glycerin) *(C)*.

Substep 3—Wash the surface with water and air-dry *(D)*.

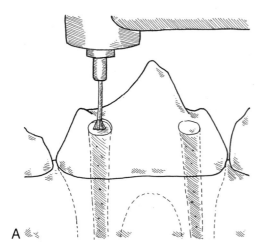

A

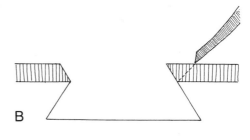

B

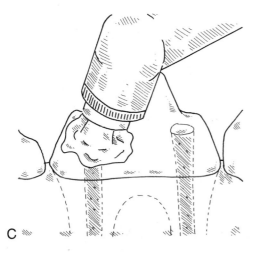

C

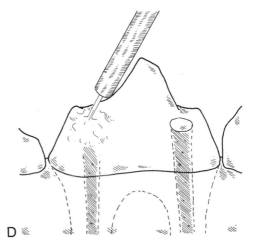

D

Substep 4—Acid-etch the enamel with 38 to 50% phosphoric acid gel for 30 to 60 seconds, according to manufacturer's instructions. Either a sponge *(A)* or a brush *(B)* may be used.

- Some authorities promote a "total etch" technique in which both the enamel and dentin are etched to improve bonding.
- On nonvital teeth, the dentin can be etched along with the enamel, using the phosphoric acid gel.
- On vital teeth, a dentin conditioner, which is a lesser concentration of etching gel (acid), can be used to etch the dentin for 10 to 15 seconds only.

Substep 5—Wash the surface with water for at least 20 seconds *(C)*.

Substep 6—Dry the surface by air-drying *(D)*.

- The area to be restored should have a chalky white appearance; if it does not, the surface should be re-etched.
- It is important to keep the surface free from chemicals, saliva, blood, and other contaminants that interfere with bonding.
- Contamination is the most common reason for restorative failure.
- If contamination occurs, the surface should be re-prepared, although a shorter etching time may be used.

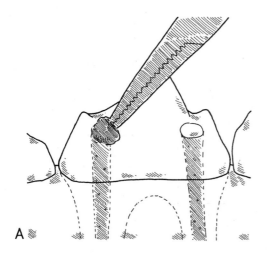

A

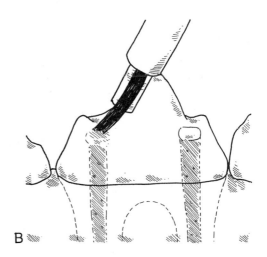

B

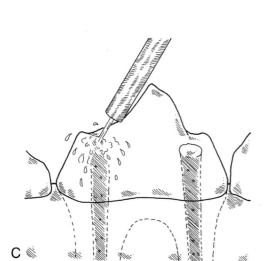

C

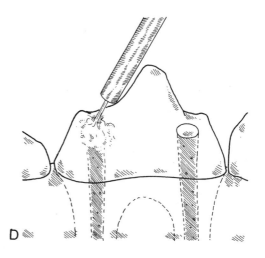

D

Step 2—Application of the Bonding Agent: Chemical Cure (Light-Cure Gun Not Available)

- The following procedure is for applying a chemical-cured bonding agent followed by applying a chemical-cured restorative resin.
- These steps vary with the manufacturer (Table 8–1). Some first apply a chemical to enhance bonding of the unfilled resin; others mix chemicals and the unfilled resin.

Substep 1—Bonding agent solution A is dropped into a dappen dish *(A).*

Substep 2—Bonding agent solution B is dropped into the same dappen dish *(B).* (Exact proportions of the two solutions are used according to the manufacturer's recommendations.) The solutions are mixed with a brush *(C).*

Substep 3—A thin coat of bonding agent is applied to the prepared surface *(D).*

Substep 4—A gentle stream of air is blown over the surface to minimize the thickness and eliminate pooling of the bonding agent.

Substep 5—The unfilled resin is placed onto a brush *(E)* and is brushed onto the tooth *(F).*

Substep 6—A gentle stream of air is directed onto the unfilled resin-covered tooth surface to thin the layer of resin and to eliminate pooling.

Table 8–1 • BONDING AGENTS

Chemical-Cured Bonding Agents	
Product	*Manufacturer*
Bonding Agent	Johnson & Johnson
Bonding Agent Self	L. D. Caulk
Cure	Schein
Etch-Prep	
Dentin Bonding Agents	
Product	*Manufacturer*
Bondlite	Kerr
Clearfil New Bond	J. Morita
Gluma	Columbus
Mirage-Bond	Chameleon
Scotchbond II	3M
Vitrebond	3M
Tenue	Den-Mat
XR Bonding System	Kerr
Dentin Conditioning Gel	Pulpdent
Confi-Bond	Confidential Products
Dentin-Protector	Vivadent
Syntac	Vivadent
Dual-Cure Bonding Agents	
Product	*Manufacturer*
Scotchbond Dual Cure	3M
Imperva Bond System	Shofu

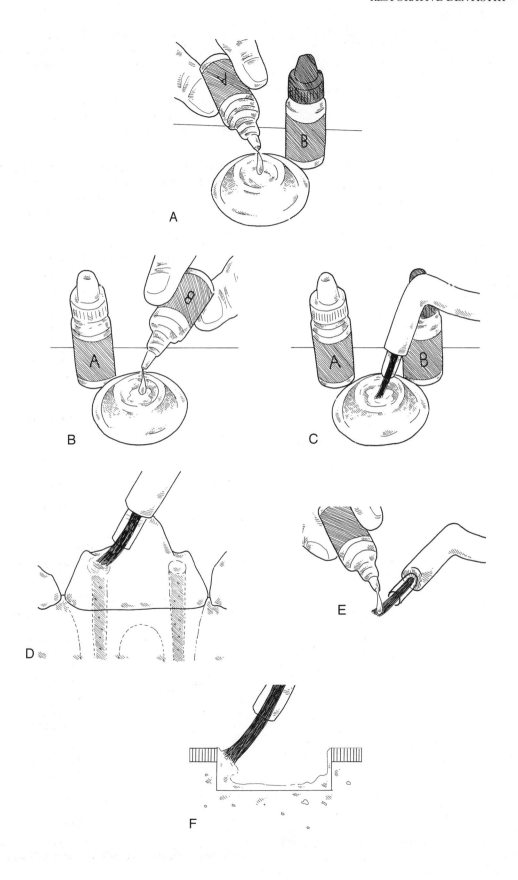

Table 8–2 • CHEMICAL-CURED COMPOSITE RESINS

Conventional Fillers

Product	Manufacturer
Concise	3M
Adaptic	Johnson & Johnson
Profile	S. S. White
Simulate	Kerr
Compolite	Darby
Profile	Mission Dental
Silar	3M
Crystalline C2	Confidential Products

Intermediate or Macrofilled Fillers

Product	Manufacturer
P10	3M
Cervident	S. S. White
Power Lite	S. S. White
Extra Smooth	Den-Mat
Ultra Bond	Den-Mat
Marathon	Den-Mat
Class II	Den-Mat

Microfilled Fillers

Product	Manufacturer
Finesse	L. D. Caulk
Silar	3M
Isocap	Viadent
Isopast	Viadent

Hybrid Fillers

Product	Manufacturer
Miradapt	Johnson & Johnson

Step 3—Application of the Restorative Agent: Chemical Cure (Light-Cure Gun Not Available)

- The chemical-cured, filled resin (Table 8–2) is mixed as directed by the manufacturer.

Substep 1—Equal portions of the filled resin are placed on a slab (A).

Substep 2—The restorative material is spatulated in a figure-of-eight spatulation method.

- The mixing should be thorough and take 15 to 20 seconds.

Substep 3—The mixed resin is transferred to the site with a plastic filling instrument (B).

- The material may also be transferred to the site using an injection syringe.*
- The injection syringe is loaded by scooping the material into the plastic tip from either the spatula or the glass slab (C).

---

*Centrix II Syringe, Centrix, Inc., 770 River Rd., Shelton, CT 06484

- The rubber plunger is placed into the plastic tip on top of the restorative material (D).
- The material is injected into the restoration site (E).

Substep 4 (optional)—A Mylar strip is placed over the site to conform the material to the tooth shape (F).

Table 8–3 • LIGHT-CURED RESTORATIVES

Conventional Fillers

Product	Manufacturer
Commend	Kerr
Nuva Fil PA	L. D. Caulk

Intermediate or Macrofilled Fillers

Product	Manufacturer
Aurafil	Johnson & Johnson
Command	Kerr
Estilux	Kulzer
Extra Smooth	Den-Mat
Ful-Fil	L. D. Caulk
Ultra Bond	Den-Mat
Prisma Fil	L. D. Caulk
P30	3M
Visio Fil	ESPE/Premier

Microfilled Fillers

Product	Manufacturer
Adaptic LCM	3M
Durafil VS	Kulzer
Heliosit	Vivadent
Heliomolar	Vivadent
Helioprogress	Vivadent
Opalux	Coe
Pekalux	Columbus
Prisma Microfine	L. D. Caulk
Silux	3M

Microhybrid Fillers

Product	Manufacturer
XRV Herculite	Kerr

Hybrid Fillers

Product	Manufacturer
Adaptic II	Johnson & Johnson
APH (All Purpose Hybrid)	L. D. Caulk
Prisma TPH	L. D. Caulk
Bis Fil P	Bisco
Bis Fil M	Bisco
Command Ultrafine	Kerr
Herculite XR	Kerr
Lumifor	Columbus
Mirage	Chameleon
P50	3M
Perfection	Den-Mat
Prisma APH	L. D. Caulk
Profile TLC	S. S. White
Occlusin	Coe
Silux Plus	3M
Ultra Bond	Den-Mat
Visarfil	Den-Mat
Z-100	3M
Crystalline L3	Confidential Products

Step 2—Application of the Bonding Agent: Light Cure (Light-Cure Gun Available)

- The following procedure is for applying a light-cure bonding agent followed by applying a light-cure restorative resin.

  Substep 1—The dentin primer is applied with a brush to the prepared surface.

  Substep 2—The dentin primer is air-dried for 5 seconds or pat-dried with a cotton pellet or paper point.

- The manufacturer's directions should be followed. In most cases complete desiccation of dental tissues should be avoided.

  Substep 3—A thin coat of bonding agent (type 1 resin) is applied to the prepared surface.

Substep 4—The bonding agent is light-cured.

Step 3—Application of the Restorative Agent (Light-Cure Gun Available)

General Comments

- Some light-cure products require mixing (substeps 1 and 2); others may be used directly without mixing (Table 8–3). Generally, light-cure products come either in a syringe or in a preloaded syringe tip.
- Dual-cure materials cure by both light and chemical reactions.
- The unfilled resin may also need light curing before application of the filled resin.
- An advantage of light-cured restoratives is the increased time for shaping the filled resin before hardening it with the light gun.

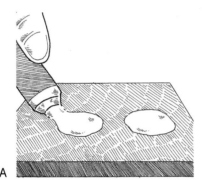

A

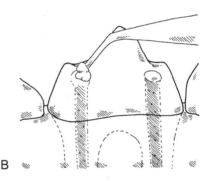

B

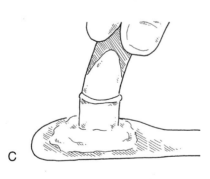

C

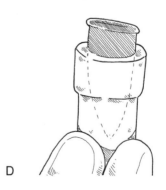

D

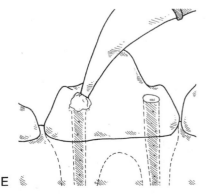

E

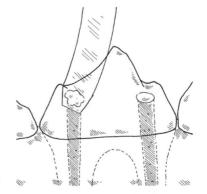

F

Light-Cure Technique

Substep 1—The filled resin is dispensed from the syringe onto a plastic working instrument (A).

Substep 2—The resin is applied to the prepared surface (B).

Substep 3—The restorative material is shaped with a plastic working instrument.

- A small amount of unfilled resin on a plastic filling instrument can be used to help shape the filled resin and prevent sticking.

Substep 4 (optional)—For some sites, a Mylar strip can be drawn taut over the site to conform the material more densely and more exactly to the tooth shape.

Substep 5—The filled resin is hardened with a light-cure gun (C). Cure the restorative material for 60 to 90 seconds according to the manufacturer's instructions. Time will vary depending on the darkness of the shade, the thickness depth of the restoration, the product used, and the strength of the cure light. The thickness of restorative material should be no more than 3 to 4 mm at a time without curing. The deeper the fill, the longer the cure time required.

Dual-Cure Technique

Substep 1—Equal portions of the filled resin are placed on a slab.

Substep 2—The restorative material is spatulated to a homogeneous consistency.

Substep 3—The mixed resin is transferred to the site with a plastic filling instrument or injection syringe.

Substep 4—The restorative material is shaped with a plastic working instrument.

Substep 5 (optional)—A Mylar strip is pulled tightly over the filling material.

Substep 6—The restorative material is cured.

- Additional layers of restorative material can be placed on top of the cured material and, in turn, cured to provide thicker restorations.

Complications/Cautions

- It is important when using light-curing units to use appropriate protective glasses or shields.
- Light-activation techniques require that light emission be close to the restoration (less than 1 mm).
- To ensure a full cure, cure the filled resin for a minimum of 60 seconds.

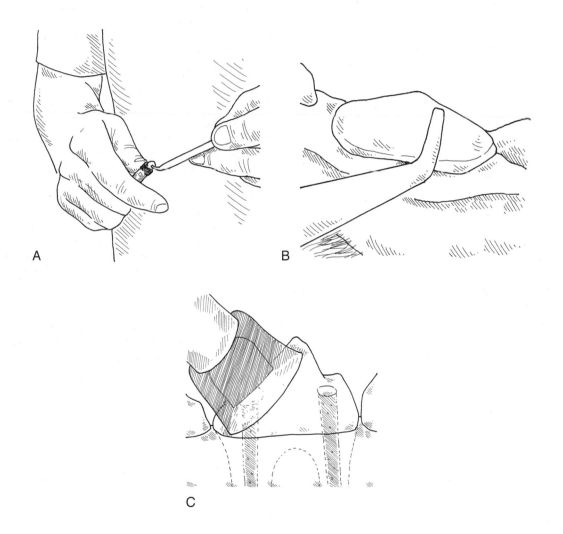

Step 4—Shaping the Hardened Restoration

- The material is shaped with finishing diamond burs, 12-blade carbide finishing burs, or fine particle stones (see pp. 46 to 47).

Step 5—Smoothing the Restoration

- The restoration is smoothed with abrasive discs, strips, or fine-particle stones.

Abrasive Discs

Description
- Plastic or stiff-paper circular discs are attached to a mandrel and driven by a contra-angle and low-speed handpiece.
- Paste lubricants/polishing agents are available to aid in smoothing.

Advantages
- Supplied in various grits and materials.
- Quick reduction of tooth surface.
- Inexpensive.

Disadvantage
- Being circular, the discs may not fit into all contours of the restorative surface.

Finishing Strips

Description
- Thin plastic sanding strips.

Advantage
- Useful in conical-shaped teeth, such as canine teeth, to smooth the surface rapidly.

Disadvantage
- Do not fit into all spaces.

Nonadhesive Strips

Description
- Do not contain adhesive to hold particles. This decreases the number of particles that break free and re-adhere to the strip, becoming captured particles.
- Captured particles have the potential to damage the surface being finished by leaving deep grooves.
- Thin, flexible strips to smooth down the tooth surface.

Advantages
- Easy interproximal access.
- Readily contour to the shape of the tooth.

Complications
- Microleakage is recognized by a black line between the restorative material and the tooth occurring some time after restoration.
- In the case of vital teeth, sensitivity can result from microleakage.
- The three main factors that cause microleakage are (1) poor technique; (2) shrinkage of the restorative material occurring with polymerization; and (3) inability of the resin to bond chemically to the tooth structure.
- Acid-etching may cause dentinal sensitivity in vital teeth. Etching dentin, when performed, should be done with the milder acids called dentin conditioners.

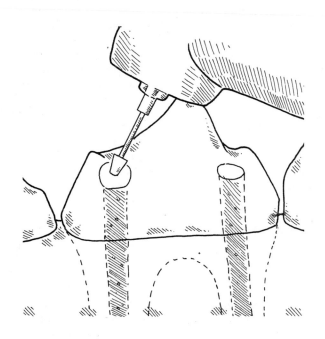

Product Options

Repair of Defective Composite Resin Restorations[6]

General Comments
- The trauma of use may cause defects in the composite resin restoration.
- The overall strength of the repair may not be as strong as the original restoration.

Indication
- Fractured composite resin restoration.

Contraindication
- Fracture of tooth that may require more than conservative restoration.

Materials
- Same as with composite restoration.

Technique
Step 1—The restoration is probed to discover any defects that may not have been visualized.

Step 2—A water-cooled, inverted-cone carbide bur is used to remove defective resin. A slight undercut may aid retention.

Step 3—A coarse diamond bur is used to roughen the entire surface of the remainder of the restoration to eliminate superficial resin that has been exposed to the oral environment.

Step 4—A phosphoric acid gel is spread over the entire preparation for 30 seconds, rinsed with water for 30 seconds, and air-dried.

Step 5—An unfilled resin is applied over the surface and blown gently with compressed air to a thin layer. (The unfilled resin is light-cured, if required.)

Step 6—The filled resin is mixed, placed into an injection syringe, and injected uniformly into the restorative site.

Step 7—The resin is allowed to cure. If using a light-cure restorative material, the curing light is held from the side in an attempt to cure from the restorative margins first.

Step 8—The surface is recontoured and smoothed as described on page 336.

Glass Ionomers
General Comments
- Glass ionomers are sold in kits that may contain powder (in various shades), liquid, measuring scoops, varnish, etching agent, and mixing pads.
- The powder is an aluminosilicate glass.
- The anhydrous form contains acid in the powder.
- The hydrous form contains acid in the liquid.
- When the powder and liquid are mixed together, chemical reactions bond the restoration to tooth structure and harden the compound.
- Light-cure and dual-cure glass ionomer restorative materials are available.
- Glass ionomers can be classified as type I (luting) cement or type II (lining, restorative, or core) (Table 8–4).
- Type I glass ionomers are finely grained and are used for cementing (luting) crowns, bridges, and other castings.
- Type II glass ionomers are used as restorative materials.
- Type II glass ionomers are coarser than type I and therefore are not suitable for cementing.
- Restorative glass ionomers can be used as a base or as the sole restorative.
- Glass ionomers are biocompatible and do not require placement of obtunding base material to protect the pulp, except in case of direct pulp exposure.
- Nonencapsulated forms are mixed with a spatula and pad.
- The encapsulated form requires a special instrument to break the internal separation between the liquid and powder, an amalgamator to mix the compound, and a special syringe to apply the mixture.
- A consideration with glass ionomer compounds is their lack of wearability. In an attempt to increase wearability, some manufacturers have added metals to the mixture. Most commonly, silver is added; gold, copper, and zinc have been suggested as possible alternatives.
- On mixing nonencapsulated forms, the material is either transferred to an injection

Table 8–4 • GLASS IONOMER RESTORATIVE MATERIALS

Type I: Luting or Cementing

Chemical-Cure

Product	Manufacturer
Glassic	Stratford Cookson
Glasslute	Pulpdent
Dentin Cement	G. C. America
Fuji I	G. C. America
Fuji Lining LC	G. C. America
Ketac Cem	ESPE/Premier
Shofu Type I	Shofu

Light-Cure

Product	Manufacturer
Vitrabond	3M
Zionomer	Den-Mat

Type II: Core

Product	Manufacturer
Glasscore	Pulpdent
Ketac Silver	ESPE/Premier
Miracle Mix	G. C. America
Shofu Base Cement	Shofu
Zionomer Core	Den-Mat

Type II: Glass Ionomers—Lining Ionomers

Product	Manufacturer
G. C. Lining Cement	G. C. America
Gingiva Seal	Parkell
Glassline	Pulpdent
Ketac Bond	ESPE/Premier
Ketac Bond Aplicap	ESPE/Premier
Shofu Lining	Shofu
Shofu Base	Shofu
3M Ionomer	3M
Zionomer Lining	Den-Mat

Type II: Glass Ionomers—Restorative

Product	Manufacturer
Chemfil II	Dentsply DeTrey
Fuji Cap	G. C. America
Fuji Type II	G. C. America
Fuji Type II LC	G. C. America
Ketac Fil	ESPE/Premier
Ketac-Fil Aplicap	ESPE/Premier
Ketac-Silver Maxicap	ESPE/Premier
Chelon-Fil	ESPE/Premier
Shofu Type II	Shofu
Vitremer	3M

syringe and squeezed into the prepared cavity or installed with a plastic placement instrument.

- Once hardened, the surface can be smoothed with a diamond finishing bur while being irrigated with copious amounts of water.
- The restoration should not be smoothed with a carbide bur.
- If water is not used, cocoa butter can be used as a lubricant.
- Without a lubricant, the material will overheat, desiccate, and weaken.
- Glass ionomer restorative materials have the advantage of forming a chemical bond as well as a mechanical bond to teeth.
- Glass ionomers release fluoride slowly.
- The expansion coefficient is the same as that of the tooth.

Indications

- Type I glass ionomers are used well for cementing (luting) crowns, onlays, and orthodontic appliances.
- Type II lining glass ionomers are used as a foundation upon which other materials, such as plastic resins, are applied.
- Core glass ionomers are used as a base or for building up material around a post to support a laboratory-manufactured crown.
- Type II can also be used as a sandwich, in combination with light-cure composites, to reduce the amount of light-cure restorative required and to decrease the potential for polymerization shrinkage.
- Type II glass ionomers are ideal for repairing cervical erosive lesions[7, 8] and for filling root canal access points on nonocclusal areas.

Contraindication

- Because these materials are less durable than other restoratives, glass ionomers are not recommended on high-wear surfaces.

Materials

- Small excavator/curet.
- Power equipment (air preferred).
- Glass or paper slab.
- Spatula.
- Centrix syringe or Jiffy tube.
- Glass ionomer.
- Placement instrument(s).

Technique for Restoration After Root Canal Therapy

Step 1—Preparation of the Surface

Substep 1—In most situations, cavity preparation will be the same as a standard preparation for composite resins *(A)*.

- In the treatment of nonocclusal, class V lesions, the creation of an undercut may not be necessary.

Substep 2—The surface is cleaned with flour pumice (without fluoride or glycerin) with a prophy cup.

- Etching/conditioning of nonvital dentin to remove the smear layer that forms during preparation is controversial. If a conditioner is supplied with the restorative kit, it should be used according to the manufacturer's instructions.

Substep 3—The cavity is dried with an air source or blotted dry with paper points.

Substep 4—The cavity preparation agent (usually a mild acid) is applied *(B)*.

Substep 5—After 15 seconds the cavity preparation agent is washed off with water *(C)*.

Substep 6—The area is dried.

- Unlike for composite resin techniques, it is important that the cavity not be "bone dry." Although there should be no pools of water in the preparation, the area should not have the chalky white appearance of a completely dried tooth.
- If overdried, the preparation should be rehydrated with water.
- Once the area has been prepared, it is important to prevent contamination. If contaminated, the area must be reprepared.

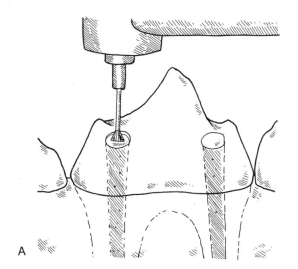

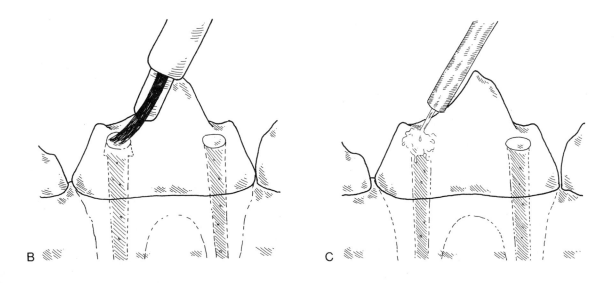

Step 2—Application of the Bonding Agent

- In this case, it is the glass ionomer applied in step 3.

Step 3—Application of the Glass Ionomer

- Glass ionomer restorative material is quickly mixed according to the manufacturer's instructions. Although the ratios may vary by manufacturer and the amounts by case, the following substeps apply.

Substep 1—The powder is "fluffed" (shaken) with the lid closed, and level scoops of the powder are measured and placed, preferably, on a heavy glass slab *(A)*.

Substep 2—The appropriate number of drops of liquid are dripped out; avoid air bubbles that may distort the measurement *(B)*.

Substep 3—The powder is divided in half, and one of the halves is divided into quarters *(C)*.

Substep 4—Half the powder is pulled into the liquid and is rapidly mixed *(D)*.

Substep 5—One quarter of the remaining powder is pulled into the liquid *(E)*, and the other quarter is mixed in *(F)*. A figure-of-eight motion is used to mix the glass ionomer *(G)*.

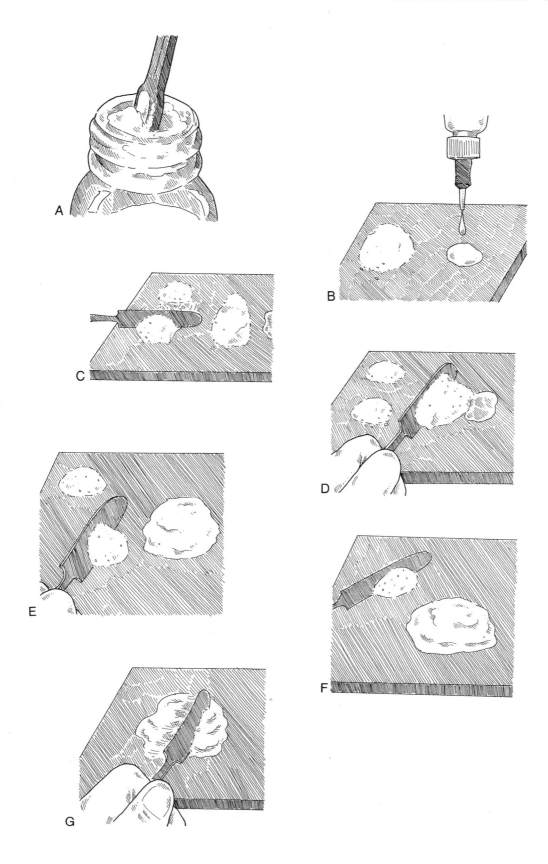

• Once the material is applied to the cavity, manipulation should be limited.

Substep 6—The mix may be loaded into the curved tip of a Centrix injection syringe *(A)*.

Substep 7—The tip is pushed down over the plug *(B)*. The tip and plug are loaded into the syringe.

Substep 8—The restorative material is injected uniformly into the defect to be filled *(C)*.

Step 4—Shaping the Restoration

Substep 1 (optional)—While the glass ionomer is setting, it is covered with a Mylar strip to prevent moisture contamination *(D)*. A condenser may be placed over the Mylar strip to conform the restorative material to the tooth structure *(E)*.

Substep 2—The overlapping edges of the material (flashing) are painted with a varnish *(F)*. If a Mylar strip is not used, the surface of the restorative material must be coated with a layer of varnish after it begins to harden.

• Alternatively, the liquid component of a light-cure resin can be painted on to protect the glass ionomer as it sets.

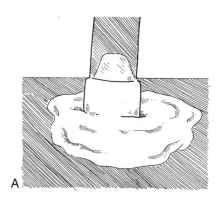

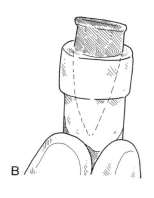

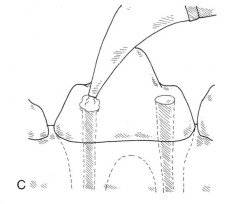

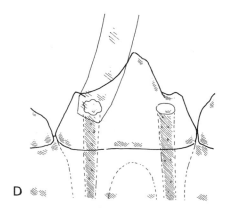

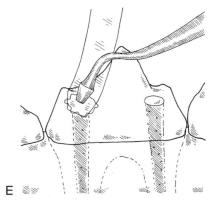

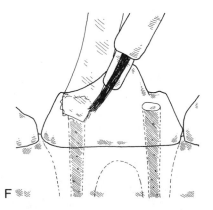

Step 5—Smoothing the Restoration

Substep 1—The restoration is carved with a fine diamond bur and coated with cocoa butter *(A)*.

Substep 2—The cocoa butter is wiped from the tooth *(B)*.

Substep 3—A coat of varnish or the liquid portion of a light-cure resin is applied as a final protective coat *(C)*.

Complications/Cautions

- The tooth conditioner may cause dentinal sensitivity, because it is a form of acid etch.
- It is important that the glass ionomer material be applied before the mixture loses its shiny appearance and thus its adherent quality. If this loss occurs, a new batch of material should be mixed.
- If the glass ionomer restoration crazes, cracks, or falls out, it is usually a problem of moisture *(D)*. Water contamination as well as overdrying can cause these problems.
- Many of the newer glass ionomer hybrids that are light-cure products contain resin, which protects them from the moisture problems of the pure glass ionomers. These may not be as technique-sensitive as the pure glass ionomer materials. They may not need cocoa butter or other protectants while shaping and smoothing.

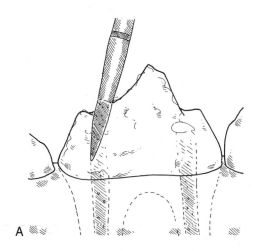

A

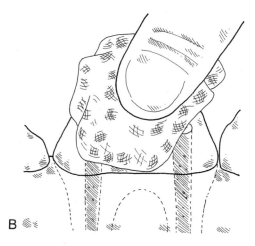

B

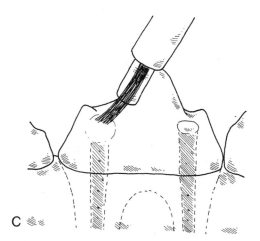

C

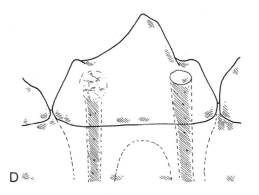

D

Feline Odontoclastic Resorptive (Cervical Line) Lesions

Etiology

- The pathogenesis of odontoclastic resorptive lesions on feline teeth is not fully understood.
- Research shows that these lesions tend to start at the gingival margin or subgingivally and progress apically and coronally.
- These lesions have been called cervical line lesion, odontoclastic resorption, neck lesion, feline neck lesion, feline caries, feline odontoclastic resorptive lesion, cavities (and "catvities").

Signs

- They are often covered with hyperplastic gingiva and are not detectable without using an explorer to probe for irregularities of the tooth surface.
- The patient usually shows signs of discomfort and pain when the lesions are probed.
- This discomfort is sometimes even evident under deep, plane II surgical anesthesia.
- The lesions may be found on any of the teeth, but molars and premolars are most frequently involved, followed by the canine teeth.
- The lesions may be covered with calculus, especially in the molar and premolar teeth, which protects them from pain.
- Lesions are found on the buccal and lingual or palatal surfaces.
- The lesions seem to be progressive, and many teeth in a patient may be affected and show different stages of destruction at any one time.
- In early stages, lesions can be so small that they are difficult to detect.
- As lesions progress, they enlarge, encompassing more and more of the root and crown.
- In advanced lesions, an overhang of enamel can be found, with the underlying dentin missing.
- Radiographs often show the affected teeth to be demineralized much more dramatically than appears on visual examination. These roots are often undergoing resorption and replacement with osteoid tissue.

Treatment Protocol

Technique for Restoration of Feline Odontoclastic Resorptive Lesions

Step 1—Before restoration is attempted, the tooth should be examined carefully to determine the amount of involvement *(A)*.

- A radiograph is a very important part of this evaluation.
- It is inappropriate service to restore a tooth whose roots are already being resorbed.
- The following classification system of feline resorptive lesions is in common usage.[9]

Stage 1—Abrasions or shallow cementum or enamel defects that do not enter the dentin.

Stage 2—Erosions that progress into the dentin through enamel or cementum.

Stage 3—Erosions that extend into the root canal.

Stage 4—Chronic resorptive lesions resulting in loss of tooth structure, complete root destructions, and ankylosis of roots.

- The following system can be used to plan treatment.

Stage 1—Thorough dental prophylaxis; fluoride gel application; home care.

Stage 2—Thorough dental prophylaxis; possible surgical gingivectomy; glass ionomer restorations.

Stage 3—Thorough dental prophylaxis and possible surgical gingivectomy; endodontic procedures and glass ionomer restorative or extraction and alveoplasty.

Stage 4—Extraction and alveoplasty; supportive care.

Step 2—Clean the lesion of plaque and hyperplastic gingiva; remove by curettage any soft dentin that may be present *(B)*.

- This is often difficult to do without penetrating the pulp chamber.
- If the pulp chamber is iatrogenically penetrated, a direct pulp capping or extraction should be performed.

Step 3—The lesion may be isolated by packing retraction cord into the sulcus *(C)*. If necessary to maintain a dry field and access to subgingival lesions, a gingival flap can be created.

Step 4—The lesion is cleaned with a prophy cup loaded with pumice. This removes debris from the cavity surface *(D)*.

Step 5—The lesion is rinsed and dried, and a restorative of either glass ionomer or a dentinal bonding agent/acrylic resin is placed.

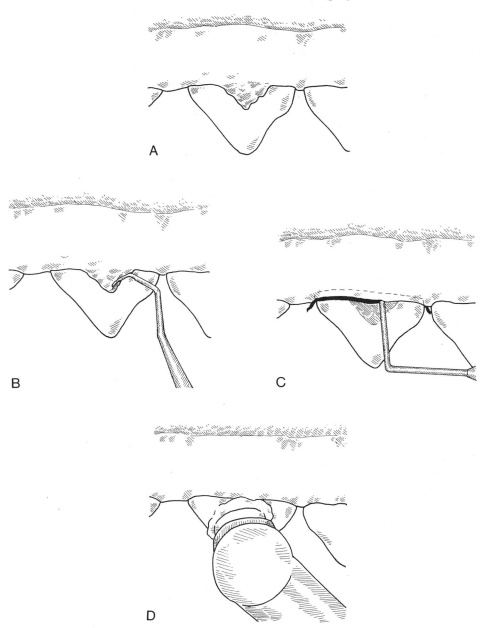

Placing a Glass Ionomer Restorative

Substep 1—A dentin conditioner is applied to the lesion with a brush *(A)* and, following the manufacturer's instructions, either actively scrubbed or left passively to perform on the surface.

Substep 2—The dentin conditioner is thoroughly washed from the tooth surface *(B)*, and the tooth is dried.

Substep 3—After mixing, the glass ionomer is inserted into an injection syringe and delivered into the defect *(C)*.

Substep 4—A Mylar strip is placed over the glass ionomer and tooth *(D)*. Pressure is placed on the Mylar strip with an instrument such as a condenser, curette, or explorer *(E)*.

Substep 5—The "flashing" (glass ionomer that has overflowed the prepared defect margin) is coated with varnish or a light-cured unfilled resin *(F)*.

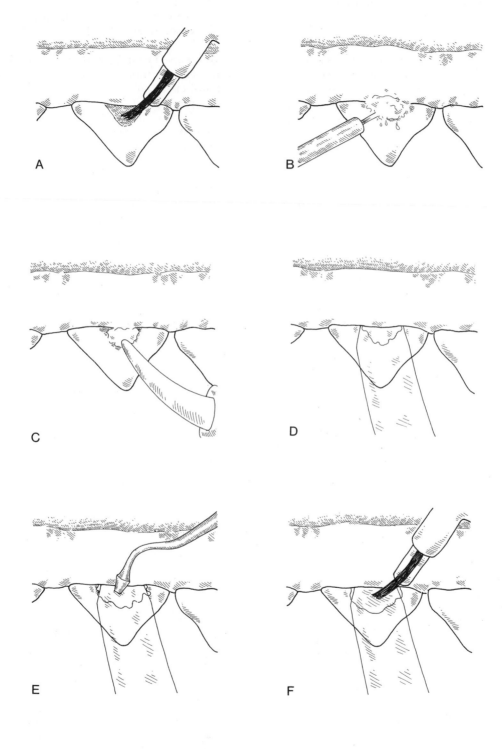

Substep 6—When the glass ionomer is hard (after 2 to 3 minutes), the Mylar strip is removed, and the excess glass ionomer is trimmed away, leaving a smooth surface and blended margin *(A)*.

Substep 7—Excess material is wiped away from the surface *(B)*.

Substep 8—The glass ionomer is recoated with varnish or light-cured unfilled resin *(C)*.

Alternative Step 5—An alternative restorative method is to use a flowable, light-cured glass ionomer material.* The lesion is pre-

---

*Vitebond and Vitremer: 3M Dental Products Division, Bldg 260-28-09, #M Center, St. Paul, MN 55144-1000; Zionomer: Den-Mat, Santa Maria, CA 93456

pared as in steps 1 to 4. The lesion is rinsed and dried but should not be overdried.

Substep 1—The glass ionomer material is mixed as directed. Using a small ball-end placement instrument, a small amount of the glass ionomer material is flowed into the defect.

Substep 2—The material is light-cured for the prescribed time. Deeper lesions can be filled and cured in layers.

Substep 3—The restoration margins are finished and smoothed.

Step 6—Home care will assist in maintaining the patient's oral health.

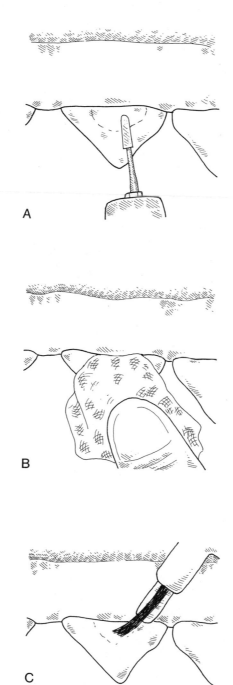

A

B

C

Amalgam

General Comments

- Amalgam is a metal alloy of mercury and silver that may also contain copper, zinc, tin, and other metals.
- Amalgam is mixed with amalgamators, which are mechanical mixing devices that have universally replaced the traditional method of mixing amalgam by mortar and pestle trituration. The mortar has been replaced by a capsule that contains the mercury alloy and by a metal or plastic ball, of smaller diameter than the capsule, that serves as the pestle. The capsule is placed in the amalgamator, and when the machine is turned on the materials are mixed.
- Depending on the alloy, it takes usually from 10 to 30 seconds to mix the amalgam. Follow the manufacturer's recommendation.
- It is important that amalgam be mixed in proper proportions; this is one of the major advantages of the premixed capsules.
- Amalgam is an easy material to work with; it is strong and able to withstand years of wear. Often the tooth will wear around an amalgam restoration, leaving a button of amalgam protruding beyond the worn tooth structure.
- Mercury is a poison, and direct contact with skin should be avoided.
- Amalgam seals by corrosion, and a black edge will be seen around the filled area at a later date. Because black discoloration is normal, clients should be told of its future appearance. Painting a varnish over the area to be restored before amalgam placement can reduce discoloration.

Indications

- Surface restoration.
- Core build-up for crown.

Contraindications

- Restorations where cosmetics are important.
- Very small teeth that will be weakened by an undercut macropreparation.

Materials

- Amalgam in capsule.
- Amalgamator.
- Amalgam carrier.
- Amalgam condensers.
- Amalgam burnishers.
- Amalgam carvers.
- Amalgam finishing cups.
- Amalgam well.

Technique

Step 1—Preparing the Surface

Substep 1—The outline and retention of the cavity are prepared using a diamond or carbide bur *(A)*.

Substep 2—Unsupported enamel is chiseled along the margins to remove the enamel overhangs *(B)*.

Substep 3—In areas within 1 mm of the pulp, resinated calcium hydroxide is placed *(C)*. (See Chapter 7, p. 258.)

Substep 4—In deep restorations, a liner of glass ionomer may be placed (see the preceding section on glass ionomers).

Step 2—Sealing Dentinal Tubules of Vital Teeth

- A cavity varnish or dentin adhesive is placed *(D)*.
- Dentin adhesives have been shown to significantly reduce microleakage around amalgam restorations.[10]
- Use only a thin layer over all surfaces, and allow to dry before placing the amalgam.

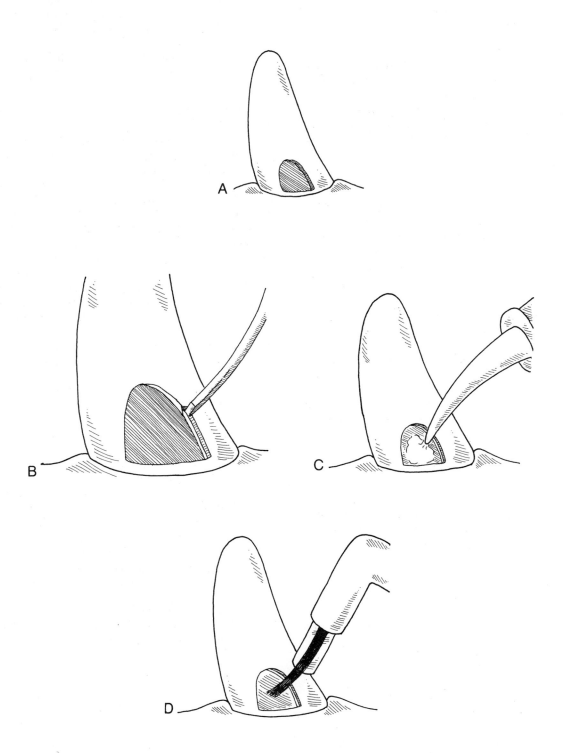

Step 3—Placing Restorative Material

Substep 1—The amalgam capsule is activated according to the manufacturer's instructions.

Substep 2—The amalgam is triturated at the time and speed directed by the manufacturer.

Substep 3—The mixed amalgam pellet is placed in an amalgam well (A). Properly prepared amalgam should appear shiny and moist. "Overmixed" amalgam appears chalky and flaky and does not condense. Undermixed amalgam appears nonhomogeneous.

Substep 4—An amalgam carrier is loaded with amalgam from the well (B).

- Caution should be used not to compact the amalgam in the carrier. If it becomes compacted, it may be necessary to replace the carrier tip or use a sharp, pointed instrument to dig out the amalgam.

Substep 5—Amalgam is placed in the restoration (C).

Substep 6—The first layer of amalgam is condensed with pressure (D). Smaller condensers are used in the early filling stage, and larger condensers are used for final condensing.

Substep 7—Subsequent layers are condensed. It is important when condensing each layer to eliminate voids. A slight overfill is desired; this is reduced in the next step.

Step 4—Carving Amalgam

- The final anatomic form is created with an amalgam carver. While carving, the operator should carve from tooth surface into the restoration to avoid "scooping" out the amalgam.

Step 5—Burnishing

- The surface of the amalgam is burnished by a burnisher (E).
- Burnishing renders the restoration more corrosion-resistant.
- The surface is rubbed lightly until it takes on a velveteen or satin appearance.[4]
- When burnishing, the instrument is directed from the restorative surface to the tooth surface.[11]
- The restoration should be polished ideally when completely set 24 hours after placement (F).

Complications

- Microleakage resulting in penetration of bacteria, bacterial products, soluble ions, and saliva into the gap between the restoration and the cavity walls.
- Microleakage resulting in pulp irritation, inflammation, and necrosis.
- Inherent characteristics of the material—such as the lack of chemical adhesion, differences in the coefficients of thermal expansion between the amalgam restoration and tooth structure, and the dimensional changes and surface texture of the amalgam after insertion into the prepared cavity—leading to microleakage or tooth fracture.
- Inadequate condensation resulting in voids along the cavity margins and in the restorative material.
- Overtrituration (mixing) resulting in overcontraction.
- Overmixing causing amalgam to set before it is placed into the cavity preparation.
- Undertrituration resulting in high-setting expansion and increased corrosion. If undermixed, the material will be dull and grainy, leading to a weak and rough surface with free mercury.
- Delay in placing the amalgam into the restoration, resulting in a partial setting of the amalgam and weakening of the restoration. Varying with the product and amount of trituration, the amalgam begins to solidify in 1 to 5 minutes.
- Careless placing of lining material on the walls, reducing macroretention of the amalgam with the tooth structure.[10]

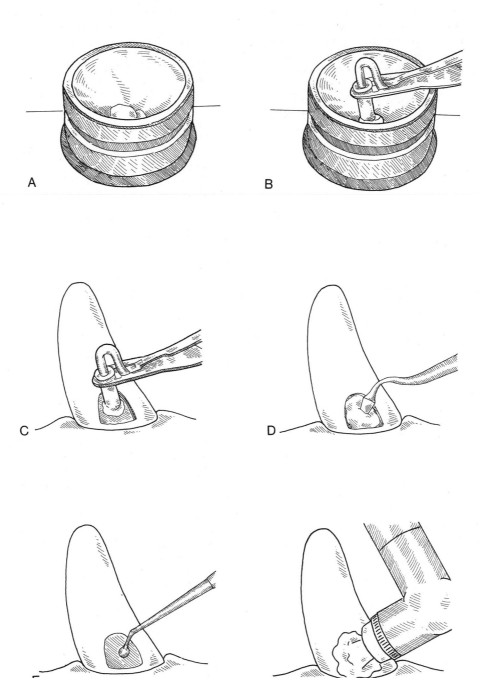

PIN RESTORATION

General Comments

- A pin-retained buildup is formed with pins placed into the dentin and covered with amalgam, composite, or a glass ionomer.
- If a minimal buildup is needed, the pin-retained buildup method may be used.
- In general, pins strengthen retention but weaken the tooth, so the least number of pins possible (minimum of two) should be used. They should be placed at least 2 mm from each other, the other walls, and the pulp. At least 1.5 mm of restorative material should cover the pin.[11]

Advantage

- Provides additional retentive surface.

Disadvantages

- Pins weaken tooth structure.
- Restoration will not withstand much lateral force.

Materials

- Power equipment.
- Low-speed handpiece.
- TMS pin kit: Minikins.*

Technique

Step 1—Appropriate endodontic or restorative preparation is performed *(A) (B)*.

---

*Whaledent, 236 5th Ave., New York, NY 10001

Step 2—With a low-speed handpiece and bur that comes with the Minikin kit, a hole is drilled in the dentin with one pass *(C)*.

- A small indentation in the dentin surface can be made with a ¼ round bur before drilling the hole to prevent wandering of the drill bit during initiation of the drilling.

Step 3—The pin is loaded into the pin instrument *(D)*.

Step 4—The pin self-taps and is threaded into the predrilled hole *(E)*.

Step 5—When the pin is set, the pin will break off at the precut location *(F)*.

Step 6—A restoration is placed (chemical or light-cure composite resin, glass ionomer, or amalgam) with a previously described technique *(G)*.

Complications

- Caution must be used for vital teeth not to penetrate into the pulp tissue; this may lead to sensitivity, infection, and failure. If penetration occurs, a small amount of calcium hydroxide may be placed in the hole, followed by the permanent restoration. The hole should not be used for the pin.
- Caution must be used to avoid perforation into the periodontal ligament space. If this should occur, a small amount of calcium hydroxide should be placed in the hole, and that hole should not be used for the procedure. Radiographs should be taken postoperatively and at 6 month intervals so that early detection and treatment planning can be made if complications arise.
- When drilling, caution must be used to make the hole as close to the size of the drill as possible (avoid drill wobble).
- Stripping threads of drilled holes will lead to an unstable pin, and the hole should not be used.

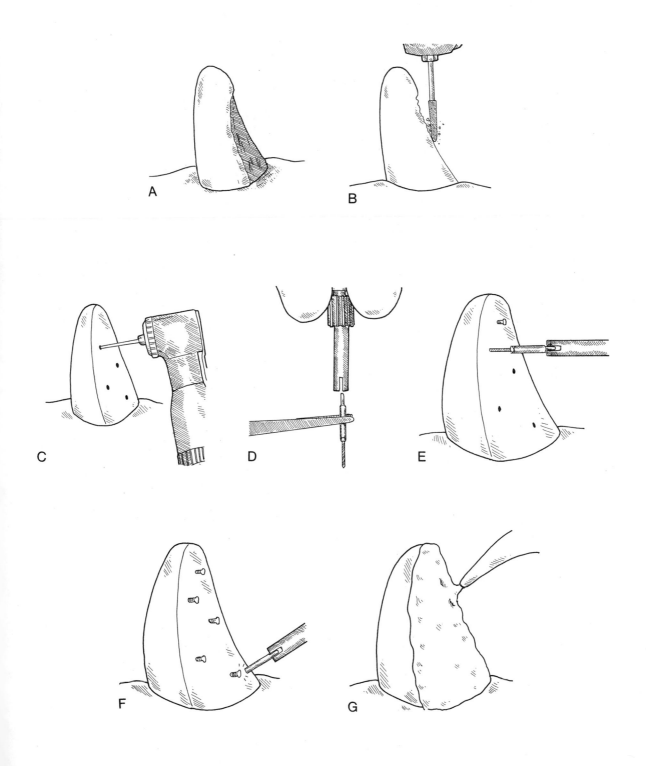

CROWN THERAPY

Crown ("Cap"): General Technique

General Comments

- A crown is an appliance that replaces the function and structure of a damaged tooth and protects the portion of the tooth that remains.
- A crown can be made to closely match the function and appearance of the tooth.
- The decision to place a crown is determined after careful consideration of the animal's lifestyle and the client's wishes.
- The replacement crown is called a full crown if it covers all of the tooth.[12]
- The replacement crown is called a partial crown if it covers only a portion of the tooth.
- The material that the crown is made of affects its appearance.
- The margin of the crown is the edge that interfaces with the margin of the tooth preparation.
- Maintenance (conservation) of tooth structure is the primary concern in crown preparation design. It is unwise to remove more tooth structure than is absolutely necessary for creating retention and integrity; at the same time, enough tooth structure must be removed to create adequate space for the restoration. The goal is to have the final restoration the same dimensions as the original unbroken tooth unless specifics of the case dictate otherwise.
- The preparation should be designed with a parallel technique of the walls and a 6 vertical taper to increase the resistance of the crown to dislodgment.
- Canine teeth in dogs and cats do not lend themselves to parallel technique as readily as do most human teeth, because canines in dogs and cats are conical and not box-like, as in humans.
- Parallelism may be accomplished by "stair-stepping" the preparation between the mesial and the distal surfaces in canine teeth. However, this is seldom necessary.
- Greater retention is achieved when most of the available surface area of the prepared axial wall of the tooth is in contact with the cast restoration.
- The restoration must have adequate occlusal clearance or it will strike other teeth.
- The margin of the restoration must facilitate good hygiene and not create areas for plaque and debris to accumulate; at the same time, it should be accessible so the veterinarian can finish it and the client can maintain it.
- Ideally, the margin placement is on the enamel surface. This is more readily accomplished when aesthetics are not a primary concern.
- If aesthetics are of paramount importance, subgingival placement of the margin is necessary.

Indications

- Enamel hypoplasia or aplasia (dentinal structures are intact, pulp is vital).
- Fractured teeth with damaged pulp and lost vitality; performed after endodontic therapy.
- Undamaged pulp: pulp vital but additional protection desired.
- When deterioration or damage has left an unstable or inadequate supragingival portion of the crown structure and the damage is not reparable by other methods.
- To protect a damaged tooth from further trauma or deterioration.

Contraindications

- Thin wall structure; always take a radiograph before performing a crown preparation.
- Nonvital teeth that have not received endodontic therapy.
- Endodontically treated tooth where practitioner is unsure of success.

Objective

- To protect the tooth and to improve the cosmetics and function of the tooth.

Materials

- A crown of semiprecious metal. The least expensive material that should be used is silver-colored. Generally, the cost of the metal is a smaller portion of the total cost of a crown.
- A premium gold alloy contains a greater percentage of gold; when the percentage is greater than 40%, the alloy produces a gold-colored crown. Crowns with 30% or less gold in the alloy are silver in color.[13]
- A crown made of a gold alloy is more malleable, resulting in easier fabrication and placement, but softer and more subject to wear.
- A tooth-colored crown can be made by fusing porcelain to a metal shell or by using porcelain alone. Porcelain by itself is extremely fragile, and its use is limited.[14]

- Porcelain fused to metal can be used to create aesthetic restorations. Unfortunately, this method requires removal of more tooth structure than does a metal crown.

Technique

- (1) Evaluation for preparation; (2) tooth reduction and margin preparation; (3) taking an impression and casting; (4) manufacture of temporary crown (optional); (5) laboratory orders and manufacture of crown; and (6) cementation of crown.
- The many alternatives and methods that can be used must be selected case by case.

Step 1—Evaluation for Preparation

- The occlusal edge or surface is evaluated for reduction to allow space for the metal in the crown.
- Anticipated wear determines space requirements and crown thickness.
- Allow a minimum of 1.5 mm of space for the areas of increased wear potential and 1 mm of space for the areas of little or no wear potential.[12, 14, 15]
- The incisor, premolar, and molar teeth that have occlusal surfaces require additional space allowance on the occlusal surface.
- The canine and premolar teeth without an actual occlusal surface usually require little reduction for space allowance but do require reduction and beveling of any sharp or thin edges.

Step 2—Tooth Reduction and Margin Preparation

- A gingival retraction cord is placed with a cord packer. The purpose of the cord is to isolate the gingiva from the tooth surface. Avoid wrapping the gingival cord in the bur while preparing the tooth surface.
- A tapered coarse diamond bur is used for initial reduction (Table 8–5).

Table 8–5 • DIAMOND BURS FOR CROWN THERAPY

Type	Use
Tapered flat end	Creates flat shoulder
Long, thin round end	Creates chamfer
Long shank with flame tip	Modifies shoulder preparation
Curettage, 55 degree bevel	Creates shoulder with bevel
12 mm flame	Creates feather
Stip-tipped	Periodontal use for curettage

- Either a chamfer or a shoulder, depending on the preference of the laboratory and the clinician, is created at the gingival edge of the preparation.
- The margin should be placed either 1 mm above or 1 mm below the free gingival margin to reduce the incidence of gingivitis.

Axial Reduction

- The tooth structure is removed by axial reduction along the long axis of the tooth. The bur is held nearly parallel to the tooth axis.
- The tooth surface should be reduced in the attempt to create walls that are nearly parallel with a 6 degree slope.
- Undercuts should be avoided, and when looking at the preparation from the coronal surface, the absence of undercuts is ensured when the entire prepared surface can be visualized.
- If possible, reduction should be made in one pass, moving in a counterclockwise direction around the tooth.
- A level margin all around the tooth should be maintained.
- A stair-step reduction of the canine tooth may be necessary to maintain parallel walls (A).

Margins

Chamfer

Description

- A chamfer is a type of margin created by removing structure to leave a gradual tran-

sition to the uncut surface (B). This may be accomplished first by gross reduction with a tapered coarse diamond bur and then by creating a finish line with a tapered medium or fine diamond bur.

Advantage

- This type of margin allows for a slip joint and is a good design for gold restorations.

Disadvantages

- More difficult to design clearly.
- Not a good design for a porcelain or a porcelain-fused-to-metal restoration because it does not give enough support to the edge of the porcelain.

Shoulder Joint

Description

- A shoulder joint is a butt joint (C). It is created at the same time as axial reduction, using a tapered-cylinder flat-end bur.
- This margin must be used for porcelain restoration to give adequate support to the edge of the restoration.
- A shoulder with an internal bevel is created at the same time as axial reduction, using a tapered-cylinder round-end bur (D).

Advantages

- The biggest advantage of this margin is that a definite finish line is created.
- For the beginner, the shoulder is more easily created.
- The diameter of the bur is an easy means by which to measure the amount of reduction performed.

Disadvantage

- Difficult to seal definitively.

Shoulder with External Bevel

Description

- The shoulder is trimmed with a flame-shaped or beveled-cylinder diamond bur (E).

Advantage

- Creates a better margin.

Disadvantage

- A steady hand is necessary to avoid destruction of the shoulder.

Additional Comments

- A metal cast crown requires a circumferential, axial reduction of 1 mm.
- A crown of porcelain fused to metal requires a reduction of 1.5 to 2.0 mm to allow additional space for the porcelain.

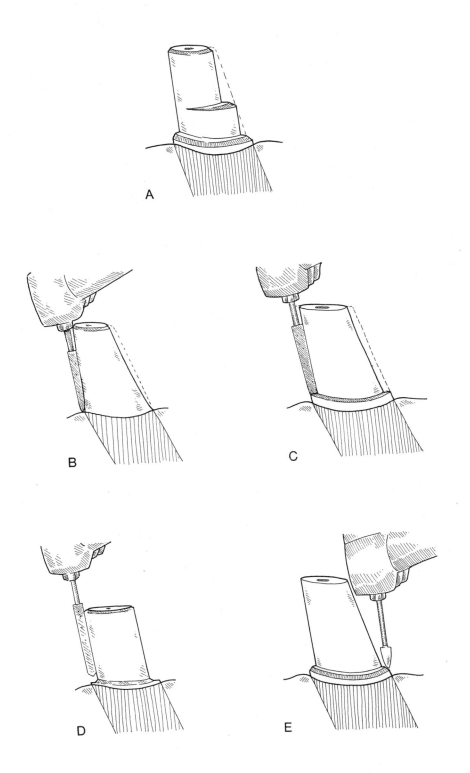

Minimal Preparation Techniques

- There are times when reduction of the crown of less than 1 mm can take place.
- This can occur when the teeth will not be hitting opposing teeth.
- Placing a crown without considering the occlusion may lead to patient discomfort and tooth wear. It makes no sense to save one tooth with crown therapy and cause damage to another tooth in so doing.

Step 3—Taking an Impression and Casting

General Comments

- Several types of materials are available for taking impressions for crowns. The alginate impressions, as used for making study models for orthodontics, do not show enough detail for crown fabrication.
- Quadrant impression trays or small custom-made trays can be used when taking an impression with a rubber-base material of a tooth that has had a crown preparation. The impression should include the tooth on either side of the prepared tooth. Full-mouth alginate impressions should also be taken.

Rubber Base

Description

- These materials are rubber-like in nature and contain large molecules with weak interaction between them. These molecules are joined together at certain points to form a three-dimensional network.[2]
- The three kinds of commonly used rubber-based materials for taking impressions are polysulfide rubber, siloxane polymers, and vinyl polysiloxane polymers.

Polysulfide Rubber

Description

- An impression material supplied as a two-part system, containing a base and a catalyst.

Use

- Impressions for crown, bridge, implant crown.

Advantage

- Good working time (although may be too long for many).

Disadvantages

- Requires thorough mixing.
- Lack of a "snap set"; curing progresses slowly.
- Impressions should be poured after 15 minutes and before 72 hours.
- Messy; unpleasant odor.

Siloxane Polymers

Use

- Crowns and bridges.

Advantage

- Accurate representation of the prepared tooth.

Disadvantage

- Poor ability of dental stone to "wet and flow" into the impression.

Vinyl Polysiloxane Polymers

Description

- These are silicone-addition–type impression materials.

- These impression materials are usually available in different consistencies: light-, medium-, and heavy-body.

Use

- Impressions for crown and bridge.

Advantages

- Accurate reproduction of detail.
- Dimensional stability; prevents longer delay before pouring.
- Excellent elasticity; enables recovery from undercuts.
- Good tear strength reduces likelihood of impression damage.

Disadvantage

- Decreased "wetability"; stone does not flow as readily into the impression.

Materials

- Orthodontic trays.
- Large paper mixing pads.
- Large spatulas.

Technique

- The crown is prepared as previously described.
- The retraction cord is pulled from the gingival sulcus just before taking the impression.

Step 1—Equal parts of the material, supplied in tubes, are placed on a paper pad.

Step 2—The material is mixed thoroughly.

NOTE: Alternatively, but more expensively, convenient premeasured materials may be purchased in tandem cartridges. The contents are joined by a mixing tip, which leads to an intraoral tip. The cartridges are placed in a dispensing gun, which delivers the material through the mixing tip and the intraoral tip to the crown site.

Step 3—If not using the cartridges, the material is placed into an impression tray.

Step 4—The filled tray is placed over the prepared tooth.

Step 5—Once set, the impression material is removed with a snapping movement from the mouth and the cast is poured.

Variation in Technique with Vinyl Polysiloxane Polymers

Step 1—The light-bodied material is mixed and placed into a curved-tip syringe or, if supplied in premeasured cartridges, it is mounted into the dispensing gun.

Step 2—The light-bodied material is injected around the prepared tooth and into the subgingival area.

Step 3—Equal amounts of the medium-bodied material are placed on the mixing pad, are mixed, and are placed in the impression tray or, if supplied in premeasured cartridges, can be injected directly on top of the light-bodied material.

Step 4—The filled tray is placed over the light-bodied material covering the prepared tooth.

Step 5—Once the impression material is set, the tray and impression material are removed, and a cast is poured in standard fashion.

Advantage

- The light-bodied material will create an impression of even greater detail.

Complications

- Organic contaminants on the teeth possibly causing roughness to the impression or bubbles and voids.
- Roughness being caused by overdessication of teeth before the impression is taken.
- Inadequate working time caused by incorrect base/accelerator ratio, with excess catalyst or when ambient temperature and humidity are too high.
- Prolonged setting time caused by incorrect base/accelerator ratio, poor storage conditions, or use of outdated materials.
- Poor mixing techniques resulting in an uneven mix, causing uneven curing that may cause distortion, loss of detail, and/or roughness of the impression as well as bubbles or voids.
- Distortion caused by poor adhesion of im-

pression material to tray; may be avoided by using the tray adhesive that comes with many impression materials.

- Distortion, from partial polymerization, caused by excessive delay in seating the tray in the mouth.
- Distortion and loss of detail due to movement of the tray after it is seated in position.
- Excessive bulk of material possibly causing marked thermal contraction on cooling, thus causing distortion.
- Loss of detail and/or roughness caused by removing the tray before full setting of the impression material.
- Prolonged removal of the tray from the mouth possibly causing prolonged stress, with distortion and loss of detail of the impression.
- After impression taken, distortion avoided by placing tray down with impression material up.
- Care must be taken to make sure material completely set before removal from the mouth.

Putty-Wash Technique with No Preformed Tray

Comments

- This technique may be useful in very large impressions for which custom trays are not available.
- The technique takes advantage of the variation between the consistency and viscosity of the vinyl polysiloxane materials and their ability to work together.

- Certain gloves may inhibit the set of the material, so a small amount should be tested with the gloves to be used.
- This technique, as with most impression techniques, must be performed on a patient intubated under general anesthesia.

Advantages

- Impressions can be made of very large patients.
- Impressions do not require tray manufacturer.

Disadvantage

- May have some distortion due to lack of a tray.

Technique

Step 1—Following the manufacturer's instructions, the putty is mixed by gloved hands. The material is kneaded until a uniform, streak-free color is obtained.

Step 2—The impression material is spread out over one hand.

Step 3—The impression material is inserted in the mouth, over the teeth and gums, and held in place with hands until set up.

Step 4—When hard, the material is removed from the mouth.

Step 5—With an automix cartridge, the extra-light material is injected into the teeth impressions of the already set-up impression.

Step 6—The material is reintroduced into the mouth, seated, and allowed to set up.

Step 7—The model is poured as with previous techniques.

Hydrocolloid/Alginate

Description
- A two-part process is performed: first, the impression material is warmed and injected around the tooth; second, as the injected material cools and solidifies, an alginate mixture is mixed, placed in a tray, and placed over the solidified material.

Use
- Impressions for crowns.

Advantage
- Superior reproduction of the crown preparation.

Disadvantage
- Requires a boiler pot to heat the hydrocolloid.

Equipment
- Boiler pot and thermometer.
- Impression trays.
- Cohere* reversible hydrocolloid.
- Large-gauge injection needles.
- Rubber bowl.
- Large spatula.
- Type II alginate (irreversible hydrocolloid).

Technique
Step 1—The syringe containing the hydrocolloid material is placed in the boiling pot,

---

*Gingi-Pak, 4820 Calle Alto, P.O. Box 240, Camarillo, CA 93011

and the water is brought to a boil for 5 minutes.

Step 2—The temperature in the pot is reduced to a constant 140 to 150 degrees F for a minimum of 10 minutes before use.

Step 3 (optional)—The teeth may be lightly sprayed with a preimpression release agent.

Step 4—A large-gauge injection needle (which comes with the hydrocolloid) is placed on the syringe, and the material is injected around the prepared tooth.

Step 5—Type II alginate is mixed in a rubber bowl and placed into the impression tray.

Step 6—A standard alginate irreversible hydrocolloid impression is made (see Chapter 9, Dental Orthodontics, p. 404).

Step 7—Once set, the alginate with the hardened hydrocolloid around the tooth is removed from the mouth, and standard casts are poured.

Complication
- Care should be taken not to burn the oral cavity by using inadequately tempered hydrocolloid (too hot).

Bite Registration

General Comment
- Bite registration allows the dental laboratory to place the models in proper articulation to avoid occlusal interference.

Indications
- Crown and bridge.
- Orthodontics.

Objective
- To obtain an accurate representation of the occlusion.

Materials
- Vinyl polysiloxane.
- Bite wax.

Technique
Step 1—The patient's vital signs are checked and anesthetic stability is confirmed.

Step 2—After all other impressions are made, the patient is extubated. The tongue may be gently rolled back over itself and placed into the pharynx. The patient should be observed to make sure that breathing is normal.

Step 3—The impression material of choice (a self-mixing injection-type vinyl polysiloxane sets rapidly and removes operator error in mixing) is placed over the canine and incisor teeth.

- If using a chemical-curing material, curing may be hastened by using a hair dryer.
- If using bite wax, the wax may be warmed with warm water or with the hair dryer and then placed between the incisors.

Step 4—The mouth is closed to a point of normal closed occlusion with the registration material between the upper and lower teeth. The mouth is opened, and the bite registration material is carefully removed.

Step 5—The tongue is placed back in the normal position, and the patient is recovered from anesthesia or, if another procedure is to be performed, reintubated.

Complications
- Respiratory obstruction with the tongue.
- Inaccurate impression.
- Recovery from anesthesia before impression material sets.
- Time for material to set may be decreased by the bite registration material being warmed.

Considerations for Making Casts for Crowns and Bridges

Material Complications
- Poor cleaning of the impression before pouring the cast may cause an inferior, rough, or chalky cast.
- Excess water in the impression may cause a distorted cast.
- Premature removal of the cast from the impression may cause the cast to break.
- Poor mixing or casting technique may cause bubbles or an inferior cast.
- Contamination of the impression surface or dental stone powder may cause a rough cast.
- Incorrect water/powder ratio for the dental stone may cause distortion of the cast. A hard laboratory stone material is preferred to plaster of Paris.
- The stone model may be toughened to reduce tooth breakage while in laboratory transit by applying Stone Die and Plaster Hardener* after the model is dry.

---

*Stone Die and Plaster Hardener, George Taub Products & Fusion Co., Inc., 277 New York Ave., Jersey City, NJ 07307

Step 4—Manufacture of Temporary Crown (Optional)

General Comments

- The prepared tooth may be protected until the final cast restoration is returned from the laboratory and placed.
- In veterinary patients, this step can make the difference between a successful restoration and a failure, because patients and clients respond variably to instructions about protecting the prepared tooth.
- A temporary restoration must be strong enough to remain in place for the time needed.
- The client should be able to clean around the temporary restoration to prevent soft tissue inflammation or deterioration of the periodontal health, which could interfere with placement of the final restoration.

Direct Acrylic Technique

Step 1—An alginate impression of the prepared tooth and of the surrounding area is taken *(A)*.

Step 2—After unseating the impression, a round-ball carbide bur is used to carve some of the alginate away from the impression of the prepared tooth *(B)*.

Step 3—The alginate is filled with a thin mix of acrylic *(C)*.

Step 4—The tooth and surrounding gingiva are lubricated with petroleum jelly *(D)*, and the alginate with the acrylic is seated in the mouth *(E)*.

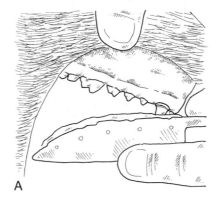

A

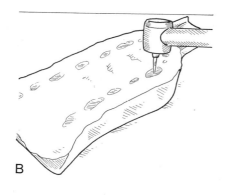

B

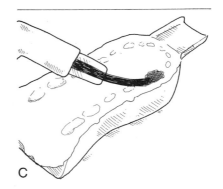

C

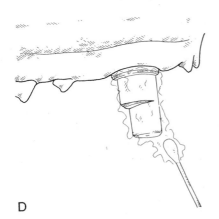

D

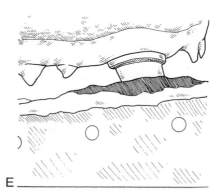

E

Step 5—When the acrylic has hardened, the alginate is removed, and the acrylic casting is removed from the alginate *(A)*.

Step 6—The casting is trimmed and shaped with acrylic burs in a slow-speed handpiece *(B)*.

Step 7—The acrylic casting is trial-fitted and trimmed again or shaped as needed.

- Because the primary function of the temporary restoration is to protect the prepared tooth, it is usually better to make it smaller so the patient will not place as much pressure or force on it.

Step 8—Once it fits properly, the restoration can be smoothed with sanding discs and polished with wet pumice on a wheel.

Step 9—A zinc oxide–eugenol temporary cement is applied to cement it in place *(C)*. The restoration is cemented in place *(D)*.

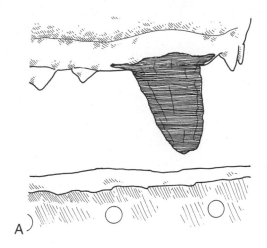

A

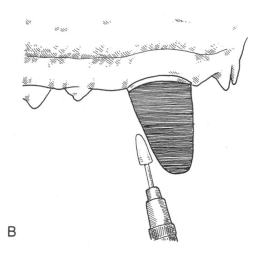

B

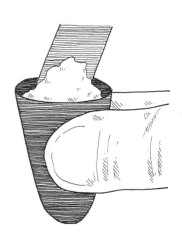

C

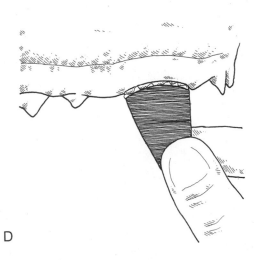

D

Step 5—Laboratory Order and Manufacture of Crown

- A written laboratory prescription is sent with the model castings and bite impression registrations.
- The prescription should include type of material to be used for the crown and color with a shade guide.
- The model and new crown are returned from the dental laboratory (A).

Step 6—Trial Placement of the Crown

Substep 1—The temporary crown and temporary filling material are carefully removed so the shape of the preparation is not altered (B). The surface is cleaned with a curette (C).

Substep 2—The crown and/or dowel core are checked for proper fit by trial seating on/in the tooth (D).

Substep 3—If there is any binding, the casting is removed, brushed with polishing rouge dissolved in chloroform, and reseated. Alternatively, occlusal chalk may be sprayed into the crown and the crown fit over the tooth (E).

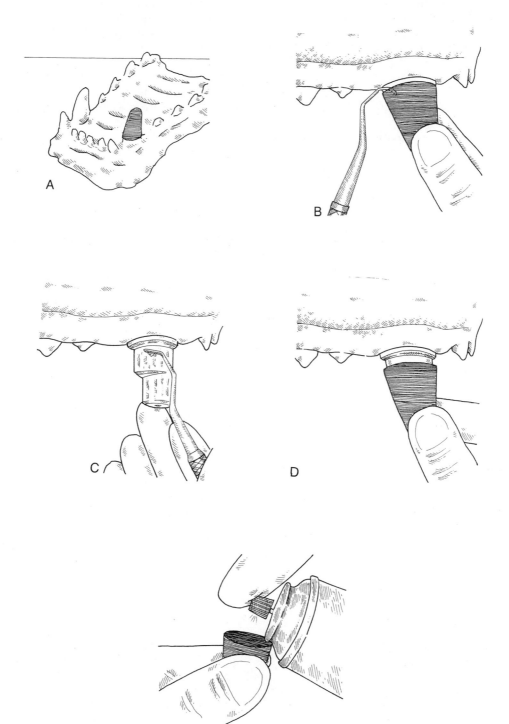

Substep 4—The casting is removed, and the teeth are examined for residue. Residue *(arrow)* indicates the areas that are binding *(A)*.

Substep 5—Carefully remove some material tooth structure from these spots with a bur and retest *(B)*.

- This process is repeated until the casting seats properly and all the rouge is removed.
- The fit should be snug, and the margins should be smooth.
- Margins are examined with an explorer by pointing the tip toward the gingiva and sliding it down the crown onto the root.
- If the explorer slides over the interface smoothly, the crown fits properly.
- This procedure is repeated in several places around the tooth.
- Pumice the inside of the crown with a prophy brush with flour pumice *(C)*.
- Pumice the tooth with a prophy brush *(D)*.

Complications
- Avoid acids, alcoholic solutions, or pure alcohol when placing the crown on a vital tooth.

- When the cement is dry, do not remove any residual cement with sonic or ultrasonic scalers, because doing so may destroy the molecular structure of the cement, weakening the bond and causing loss of the crown.
- Use spatula/hand scaler/curette to remove excess cement.
- If the tooth is damaged to a degree that little structure remains, the surface area is increased with additional cuts of box shapes or grooves, or a combination of the two, in the wall of the tooth.
- Teeth with shortened coronal height may be built up using a dowel-core technique or post-retained buildup, or the crown can be lengthened surgically.
- Although preservation of tooth structure is important, enough space must be created to allow for the thickness of the metal. If the metal is too thin, the restoration will flex or bend under occlusal forces, and the restoration will deteriorate or fail. Bulk can be added at margins where rigidity and reinforcement are needed.

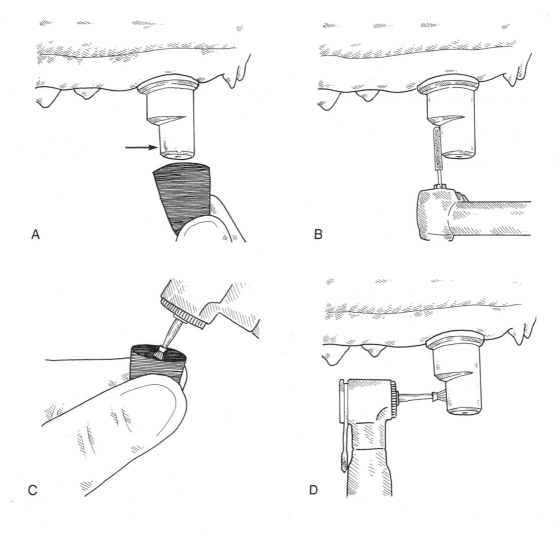

A

B

C

D

Step 7—Cementation of Crown

Technique

Substep 1—The prepared tooth crown is rinsed well with water *(A)*.

Substep 2—The prepared tooth crown is dried according to the type of cement used *(B)*. Some cements require the surface to be bone-dry, whereas others (glass ionomers) require a slight amount of moisture (see the following section).

Substep 3—The manufacturer's directions are followed in mixing the cement *(C)*.

Substep 4—The cement is placed into the crown with a spatula *(D)*.

Substep 5—The crown is seated and held in place firmly until the cement hardens *(E)*.

Substep 6—Excess cement is trimmed from the crown *(F)*.

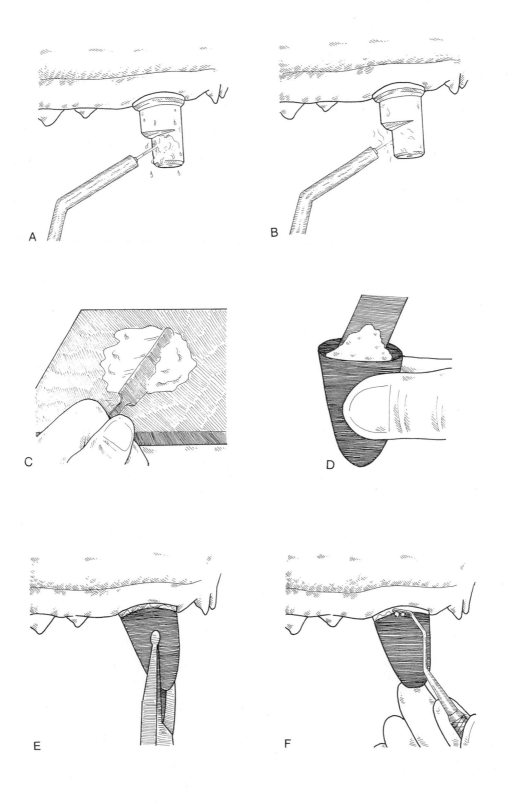

Cementation Materials for Crowns

- Most dental cements have a similar background, and their basic chemistry is derived from a powder, either zinc oxide or aluminum silicate, and a liquid, either phosphoric acid or polyacrylic acid[16] (Table 8–6).
- Cements are also made from composite resins.

Zinc Phosphate

Description

- A mixture of zinc oxide and phosphoric acid.
- This cement has been used for a long time in human dentistry.

Use

- Luting cement for seating permanent prosthesis, crown, or bridge.

Advantage

- One of its primary advantages—excellent thermal insulation—may not be applicable in veterinary medicine, because most veterinary patients are not fed food that has a wide range of temperature.

Disadvantage

- Very poor adhesive properties limit its use to temporary crowns or techniques that use mechanical retention.

Zinc Oxide–Eugenol

Description

- A mixture of zinc oxide and eugenol.

Uses

- As a temporary luting agent for crowns and bridges or as a temporary filling material.
- As a root canal sealant.

Advantage

- Soothing effect on the pulp.

Disadvantage

- Poor retentive and other physical properties limit its use in veterinary dentistry.

Zinc Polycarboxylate

Description

- The liquid is an aqueous solution of polyacrylic acid and copolymers; the powder is zinc oxide with some magnesium or stannous oxide.
- Stannous fluoride may be added to increase the strength of the cement.

Table 8–6 • CEMENTS

Zinc Phosphate	
Product	**Manufacturer**
Hy-Bond Zinc Phosphate	Shofu

Zinc Polycarboxylate	
Product	**Manufacturer**
Durelon	ESPE/Premier
LivCarbo	G. C. America

Zinc Oxide–Eugenol	
Product	**Manufacturer**
Hy-Bond Zinc Oxide Eugenol	Shofu
Temerex Cement	Interstate
ZOE 2200	L. D. Caulk
Temp Bond NE	Kerr

Glass Ionomers	
Product	**Manufacturer**
Biocem	L. D. Caulk
Cement/Liner	Parkell
Chem-Fil	Dentsply DeTrey
Everbone	Kerr
Fuji Ionomer Type I	Fuji
Lining Cement	G. C. America
Ketac-Cem	ESPE/Premier
Shofu 1	Shofu

Composite Resin Cements	
Product	**Manufacturer**
Comspan	L. D. Caulk
Conclude	3M
Flexi-Flow	Essential Dental
Panavia	J. Morita
Panavia 21	J. Morita
Resiment	Septodont
Porcelite Dual Care	Kerr

Bridge Cements	
Product	**Manufacturer**
Resin Bonded Bridge Cement	Kerr
MD Bridge Cementation Cement	Den-Mat
Maryland Bridge Adhesive	Getz

Use

- Luting crowns (very clean metal casting required for adhesion of cement to crown).

Advantage

- Adhesion to tooth structure.

Disadvantage

- Short working times.

Glass Ionomer

Description

- The glass ionomer cements have been modified to provide radiopacity and handling properties suitable for lining or cementing purposes.

Advantages

- Cariostatic activity.
- Bonds to dentin.
- High strength.

Disadvantages

- Dental hypersensitivity reported in humans; may be avoided by using proper technique.
- In vital teeth, pulp sensitivity and possible necrosis caused by chemical irritation from the material and leakage may be a problem.[17]
- Glass ionomers initially have a low pH.

Complications

- The tooth should not be overdried, but rather dried with a gentle stream of air or simply blotted dry with a gauze pad or cotton pellet.
- Observe mixing ratios recommended by the manufacturer; otherwise, excessive free acid will remain in the tooth structure and cause sensitivity.
- Avoid excessive hydraulic pressure by creating channels in the crown for excess cement to flow out or by seating the crown with a slow, steady pressure when cementing it in place.

- Prevent contamination with saliva or water in the early setting stages by using varnish, cocoa butter, or light-cure bonding agent on the marginal surface.
- If recommended with the particular luting agent, use a dentin conditioner before placement.

Composite Resin Cements

Description

- Some of the newer composite resin cements* bond chemically to metals, porcelain, tooth enamel, and unetched dentin.
- Panavia sets in an oxygen-free environment.

Advantage

- Virtually insoluble in water.

Disadvantages

- Irritating to pulp; therefore, pulp must be protected by calcium hydroxide.
- Poor manipulative characteristics; limited working times.

*Panavia-21: J. Morita USA, Inc., 14712 Bentley Circle, Tustin, CA 92680; C.B. Metabond, Parkell, 155 Schmitt Blvd., Box 376, Farmingdale, NY 11735

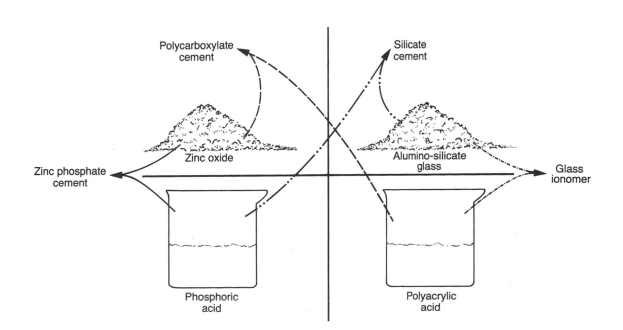

Special Situations

Crown–Dowel-Core Buildup

General Comment

- The minimum distance for dowel length is equal to the crown length.

Indication

- If the crown to be prepared has little remaining retentive surface area, a dowel-core buildup is necessary.

Contraindications

- Vertical root fractures.
- Teeth with inflammatory resorption.
- Teeth subject to excessive forces.

Objective

- To build up a crown to enable restoration of the tooth.

Materials

- Crown preparation instruments and materials.
- Peeso reamers.

Technique

- Before axial preparation, the root canal chamber is prepared.

Step 1—The endodontic filling in the coronal portion of the canal is removed (A). Ideally, two thirds to three quarters of the length of the canal is used for the post/core (B).

- The natural curve of the canine tooth usually precludes access to the desired depth of two thirds to three quarters of the length of the root.
- The preparation is extended to the greatest length possible in a straight line.
- If the dentinal wall at the curve is thick, reduction of this area can lengthen the preparation.
- Care is exercised to avoid penetration through the root wall.
- Initially, Peeso reamers are used to remove the gutta-percha and to enlarge the canal.
- Peeso reamers have a flexible shank and easily follow the gutta-percha.
- The graduated sizes of Peeso reamers offer gradual canal enlargement.
- In mature teeth, the walls are shaped parallel to aid in retention.
- If increased length is required, or the canal is larger than the Peeso reamers, a tapered fissure bur is used.
- Undercuts are carefully avoided.

Step 2—A contrabevel is placed around the periphery of the occlusal portion of the tooth (C).

Step 3—Axial reduction, as with crown preparation previously described.

Step 4—The post is trial-fitted (D); there should be no wobble. In long canals, a K-wire or other stainless steel pin should be used and bent to conform to the length of the canal. In this situation, the pin will conform to the natural canal, rather than a track drilled by the Peeso reamer. If using a K-wire or stainless steel pin, it should be notched and grooved with a bur for venting and retention.

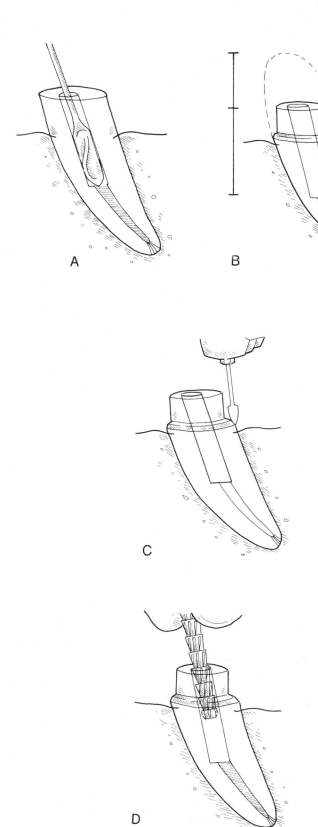

A

B

C

D

Step 5—The cement is mixed and placed on the post (A).

Step 6—The post is placed in the canal and held until the cement sets (B).

Step 7—Core material is mixed according to the manufacturer's instructions and is placed over the post and tooth (C).

Step 8—Once the core material has set, a standard crown preparation is performed (D).

- The axial preparation of these teeth is much the same except fewer, if any, "stair steps" are needed.

- The shoulder is formed around the tooth, and the axial reduction is performed.

Complications

- Perforation while preparing the root canal for dowel; the treatment is to seal the perforation with calcium hydroxide paste.[18]
- Perforation of the root canal; happens mostly on the mesial side of the tooth curvature.

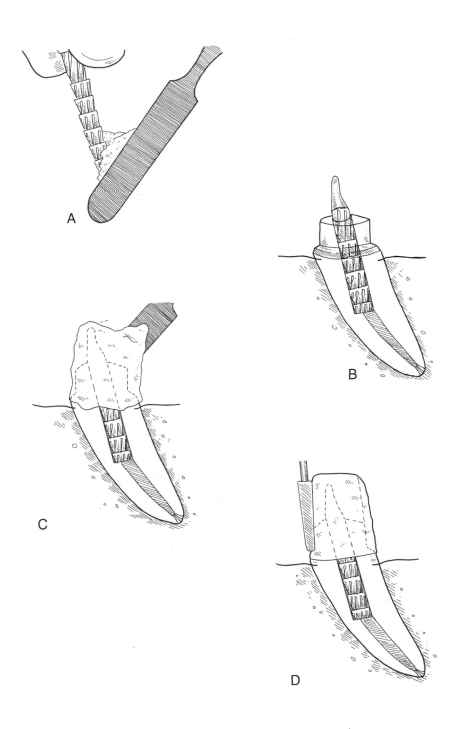

Crown: Cast Dowel Core

- A dowel core is a custom-cast post and coronal buildup.
- One of the strongest methods of crown replacement is the use of a dowel-core casting.
- Ideally, the dowel should be two thirds to three quarters the length of the root and should leave no less than 3 mm of the endodontic filling material at the apex of the tooth.
- The path of insertion becomes important when placing the crown.
- The path of insertion is the line that coincides with the long axis of the preparation; this is not necessarily equal to the long axis of the tooth.
- The crown will be placed on the prepared tooth along this line, and no other oral structures can restrict the placement of the crown along this line.
- The path of insertion must always be determined before starting the preparation.
- Any retentive grooves or boxes must be oriented in the same direction as the path of insertion.
- The path of insertion of the dowel core and that of the crown do not necessarily need to be the same. The canal is prepared with a Peeso reamer as previously described.

Step 1—The prepared canal is lubricated with a small Peeso reamer and cotton ball covered with petroleum jelly.

Step 2—A plastic sprue, notched or roughened to prevent it from pulling out of the final acrylic pattern, is trimmed to fit into the canal to the apical limit of the dowel preparation.

Step 3—Acrylic is mixed in a dappen dish to a thin consistency.

Step 4—The acrylic is placed in the prepared canal without any voids.

Step 5—A plastic sprue is seated in the canal, and the acrylic is added as needed to encompass the bevel on the occlusal margin of the preparation.

Step 6—As the acrylic reaches a pliable polymerization stage, the pattern is moved in and out of the canal to prevent it from locking.

Step 7—After the acrylic is polymerized, the pattern is removed, and the dowel is inspected for voids and adequate extension into the canal.

Step 8—If needed, another mix of the acrylic can be used to finish the dowel.

Step 9—When the acrylic has polymerized, it is seated, and more acrylic is placed on the tooth around the sprue.

- This acrylic becomes the foundation for the buildup.

Step 10—The pattern is seated in the tooth and shaped to fit the pulp chamber/root canal.

Step 11—The final reduction should closely replicate the desired final form of the dowel.

- An alternate method of obtaining an accurate representation of the canal is to coat the canal with K-Y jelly by coating it on an absorbent point and inserting it into the canal. Then, coat the plastic sprue with polyvinyl siloxane impression material and insert it into the canal, removing it after it sets. The procedure can then be resumed at step 9.
- The prosthodontic laboratory will use this pattern to cast the post or dowel.

Step 12—The post dowel and core are seated in the tooth, and the gingival retraction cord is placed in the gingival sulcus.

Step 13—An impression is taken (see step 3 in the preceding section on Crown Therapy).

- When the impression material has set, it is removed and examined.
- The margin of the preparation must be accurately reproduced and free of flaws.
- The pattern (dowel and core) and impression are sent to a prosthodontic laboratory for preparation of the final castings.

Step 14—Temporary cavity filling material is placed in the coronal orifice of the endodontic canal to protect it until the castings are returned from the laboratory.

Step 15—After the custom dowel and crown are returned from the laboratory, the castings are inspected for fit as with the crown technique.

Step 16—The cement is mixed and placed in the canal and on the dowel.

Step 17—The dowel casting is seated slowly, allowing excess cement to escape, and is held firmly in place until the cement has hardened.

Step 18—Excess cement is removed from the margin.

Step 19—The cast crown is trial-seated.

Step 20—The same process of checking fit, precision fitting, and cementing is repeated with the crown casting.

Surgical Crown Lengthening[19]

General Comments

- When teeth are fractured at or near the level of alveolar bone, insufficient crown length may prevent enough retentive surface from being available.
- By decreasing the root length and increasing the crown length, retention may be obtained.

Indications

- Tooth fractured at, near, or below gingival crest.
- Tooth fractured below alveolar crest.
- Inadequate retentive coronal surface.
- Gingival tissue overlying coronal surface.

Contraindications

- Patient will place excessive force on the teeth.
- General health of patient does not allow multiple anesthetic procedures.

Objective

- To expose more tooth surface for crown retention.

Materials

- Materials previously described for crown preparation.
- Oral surgical pack.

Technique

Step 1—The tooth and surrounding tissues are examined for pockets, the depth of keratinized gingiva is measured, and the tooth and surrounding area are "sounded" with an explorer to determine the level of bone and extent of fracture.

Step 2—An inverse-bevel scalloped incision and/or gingivectomy with or without mesial and distal incisions are performed as necessary, as described in Chapter 5, Periodontal Therapy, page 184. The gingival collar is removed.

Step 3—Using both high-speed and hand instrumentation, bone is carefully removed around the tooth to expose the apical level of the tooth fracture.

Step 4—The bone is smoothed and reshaped.

Step 5—The elevated flap is repositioned apically.

Step 6—The crown margins are prepared, built up if necessary, and finished in routine fashion.

Special Teeth

Canine Teeth

Step 1—Axial reduction is started on the mesial surface. The surface is reduced to the desired amount, and a straight surface is created.

Step 2—The labial and lingual surfaces are reduced until the prepared surfaces approach the 6 degree taper.

Step 3—On the distal surface, the preparation may be "stair-stepped" to create parallelism with minimal tooth reduction.

- The first "stair step" starts at the gingival edge and extends coronally as the tooth is reduced.
- The shoulder at the gingival edge is as much as 0.5 mm deeper than others in the preparation.
- When the natural shape of the tooth is tapered to the point that parallelism is not achievable, the next "stair step" is cut.
- Moving coronally, parallelism is created to the limits allowable by the natural shape of the tooth, without excessive tooth reduction, to create a shoulder close to the same dimension as the first shoulder.
- As the preparation is continued coronally, "stair steps" are created as needed.

Step 4—The final margin is finished by creating a bevel at the edge of the shoulder.

- This is best done with a flame-shaped diamond bur, using the beveled end of the bur as a gauge for cutting the tooth.
- The bur is held parallel to the tooth, and the beveled end is moved around the shoulder.
- The final bevel on the tooth is approximately the same size as the beveled end of the bur.
- When a fracture has shortened a tooth, fewer "stair steps" are needed.

Molars and Premolars

- The technique used for molars and premolars is similar to that used for canines and incisors.

Step 1—A tapered diamond bur is used for occlusal and axial preparation of premolars and molars.

- Occlusal reduction is performed only in areas that are actually in occlusion.
- Those surfaces or areas in occlusion with the opposing tooth need to be reduced sufficiently to allow 1 to 1.5 mm of clearance between the restoration and the opposing tooth.
- Sharp edges of cusps are reduced and beveled to facilitate the casting process in the laboratory.
- Axial reduction is created with a round-end diamond bur and is initiated by creating a shoulder at the gingival edge.

Step 2—When the axial reduction is adequate, the edge of the shoulder is beveled with a flame-shaped diamond bur.

- Retention is achieved with creation of parallelism and reduction for space requirements of the crown.
- An adequate approximation of parallelism is easily achieved on the lingual-to-buccal axis.
- The shape of the fourth premolars makes the achievement of parallelism on a mesial-to-distal axis difficult (A).

Step 3—Additional retention is achieved in endodontically treated teeth by preparing the pulp canals, beginning with removal of the gutta-percha with a Peeso reamer to a depth at least equal to the height of the crown (B) (C).

- The canals are prepared with a flat-end tapered diamond bur so the "line of draw" coincides with the long axis of the prepared tooth (D).
- As the bur is moved from one canal to the next, it is held steady so each canal is prepared parallel to the other.

Step 4—The coronal edge of the canal is expanded (beveled outward) to prevent binding as the restoration is seated.

- The remainder of the preparation is identical to that of preparations in canine teeth (E) (F).

Gingival Retraction

Description

- The gingiva may be retracted away from the tooth by using a gingival retraction cord.
- The cord may be precoated with a hemostatic agent or may be dipped into the hemostatic agent.

Use

- Crown therapy.
- Adhesive restorations close to gingiva.
- Hemorrhage control.

Advantage

- Allows better visualization and working space.

Disadvantage

- May occasionally interfere with working space.

Materials

- Gingicord, GingiAid*
- Gingicord packer, Nemitz no. 3.*

Technique

Step 1—The cord is cut to the length of the gingiva to be packed.
Step 2—The cord is packed into the gingival sulcus with a Gingicord packer.

Complications

- Care should be taken not to cut the gingiva.
- Hemorrhage may be controlled by a pinpoint electrocautery.

---

*GingiPak, 4820 Calle Alto, P.O. Box 240, Camarillo, CA 93010

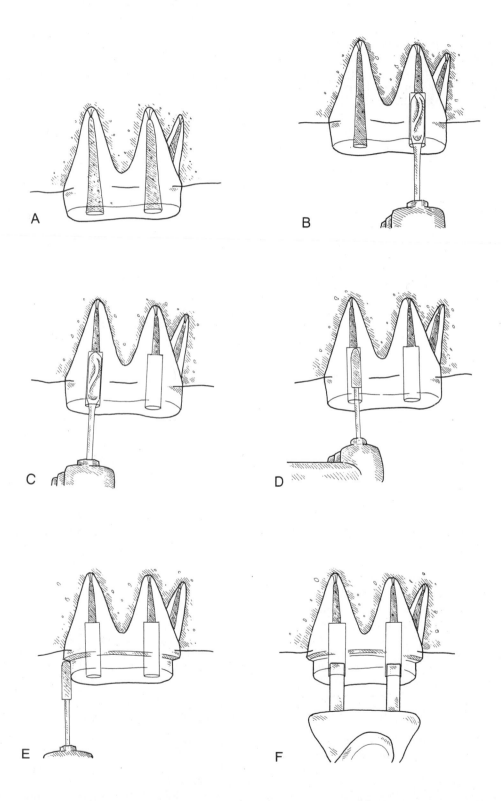

Die Stone

Description

- A harder stone is created by mixing gypsum stone with water, letting the mixture set and dry, and then grinding it again. Die-stone hardener can then be painted on the model to make the molded teeth even harder.

Use

- Restorations.

Advantages

- The stone is harder; gives a better chance to remove from the impression without fracture.
- When mixed in proper weight/volume proportions as directed by the manufacturer, it is more accurate.

Materials

- Mixing bowl.
- Spatula.
- Scale.
- Syringe/measuring cup to measure volume.

Technique

- Mix according to instructions in Chapter 9, page 408.

Improving Metal-to-Cement Adhesion

- Roughening the inside of metal crown surface may improve cement adhesion to the metal. This may be accomplished in the office by using a Micro-etcher.*
- Diamond roughening is not a good way to roughen the crown.
- Chemical-etching is messy, possibly dangerous, and not a good technique.
- The prosthodontic laboratory may be able to sandblast the crown or bridge. In this case, the restoration may be returned in a liquid environment. The crown is protected in this environment until ready for cementation.

---

*Danville Engineering, 1901 San Ramon Valley Rd., San Ramon, CA 94583

Table 8–7 • LINING/BASE MATERIALS

Calcium Hydroxide Cements	
Product	**Manufacturer**
Advanced Formula II Dycal	L. D. Caulk
Life	Kerr
Cavitec	Kerr
Alkaliner	ESPE/Premier
Reocap	Vivadent
Reolit	Vivadent
Prisma VLC Dycal	L. D. Caulk
Handi-Liner Kit	Mizzy
Care	Viadent

Glass Ionomer Liners	
Product	**Manufacturer**
Aqua Cem	Dentsply DeTrey
Fuji Dentin Cement	Fuki
Ketac-Bond	ESPE/Premier
Ketac-Cem	ESPE/Premier
Ketac Silver	ESPE/Premier
Lining Cement	Fuji
Miracle Mix	Fuji
XR Ionomer	Kerr
Shofu Base	Shofu
Shofu Lining	Shofu
Zionomer	Den-Mat

Restorations over Vital Teeth

General Comments

- Restorations placed over vital teeth require special considerations so the pulp tissue is not damaged at the time the restoration is placed or at a later date.
- Lining and base cement materials are used in restorative dentistry as pulp-protection agents (Table 8–7).
- Liners and bases provide insulation under metallic restorative materials and a chemical barrier under plastic restoratives.

Calcium Hydroxide

Description

- Calcium hydroxide lining cements are commonly used to promote pulpal protection and healing.

Advantage

- The alkaline environment encourages remineralization and antibacterial activity.

Disadvantages

- Low strength properties, leading to a weak structure.
- High solubility, leading to resorption of the material.

Resin-Based Calcium Hydroxide

Description

- Calcium hydroxide is incorporated into a resin base.

Advantage

- Easy to use.

Disadvantage

- Little is known of its relative properties and clinical performance.

INDIRECT RESTORATIONS

- An indirect restoration is one that has been fabricated by an outside laboratory.

Indications

- Teeth with large defects that require extensive restoration.
- Desire to use materials that require fabrication beyond the scope of the clinic's facilities or the clinician's expertise.

Examples

- Full- or partial-coverage metal or porcelain-fused-to-metal (PFM) crowns described on the previous pages.

Onlays

Inlays

- In addition to the metal and PFM materials, a very tough, impact- and abrasion-resistant composite has been developed: In-Ceram.*

Uses

- Reconstruction of large carnassial buccal slab fracture defects.
- Reconstruction of distal canine cage biter defects.
- Full-coverage crowns.

Clinical Tips

- Rubber-base impressions of the tooth to be restored and of the two adjacent teeth, along with full-mouth laboratory stone

---

*Vident, 3150 East Birch St., Brea, CA 92621

models and wax bite registers, are requested by most laboratories.
- For crown preparation, a flat-end diamond bur is preferred. Consult with your laboratory for the technician's preference in tooth preparation design for specific restorations.
- For onlay preparation, a 45 degree bevel, diverging from the dentin to the surface of the enamel margin, is preferred. As with any indirect restoration, all undercuts should be avoided.
- A good crown cement is recommended for installation.

Advantages

- Can be used on vital as well as nonvital teeth.
- Can use stronger restorative materials than available to the clinician for direct, in-house use.
- Can reconstruct teeth to original size and shape, which would not be possible by direct restorative techniques.
- Onlays will support and strengthen the crown beneath the fabricated restoration, as a splint would support a long bone.

Disadvantages

- More than "one-stop shopping" for the client, requiring two stages and general anesthetics.
- Expense. Laboratory charges will be similar to those for metal and PFM crown fabrication.

BLEACHING OF NONVITAL TEETH

General Comment

- Stained teeth may be whitened by using concentrated hydrogen peroxide solutions.

Indication

- Bleaching of nonvital teeth.

Contraindication

- Is not to be used on vital teeth.

Materials

* 35% hydrogen peroxide* (active and walking techniques).
* Peroxyborate monohydrate (walking technique).

Techniques[20, 21]

Active Technique

Step 1—Root canal therapy is performed; a liner is placed over the gutta-percha in the root canal to prevent penetration of the hydrogen peroxide into the apex.

Step 2—The gingiva is coated with petroleum jelly.

Step 3—A rubber dam is placed over the tooth.

Step 4—A clamp is placed.

Step 5—The rubber dam is ligated with floss.

Step 6—The pulp chamber and surface of the tooth are acid-etched for 60 seconds with phosphoric acid.

Step 7—The pulp chamber is thoroughly rinsed with water for 1 minute and dried.

Step 8—Cotton pellets or paper points are saturated with 35% hydrogen peroxide.

Step 9—The saturated paper points or cotton pellets are placed into and around the tooth. Alternatively, the cotton pellets or paper points may be placed in the canal before saturating the canal with hydrogen peroxide.

Step 10—Heat is applied to the tooth surface with a heating unit, Heat 'N Touch unit, or hair dryer. Heat should be applied to each surface for 60 seconds.

Step 11—The pellets and cotton points are replaced several times, for a total of four to six cycles.

Step 12—If bleaching is obtained, the pulp chamber is rinsed thoroughly for at least 1 minute with water and dried with paper points.

Step 13—The coronal portion of the canal and the access site are restored.

Walking Technique

Steps 1 through 11—The tooth is prepared as in the active technique.

Step 12—Peroxyborate monohydrate is mixed with 30% hydrogen peroxide to form a thick paste.

Step 13—The paste is placed into the pulp chamber, leaving space for the temporary filling material.

Step 14—A cotton pellet is placed over the paste.

Step 15—The access opening is sealed with a glass ionomer or zinc phosphate base.

Step 16—The patient is returned for re-examination and replacement of the walking paste as needed.

Step 17—Once the tooth is bleached, a restoration is placed.

Complications

* Leakage of hydrogen peroxide under the rubber dam.
* Irritation/burning of the gingiva.
* Safety goggles must be worn at all times during bleaching procedures by all staff in the dental area; extremely caustic agents are used.

Aftercare

* Tooth-whitening pastes may be beneficial in keeping the tooth bleached.

REFERENCES

1. Basrani E. Fractured Teeth. Philadelphia: Lea & Febiger, 1985.
2. Phillips RW. Skinner's Science of Dental Materials, 8th ed. Philadelphia: W.B. Saunders Co., 1982:646.
3. Zwemer TJ. Boucher's Clinical Dental Terminology, 3rd ed. St. Louis: C.V. Mosby Co., 1982.
4. Leinfelder KF, Lemons JE. Clinical Restorative Materials and Techniques. Philadelphia: Lea & Febiger, 1989:359.
5. Tholen M. Veterinary restorative dentistry: Basic principles. Veterinary Medicine Small Animal Clinic 1983; 12:1875–1880.
6. Croll TP. Repair of defective class I composite resin restorations. Quintessence Int 1990; 21(9).
7. Eisner ER. Chronic subgingival tooth erosion in cats. Vet Med 1989; 84:378–387.
8. Emily P. Restoring feline cervical erosion lesions. Vet Forum 1988; 10:22–23.
9. Lyon KF. Subgingival odontoclastic resorptive lesions. Vet Clin North Am 1992; 22:1417–1432.
10. Ben-Amar A. Reduction of microleakage around new amalgam restorations. J Am Dent Assoc 1989; 119:725–728.
11. Marzouk MA, Simoton AL, Gross RD. Operative Dentistry. St Louis: Ishiyaku, 1985.
12. Shillingburg HT, Sumiya H, Fisher DW. Preparations for Cast Gold Restorations. Die Quintessenz 1974:16, 25, 31, 147.

---

*Superoxol, Union Broach Dental Products, Division of Moyco Industries, 589 Davies Dr., York, PA 17402

13. Craig RG, O'Brien WJ, Powers JM. Gold and Nonprecious Alloys. In: Dental Materials, Properties and Manipulation, 6th ed. St. Louis: Mosby, 1996:214–229.

14. Johnson JF, Phillips RW, Dykema RW. Modern Practice in Crown and Bridge Prosthodontics. Philadelphia: W.B. Saunders Co., 1971:59, 374.

15. Coelho DH, Rieser JM. A Complete Fixed Bridge Procedure. New York: New York University Press, 1963:29, 38.

16. Seluk LW. Successful Glass Ionomer Techniques. Palo Alto: Shofu Dental Corporation, 1989.

17. Smith DC, Ruse ND. Acidity of glass ionomer cements during setting and its relation to pulp sensitivity. J Am Dent Assoc 1986;119:654–657.

18. Fahrenkrug P. Crowns: Indication, Preparation, Proceedings. Meeting of the Academy of Veterinary Dentistry and the American Veterinary Dental College. New Orleans, 1989.

19. Limardi RJ. A Surgical Approach for Increasing Crown Length. Meeting of the Academy of Veterinary Dentistry and the American Veterinary Dental College. Las Vegas, 1990.

20. Golden AL. Vital and Non Vital Bleaching Techniques. New Orleans: Nabisco, 1988.

21. Wiggs RB, Lobprise HB. Veterinary Dentistry Principles and Practice. Philadelphia: Lippincott-Raven, 1997.

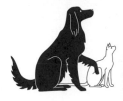

Chapter 9

DENTAL ORTHODONTICS

OCCLUSAL (BITE) EVALUATION

- Bite evaluation involves more than just the relationship of the incisors to each other and number of teeth. The entire mouth and dentition are used to evaluate occlusion properly.

  Step 1—Observe the symmetry of the head, face, and dentition.

- The midpoints of the mandibular and maxillary dental arches should be in alignment with the midsagittal plane of the head.

  Step 2—Count the teeth.

- All teeth should be present.

  Canine Dental Formula

Primary (Deciduous)

$$2\left(i\frac{3}{3}c\frac{1}{1}p\frac{3}{3}\right) = 28$$

Secondary (Adult)

$$2\left(I\frac{3}{3}C\frac{1}{1}P\frac{4}{4}M\frac{2}{3}\right) = 42$$

Feline Dental Formula
Primary (Deciduous)

$$2\left(i\frac{3}{3}c\frac{1}{1}p\frac{3}{2}\right) = 26$$

Secondary (Adult)

$$2\left(I\frac{3}{3}C\frac{1}{1}P\frac{3}{2}M\frac{1}{1}\right) = 30$$

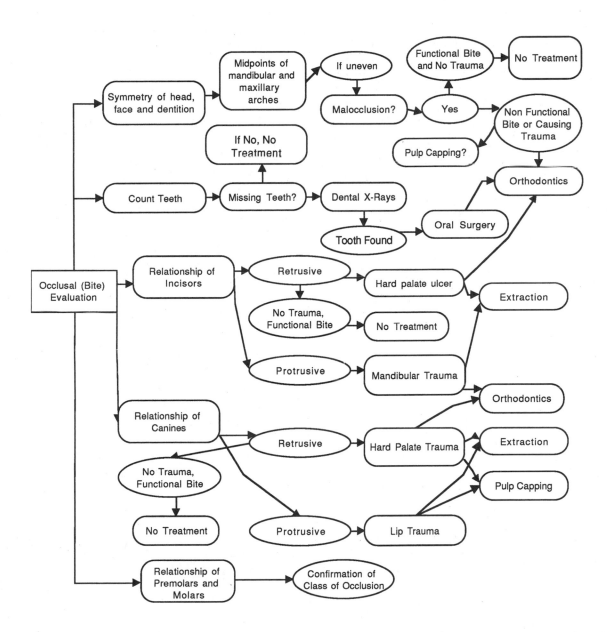

Step 3—Evaluate the occlusion of the incisors *(A)*. The normal head type in feral dogs is the mesocephalic head as seen in the German shepherd. The line of the teeth is seen as a smooth, symmetrical curve not broken by rotated or misplaced teeth. All other relationships, for scientific purposes, must be considered to be in malocclusion to a greater or lesser degree.[1] The normal incisor occlusion has the large cusps of the lower incisors occluding near the cingulum on the lingual side of the upper incisors *(B)*. The large cusps of the central incisors should be centered with each other. The second and third incisors lose their centered relationship, and the large cusp of the third mandibular incisor should be in the interproximal space between the second and third maxillary incisors.

Step 4—Observe the relationship of the canine teeth *(C)*.

- The mandibular canine tooth should occlude buccal to the gingiva of the maxilla and should be equidistant between the maxillary canine tooth and the maxillary third incisor.
- This is the most reliable reference point in the mouth.[2]

Step 5—Observe the relationship of the premolars *(D)*.

- The large cusp on the lower fourth premolar should divide the space between the upper third and fourth premolars, the central cusp pointing interproximally between the two teeth.

Step 6—Observe the occlusal plane of the upper and lower arches *(E)*.

- The premolars should interdigitate from the second premolars back to the cusps of the upper fourth premolar, and there should be overlapping of the cusp tips.
- The molars should occlude to allow the cusps to function in crushing.
- The premolars and molars should be aligned mesial to distal in a smooth curve, with none of the teeth rotated.

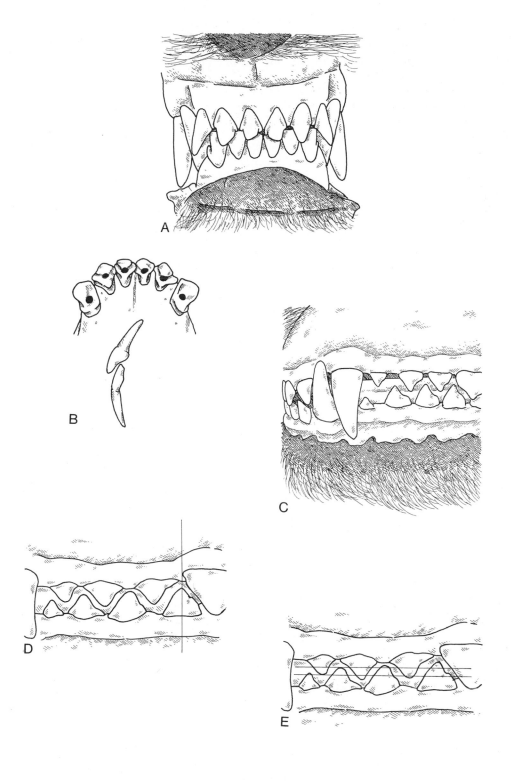

Classes of Occlusion

Normal

- Scissor bite: normal occlusion pattern in which the lower incisors occlude on the cingulum on the palatal surface of the upper incisors. The upper and lower premolars are in an anisognathic, shearing relationship with the maxillary teeth buccal to the mandibular teeth. The upper and lower arches are symmetrical.

Class 1

- Patients with class 1 malocclusion have a normal occlusion with one or more teeth out of alignment or rotated. It may present in any one of four basic formats: (1) a shift in the interdigitating relationship of the maxillary and mandibular premolars; (2) an anterior crossbite (see below); (3) a base narrow mandibular canine tooth or teeth; and (4) posterior crossbite of the premolars or molars.
- Anterior crossbite: a common abnormal occlusion in which one or more of the lower incisors are anterior to the upper incisors *(A)* and, most importantly, the rest of the teeth occlude normally.
- Base narrow or lingually displaced canine teeth: one or both of the tips of the mandibular canine teeth are displaced lingually and occlude on the hard palate *(B)*. Similar trauma may also occur in class 2 malocclusions.
- Rostrally angled maxillary canine teeth: these can be unilateral or bilateral and are most frequent in the Shetland sheepdog. The maxillary canine tooth erupts at an angle creating interference with the mandibular canine tooth, whereas the rest of the occlusion is generally normal. This occlusion is also known as lance tooth or spear tooth and can be seen in other breeds and in cats.

Class 2

- Patients with class 2 occlusion have the lower premolars and molars positioned caudal (distal) to the normal relationship *(C) (D)*. This occlusion is also known as mandibular brachygnathism, overshot, retrusive mandible, or distal mandibular excursion.

Class 3

- Patients with class 3 occlusion have the lower premolars and molars positioned rostral (mesial) to the normal relationship *(E)*. This occlusion is also known as prognathism, undershot, protrusive mandible, or mesial mandibular excursion. A level bite (often called an "even" bite by breeders) is a mild form of class III malocclusion. A reverse scissor bite is a class III occlusion that is a little more pronounced. In that case, the incisal edges of the maxillary incisors make contact with the lingual surface of the mandibular incisors. A true underbite is one in which the mandibular incisors are rostral to the maxillary incisors and not in contact with them.
- Level bite: an abnormal occlusal pattern in which the upper and lower incisors occlude cusp to cusp (edge to edge). This is a very punishing malocclusion, resulting in premature wear to the incisors, a predisposition to inflammatory periodontal problems and, to a lesser extent, endodontic disease.

Unclassified

- Wry bite: an abnormal occlusion caused by a difference in length of the two maxillae and mandibles. This abnormal occlusion is reported to be genetically created and can result in a variety of different jaw relationships. It is characterized by asymmetry of the head in which the midline of the maxilla does not align with the midline of the mandible.

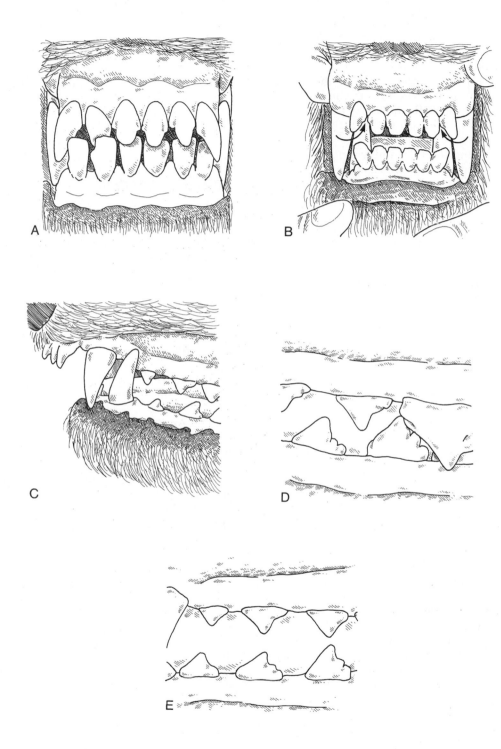

Orthodontic Fundamentals

- Tooth roots are held in the alveolus by the periodontal ligament (PDL), which attaches to the cementum on the tooth and the alveolar bone of the dental arch.
- Osteoclasts and osteoblasts occur in the alveolar bone.
- Forces applied to the crown of the tooth are transmitted by the PDL to the bone.
- Stretching the PDL applies a pull on the alveolar bone and stimulates the osteoblasts to deposit new bone.
- Compressing the PDL and compressing the periodontal space applies compressive pressure to the alveolar bone and stimulates osteoclasts to resorb bone.
- The magnitude of the force applied to the crown of the tooth is critical. If the force exceeds the capillary blood pressure in the PDL, then the PDL will necrose or hyalinize and become cell-free. Osteoclasts then remove bone in the hyalinized area, and tooth movement continues again.
- Types of movement are created by the way the force is applied to the tooth:

  Tipping: one part of the tooth moves a greater distance and direction than another *(A)* (requires light force).

  Translation or bodily: all parts of the tooth move the same distance in the same direction in the same amount of time *(B)* (requires twice the force of tipping).

  Rotational: tooth is rotated around its axis *(C)* (requires light force).

  Intrusion: tooth is moved into the alveolus *(D)* (requires the greatest amount of force).

  Extrusion: tooth is moved out of the alveolus *(E)* (requires the least amount of force).

- Duration of the force also influences the response. The three classes of duration are:

  Continuous: force gradually diminishes (but does not reach zero) between adjustments.

  Interrupted: force is reduced to zero between adjustments.

  Intermittent: force drops to zero when a removable appliance is removed and regained when the appliance is replaced.

- Anchorage is resistance to unwanted tooth movement.[3] The object is to create a platform from which an orthodontic force may be exerted that will move the active tooth and only minimally move the anchorage tooth/teeth (unless one also wants to move the anchorage).
- Once tooth movement to the desired position has been obtained, the tooth or teeth must be maintained in their desired position; in veterinary orthodontics this is usually 2 to 4 weeks. This is known as the retention period.

Legal and Ethical Considerations

Before accepting a patient for orthodontic correction, the client should be advised of the potential legal and ethical implications of these procedures. A release, approved by the practitioner's attorney, should be signed by the client. The following release is a sample only.

Agreement and Consent for Orthodontics

The correction of malocclusions in animals has moral, ethical, and legal implications. In addition, the rules of many breed clubs and organizations state that any animal that has been altered is subject to disqualification from showing.

Because many orthodontic conditions are inherited, we strongly recommend that such animals treated for orthodontic conditions not be used for breeding purposes. Such an animal should be neutered, rendering it incapable of being shown in conformation classes.

We believe that all pets are entitled to a comfortable, functional bite. There is nothing wrong with the correction of an acquired malocclusion, but please do not ask us to be an accomplice to fraud.

My signature authorizing treatment indicates that I have read and understand the above information.

Signature of Client/Owner and Date

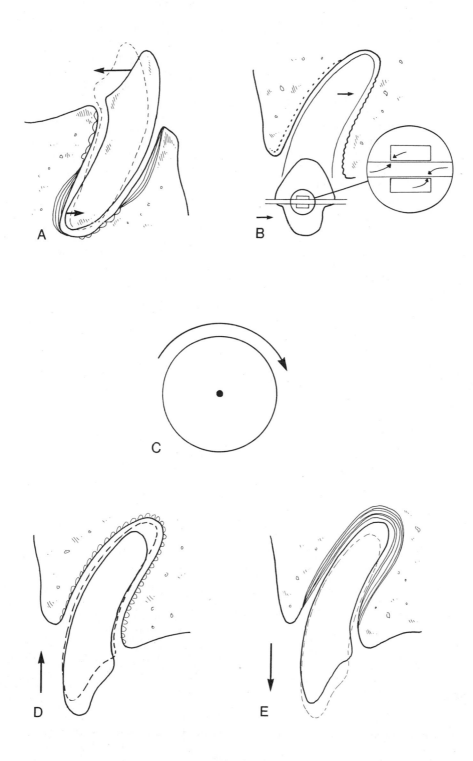

GENERAL ORTHODONTIC TECHNIQUES

Making an Impression Tray

General Comment

- There are several styles of premade impression trays of various sizes designed for use in cats and dogs. Human impression trays have been used but do not allow access to the caudal teeth, which are important when evaluation of the entire occlusion is desired and when making models that are to be placed on an articulator for the proper occlusal relationship.

Indication

- When a preformed impression tray is not available or is not of the correct size for the patient.

Contraindication

- Do not use soft flexible materials that will allow distortion of the alginate before pouring of the casts.

Materials

- Formatray.*
- Easy Tray.†
- Hydroplastic (thermomalleable material) custom-molded material.

Technique

Step 1—Follow manufacturer's instructions for preparing material. You may soften material with warm water or mix powder and liquid (Formatray).

Step 2—Shape material to desired form on model or in patient's mouth.

Step 3—Allow to harden.

Step 4—Trim rough edges before use.

Complications

- Material setting too quickly.
- Acetone odor of Formatray very strong.

---

*Kerr Corporation, 1717 West Collins, Orange, CA 92867

†Oral Dynamics, 2209 North 56th, Seattle, WA 98103

Creating the Impression

General Comments

- A good impression and model are necessary for many dental procedures.
- They allow a practitioner to study and measure the oral architecture, to confer with a colleague or laboratory, and to fabricate prostheses and appliances.
- They are an excellent medical record.
- An impression must be an accurate representation of the structure studied.
- Sedating the patient heavily or submitting the patient to general anesthesia is required for making accurate impressions.

Indication

- Any time a model is needed for study, treatment planning, or appliance fabrication.

Contraindication

- Uncooperative patient or patient unable to undergo general anesthesia.

Materials

- Impression tray (do not use styrofoam cups, cut soft plastic bottles, etc. as trays because they are too unstable).
- Alginate.
- Bowl and spatula.
- Room-temperature water.
- Bite-registration material.

Technique

Step 1—Select an impression tray that fits over all the teeth loosely (A).

Step 2—The alginate is "fluffed" by gently rolling or shaking the container. The powder is allowed to settle to avoid a particle dust cloud when the container is opened (dustless alginate is available).

Step 3—The alginate is measured into the mixing bowl with the measuring spoon provided with the alginate (B). The amount will depend on the size of the tray used. Experiment until you know how much alginate a particular tray size needs (generally two to three scoops for small breeds or anterior teeth only, and four to six scoops for a full tray). The alginate is placed in the rubber mixing bowl (C).

Step 4—Water is measured with the container provided with the alginate *(D)*. If tap water is too cold or too hot, water is used from a storage flask at room temperature to avoid variations in setting time caused by water temperature. Water temperature affects the setting speed of the alginate (warmer water increases setting time; colder water decreases it). All the water is poured into the bowl with the alginate at the same time *(E)*.

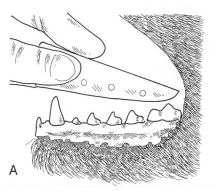

A

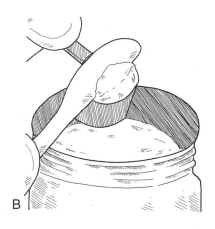

B

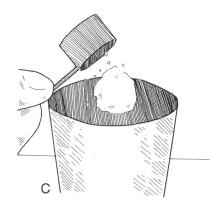

C

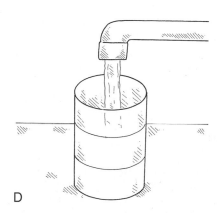

D

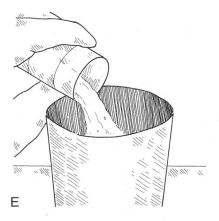

E

Step 5—The alginate and water are mixed with the spatula *(A)*. Incorporate all the powder first by mixing in the center of the bowl. Smooth the mix by spatulating the mixture against the sides of the bowl *(B)*. The bowl is held in one hand, and the spatula is used to spread the mixture vigorously onto the sides of the bowl. Turn the bowl while spatulating to get a more homogeneous mixture. The entire mixing procedure should be completed in 30 to 45 seconds. The mixing is finished when all the lumps are removed and the consistency is homogeneous.

Step 6—The alginate is placed in the tray; any air bubbles or voids are removed *(C)*.

- The surface is smoothed and lightly dampened with water.

Step 7—With the patient in sternal recumbency for the maxilla and dorsal recumbency for the mandible, the tongue is rolled back into the pharynx and the lips are held back; while the patient's mouth is held open, the tray with the alginate is carefully placed in the mouth *(D)*. Contact with the teeth is first made in the caudal portion of the mouth, and the tray is gently rocked forward to incorporate the teeth in the anterior portion of the mouth *(E)*.

- Once the tray is in position, it is held steady until the alginate has set. The amount of time depends on the alginate used and the temperature of the water (usually 3 to 7 minutes).
- The setup is tested by pressing a finger on exposed alginate. When the finger does not stick or leave an indentation, the alginate has set.

Step 8—The tray with the alginate is removed from the mouth by firmly snapping the tray off the teeth *(F)*.

- The impression is examined for voids, flaws, or bubbles. If there is an imperfection in the impression in a critical area, the impression should be retaken. If the model is not going to be poured immediately, wrap the alginate and tray in a damp paper towel *(G)*. (Do not soak the tray and alginate in water because it will absorb water and distort the impression.) For accurate representation, laboratory stone should be poured into the alginate impressions within 30 minutes.

Step 9—Bite registration is critical for helping the dental laboratory determine the proper relationship of the two jaws so as to be able to manufacture an appliance or a crown. To record the correct articulation after the impressions are made and just before the patient is awakened, the patient is extubated, and the bite registration is taken. A sheet of bite wax, which is often made of beeswax, is softened in warm water, placed in the mouth, and the patient is made to bite down on it. As an alternative to the bite wax, special bite impression registration materials are available that can be injected into the occlusal space.

Complications

- Inadequate mixing will leave lumps and voids in the alginate. To prevent this, mix the alginate thoroughly.
- Too thin a mixture will not have enough body and will tend to run out of the tray and not stay around the teeth. Follow the manufacturer's instructions on the mix and adjust only if necessary, in small increments.
- Too firm a mixture will not conform to the teeth and mouth well and, thus, will provide poor detail. Correct by creating a thinner mix.
- If the tray is not filled properly, voids (bubbles) may be incorporated into the impression. Fill the tray completely and smoothly.
- Bubbles can be trapped when the tray is placed in the mouth. To prevent bubbles, slowly place the tray caudally to rostrally.
- Movement while the alginate is setting will cause distortion. Because movement is generally caused by the patient, adequate sedation or general anesthesia of the patient is suggested.
- The alginate may tear when removed from the mouth. This is especially a problem in the mandibular canine teeth, which are splayed at their coronal end. Slow removal of the impression as well as a slight rotational movement will help prevent tearing. A minimal tear may not cause distortion and can be corrected on the model later.
- Alginate will become distorted if the water content changes between the time when the impression is taken and when the model is poured. Alginate will become distorted also if the tray is not solid.

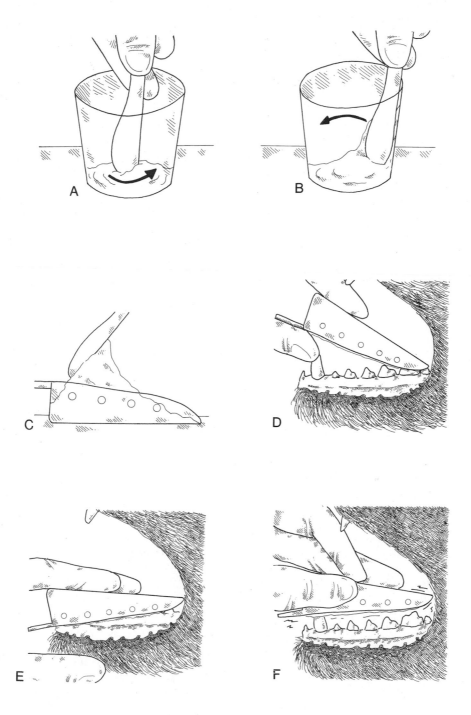

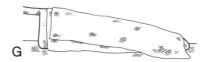

Making a Model

General Comment

- Once the impression is made, a model should be poured as soon as possible.

Indications

- The model is used as part of the medical record.
- With a model, oral structures can be evaluated extraorally, orthodontic bite evaluation can be made, and a treatment plan can be created for orthodontic appliances or crown and bridge fabrication.
- The model or a copy of the model may be used to fabricate appliances or may be used in oral surgery for production of an acrylic splint.
- The model may be used to facilitate communication with colleagues or laboratory personnel.
- The model may be used as a visual aid in discussing the case with the client, showing the indicated treatment and how the appliance will function.
- The model may also be used for forensic documentation and evaluation.

Materials

- An accurate impression.
- Die stone. There are several types of plaster and dental stone, depending on the manufacturing process. Type II plaster has low strength and hardness and is often used as the base for models. Type III dental stone has moderate strength and is often used for fabrication of dentures. Type IV stone (die stone) has high strength and hardness with minimal setting expansion and is the preferred stone in veterinary dentistry. Type V stone has high strength and a high setting expansion and is for use with alloys.
- Mixing bowl and spatula.
- Vibrator.
- Scale.

Technique

- It is often beneficial to mix a small amount of stone with a more fluid consistency first to allow flowing of the stone into the indentations made by the teeth when placed on the vibrator. When these areas are filled, a second, thicker batch of stone can be used for the rest of the model.

Step 1—The water is measured and placed in the bowl *(A)*.

Step 2—The stone is measured, ideally by weighing *(B),* and added to the water all at once.

Step 3—Mixing is started in the center of the bowl *(C)*. After all the water is incorporated into the stone, the mixture is spatulated on the sides of the bowl to remove air bubbles and to remove lumps of unmixed powder. The bowl is turned, and spatulation is done in one direction to minimize bubbles.

Step 4—The bowl with the stone can be placed on the vibrator during this process to help remove air bubbles *(D)*.

Step 5—The impression is rinsed gently with water. Excess water is removed with compressed air.

Step 6—An edge of the tray with the impression is placed onto the vibrator *(E)*.

- A small amount of mixed stone is placed in the center of the impression with a small spatula.
- With the aid of the vibrator, the stone is made to flow into the voids made by the teeth. Take enough time to allow the stone to move into the voids without trapping air. This is the most critical part of the process.
- For smaller teeth, a disposable brush may be used to place a small amount of mixed stone into the individual teeth impressions; avoid bubble formation, especially at the cusps of the teeth.

Step 7—After the stone is spread into the intricacies of the impression and any air bubbles have been vibrated out, the vibrator can be turned off, and additional stone of a thicker consistency is placed on the impression to make the model thick enough to minimize fragility *(F)*.

- Two options are available to make the base of the stone. The first layers of stone that fill in the impression tray can be allowed to harden slightly, and additional stone or plaster is placed on this first layer to create a base as described below. If sufficiently thick stone is used, a one-step model and base can be made without waiting for the stone to initially set.

Step 8—The impression is placed, with the stone in it, on a flat surface and allowed to set for 10 to 15 minutes *(G)*. Additional stone can now be added to the model to create a base. Start by mixing another batch of stone or plaster the same way as previously described.

- Place a layer of the stone onto the bottom of the hardened stone (*H*). It can be shaped to form a flat base, or the prehardened model can be placed upside down onto a block of plaster on a glass slab or countertop and leveled. Excess stone can be re-

moved before it hardens to provide a shaped model when removed from the impression tray, if a model cutter is not available. The stone should be allowed to set for at least 45 minutes.

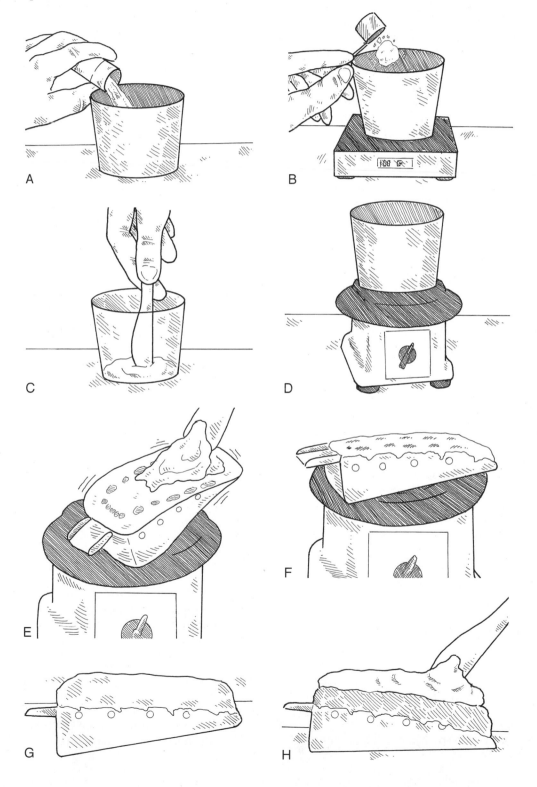

Step 9—The hardened stone is removed from the alginate impression after 45 to 60 minutes *(A)* (usually after the model has cooled following the exothermic cycle of setting). If the alginate is too dry, separation is more difficult. A laboratory knife can be used to free the margins. The model is gradually separated upward from the alginate. Do not rock the model as this may lead to fracture of a canine tooth on the model.

- Another technique is to remove the impression tray first. With the stone down and the alginate on top, a sagittal wedge of alginate is removed with a laboratory knife from the center of the impression. Transverse cuts are then made so that the alginate can be removed segmentally with the knife.

Step 10—After the alginate is removed from the models, the edges of the stone can be trimmed with a model trimmer. The models are placed in occlusion with the bite registration in place, and the caudal aspect and sides of the models are placed against the moving trimmer wheel to align the caudal edges of the upper and lower models. To realign the models, they can be stood on their caudal aspect and gently slid together.

Step 11—Label the model with the patient's and client's name, date made, and the clinic's name.

Complications

Incorrect Mix Ratios

- The stone will not flow if the mixture is too thick. Correct by using a thinner mixture, but changing the proportions from the manufacturer's instructions may cause distortion. A swab stick may be used to stir the thinner mix to help it fill the cusps of the teeth.
- Too thin a mixture will be weak and not as dimensionally stable. Correct by mixing more thickly.

Inadequate Mixing

- Lumps of unmixed stone will be found in the mix. Mix more thoroughly.

Air Bubbles

- Mixing can incorporate air into the stone mixture. Correct by spatulating against the sides of the bowl.
- Air can be trapped in the intricacies of the impression. This usually happens when the stone is placed in the impression too rapidly and is not allowed to flow into the small voids of the impression. Correct by placing small amounts of stone on the impression and allowing it to spread slowly, using the vibrator.
- In deep voids, such as those made by the canine teeth, a small amount of water left in the void will aid in prevention of trapping air.

Flexible Trays

- Allow the impression to become distorted before the stone is poured or set.

Desiccation of the Alginate

- The time between taking the impression and pouring the stone is too long. The stone should be poured quickly after the impression is taken. Wrapping the impression in a damp paper towel until it is poured or when sent to a dental laboratory will diminish this distortion. If the impression is sent to a laboratory before the stone is poured, the alginate wrapped in a damp paper towel should then be placed in a plastic bag until picked up by the laboratory. This will allow the delay of pouring the stone.

Fracturing of Crowns on Model Teeth

- This is often caused by trying to remove the stone from the impression too early *(B)*. Be patient. Even the most patient practitioner will occasionally break a crown as the model is removed from the impression. Most of the time the fractured piece can be placed back in position and cemented. Allow the model and fragment to dry completely.
- After the model is dry, the fractured piece can be repaired either with a glass ionomer cement or with polymethacrylate *(C) (D)*.
- For very long teeth with narrow diameters, a small piece of orthodontic wire (24 to 26 gauge) may be placed into the impression before pouring the model. This will support the teeth and will prevent fracture.
- The dry model may also be coated with a liquid model hardener to reduce breakage during shipment and handling.

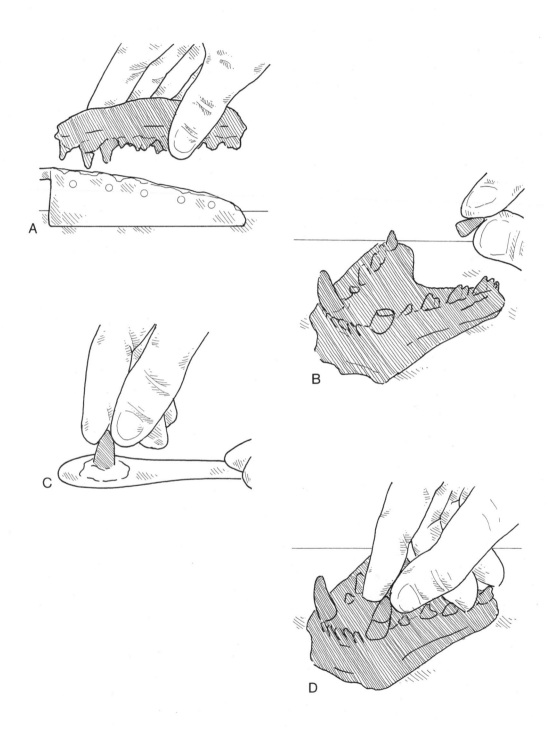

Direct Bonding of Bands, Brackets, and Buttons

General Comments

- Brackets or buttons are bonded to teeth to attach devices for applying forces to achieve orthodontic movement.
- Bands can be used alone for attachment of elastics or arch wires or are incorporated into an appliance for fixation to the teeth.

Indications

- Attachment of fixed or removable acrylic or metal appliances.
- Attachment of lingual or labial arch wires.
- Attachment of acrylic or metal appliances.
- For orthodontic movement with elastics.

Contraindication

- Patients that cannot be controlled or that chew on hard objects.

Materials

- Bands, brackets, and/or buttons.
- Orthodontic bonding agent or light-cured composite resin with bonding agent.
- Spatula.
- College pliers.
- Scaler.
- Flour pumice, prophy cup.

Technique

Step 1—The teeth that are to have brackets attached are scaled to remove any calculus (A).

Step 2—A flour pumice is used to polish and remove any plaque (B).

- Do not use prophy paste because it may contain fluoride, waxes, essential oils, and glycerin that may inhibit the bond.

Step 3—The bracket or button is chosen and trial-placed on the tooth (C). The baseplate should fit the contour of the tooth. If it does not fit, three-pronged pliers are used to bend the bracket or button baseplate to conform to the tooth surface.

Step 4—Phosphoric acid gel is placed on the tooth to etch the surface for 30 to 60 seconds (D). The time depends on the acid concentration and whether the "active" or "passive" technique is used. With the active technique, the operator scrubs the tooth surface with a sponge or brush and acid-etches for a prescribed time. The passive technique allows the phosphoric acid to coat the tooth undisturbed for a prescribed time. Using the active or passive technique depends on the manufacturer's instructions for the bonding agent. These instructions should be followed.

Step 5—Using a three-way syringe, water is used to rinse off the acid (E). It is best to make sure rinsing is complete by continuing the rinsing for 45 to 60 seconds.

Step 6—The tooth is dried using air from the three-way syringe (F) or from a hand-held hair dryer on a low setting. It is critical that this air be free of moisture and oil.

- At this point the area on which the bracket will be placed should have a dull, chalky appearance.
- If contamination of the prepared tooth surface occurs from saliva, blood, oil, or other substance, the preparation should begin again from step 2, but reducing the etching time by 75%. This is a contest between the operator and the environment—if contamination occurs first, the operator loses.

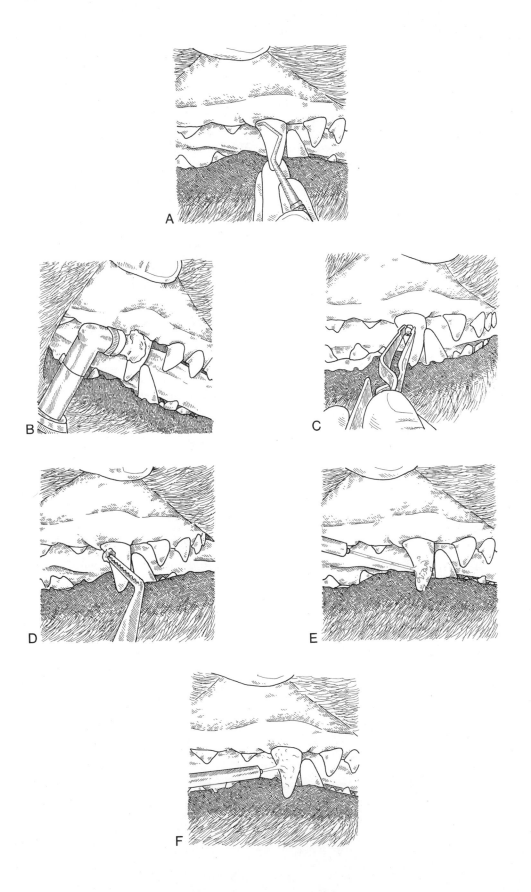

Step 7—The unfilled bonding agent is mixed and applied to the surface of the tooth (A) and to the baseplate of the button or bracket (B).

Step 8—The filled bonding agent is mixed (C) and is placed on the back side of the bracket (D). (Each manufacturer of bonding agents has specific instructions on the way its products should be mixed and handled. These materials are very technique-sensitive.)

Step 9—The bracket is placed on the tooth in the position desired and pressed firmly against the tooth so that some of the bonding agent extrudes around the edges of the bracket (E).

Step 10—Excess bonding agent is removed with a hand scaler before it has set (F). Wait to put a force on the bracket until the bonding agent has had the required time to finish polymerizing (G). The time is stated in the package insert of the bonding agent.

- Test the strength of the bond by putting pressure on the bracket with college pliers. If the bond is not sufficient, it is preferable to have it tested and to rebond it while the patient is under anesthesia than to have the procedure fail, requiring a subsequent visit and additional anesthetic.[2]

Complications

Brackets or Buttons Come Off when Force First Applied

- Usually, directions were not followed meticulously.
- The tooth must be clean, etched, and absolutely dry.

Brackets or Buttons Come Off Later

- Oral abuse, such as chewing on hard objects, can shear brackets or buttons off. Also, long hair, carpet yarn, or strings tangled on the appliance will pull them off. Improper placement of buttons or brackets may result in occlusal interference with the appliance and displacement of the bracket.
- Clients must be advised to protect their investment: during the time of orthodontic treatment, the patient must not be allowed to chew on hard objects.

Discoloration of Tooth when Brackets are Removed.

- This happens when the brackets are not kept clean; cleaning the brackets is one of the reasons for the practitioner to schedule visits for monitoring the patient.

Excess Tension Placed on Active Tooth with Elastic Apparatus Attached to Brackets (or Increased Amount of Pressure or Frequency of Adjustments)

- Pulpitis. The client has changed the elastics and has applied too much pressure on the active tooth.
- Pain and irritability, noted by patient pawing at face or rubbing face on wall or carpet or displaying other neurotic signs. Client or clinician has applied too much tension on the active tooth.

Aftercare

- Routine progress examinations will be needed to evaluate tooth movement and to ensure that proper oral hygiene is being performed.

Removing Buttons and Brackets

- When the treatment is completed, edgewise brackets are easily removed by squeezing the flanges of the bracket with a Howe pliers, snapping the bracket from the tooth.
- Buttons can be removed by grasping the protruding button with a pliers and gently torquing it to release the bond to the tooth.
- The residual cement is removed with a scaler, and the tooth is polished with a fluoride prophy paste.

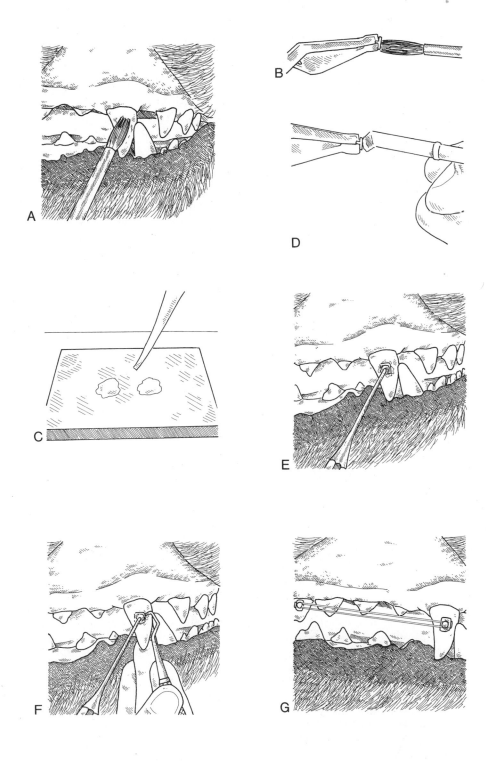

ORTHODONTIC APPLIANCES

Making Bands

General Comments

- Orthodontic bands may be used as alternatives to buttons or brackets.
- Because orthodontic bands wrap around the entire tooth, they provide more bonding surface area and mechanical retention and are more durable than buttons and brackets.
- The bands may have brackets, buttons, pegs, or hooks soldered to them, or bands may be incorporated into arch wires.

Indications

- Orthodontic tooth movement.
- Lingual or labial arch wires.
- Attachment of acrylic or metal appliances.

Contraindication

- Poor client/patient compliance with oral hygiene.

Materials

- Patient's dental model.
- Band material; suggested sizes: 0.150×0.003 inch, 0.150×0.004 inch, 0.180×0.005 inch, and 0.180×0.006 inch.
- Flux; this should be a flux recommended for orthodontic work.
- Silver solder.
- Gas torch.
- Welder (optional).
- Orthodontic bonding material or luting cement (acrylic, composite resin, zinc oxide–eugenol, or glass ionomer).

Technique

Step 1—A dental stone model is manufactured as previously described in this chapter.

Step 2—The band material is contoured to conform to the tooth shape on the model at the location where the band will be placed.

Step 3 (optional)—The band material is clamped to secure its shape with hemostats and is removed from the model. The band material may be spot "tack" welded to hold it in place. The band material is replaced on the model.

Step 4—The ends of the band material are bent along the portion of the band circling the tooth.

Step 5—Excess band material is trimmed and removed.

Step 6—Flux is applied to the band in the area to be soldered.

Step 7—The band is soldered.

- Arch wires or buttons may be soldered or welded onto the band.

Step 8—The tooth to be banded is prepared for button or bracket placement.

Step 9—The orthodontic bonding cement is mixed and applied to the inside of the band *(A)*.

Step 10—The band is placed over the crown of the tooth to be banded *(B)*.

Step 11—The band is firmly seated with pliers *(C)* or a band pusher. Excess cement is removed with a curette.

Complications

- Excess heat applied to the band may melt and destroy the band.
- Poor cementing technique may cause the band to detach from the tooth or may create voids that lead to microleakage, causing decay beneath the band, observed as a black stain in the tooth enamel when the band is removed.

Removing Bands

- Bands can be removed by using band-removing pliers, which have a narrow edge that catches the apical edge of the band while the opposite jaw has a cup that is placed on the cusp tip. The pliers are squeezed, the cement seal is broken, and the band is dislodged. Excessive force may damage the cusp tip. It may be necessary to cut cast bands with a diamond bur.
- Remnants of cement are removed with a hand or ultrasonic scaler, sonic scaler, or finishing bur (glass ionomer cements are more easily removed than composite luting cements). Some crown cements may have more bonding strength than desirable.
- The tooth is polished with a fluoride prophy paste.

Indirect Bonding of Brackets

General Comment

- Allows precise placement of brackets on teeth.

Indications

- Correction of rotated teeth.
- Placement of an edgewise appliance.

Contraindications

- Inadequate home care.
- Oral abuse by the patient.

Materials

- Brackets.
- Silicone high- and low-viscosity impression material.

- Alginate.
- Die stone.
- Laboratory knife.
- Water-soluble adhesive.
- Bonding material.

Technique

Step 1—Impressions are taken and models are made as previously described.

Step 2—The bracket location is marked on the model with a pencil (*D*).

Step 3—A line is drawn to mark the long axis; the exact location of bracket is determined on these two lines (*E*).

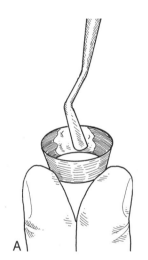

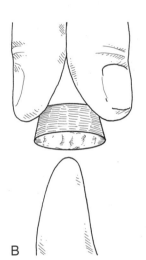

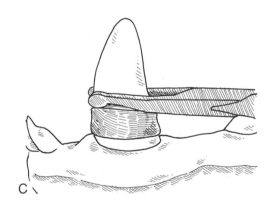

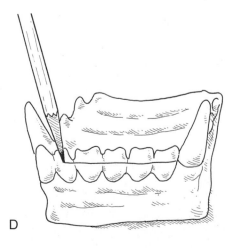

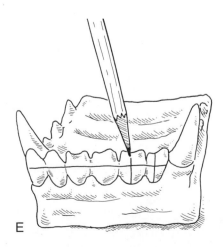

A   B   C

D   E

Step 4—A small dot of water-soluble adhesive (a sticky piece of candy does well) is applied to the marked bracket location, and the brackets are placed on the model *(A)*.

Step 5—Proper orientation of the brackets is checked.

Step 6—A low-viscosity silicone impression material is mixed.

Step 7—The material is applied around each bracket *(B)*.

Step 8—A high-viscosity material is mixed and applied.

Step 9—Impression material is peeled away from model, leaving brackets in position in the impression *(C)*.

Step 10—The tooth surface is prepared (see p. 412).

Step 11—Bonding material is mixed and applied to brackets *(D)*.

Step 12—Impression material with brackets is placed on patient in proper position; brackets are pressed against the teeth *(E)*.

Step 13—After bonding material has set, impression material is removed, and a wire is placed as needed *(F)*.

Complications

- Incorrect placement of brackets.
- Removal of brackets with impression material.

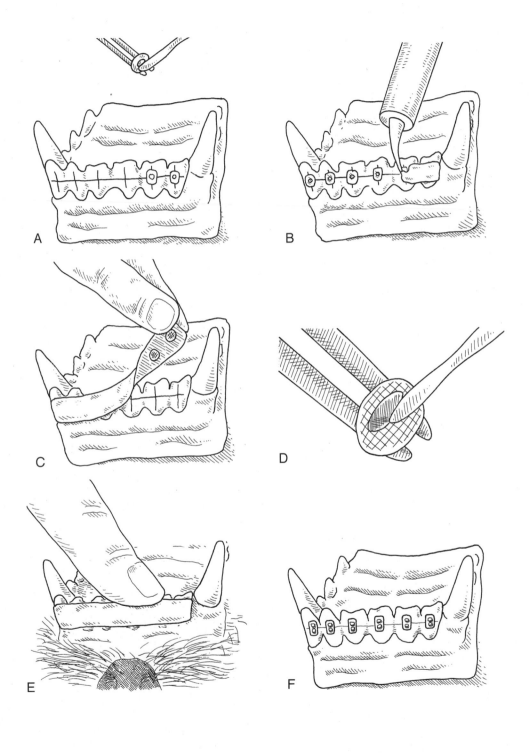

A

B

C

D

E

F

Orthodontic Wire

General Comments

- Orthodontic wire is measured in thousandths of an inch. The higher the number, the greater the cross-sectional area and relative rigidity of the wire.
- The annotation 18-8 indicates that the wire consists of 18% chromium, 8% nickel, and the rest iron.
- Elgiloy wire also contains cobalt and molybdenum. The ends of the wire have paint on them to indicate various wire characteristics: (1) red paint indicates greater spring in the wire, but that the wire is brittle, and therefore no sharp bends should be made; (2) green paint indicates good spring temper, but the wire should not be used for welding or soldering; (3) yellow paint indicates the wire is ductile, that it has good spring, and that it bends easily; and (4) blue paint indicates the wire has soft and regular temper, can be soldered, and can be welded with low heat.
- All Elgiloy wire can be heat-treated to increase spring quality.
- Proportional limit, a property of wire, is the wire's ability to return to its original position when it is bent and released. If pressure continues to be applied, the wire will reach a stress point and not return to its original position because permanent deformation has occurred.
- The bird-beak pliers is a universal pliers in orthodontics; the conical tip creates a uniform curvature. The pyramid tip bends or adjusts loops at sharp angles. The actual bends are made by applying pressure with fingers.

Techniques

- To cut the wire, the wire should be held in one hand, grasping and controlling both ends as the cut is made. The cutters should be held firmly in the other hand (A).

- To create a smoothly curved arch, the wire is held with the pliers in one hand, and the thumb or index finger is drawn over the wire against the conical tip in a downward motion (B). Repeating the process will draw the curve tighter.
- To create a right-angle bend, the wire is held in the bird-beak pliers, and bent over the pyramid tip.
- Smaller bends and loops are made with the conical beak, with the position of the wire on the cone determining the diameter of the loop.

Soldering Techniques

General Comment

- Flux protects metal and solder from oxidation.

Technique

- In this technique, a smaller wire will be soldered to a larger wire.

  Step 1—Place flux on tip of the smaller wire (C).

  Step 2—The wire is heated by bringing it to the top of the flame (D).

  Step 3—Solder is touched to the wire, and the solder is fed from a coil to make a 2 mm–diameter ball of solder and flux (E).

  Step 4—To weld the wires together, the larger wire is held in flame and heated (F).

  Step 5—The wire with solder is then touched near the larger wire. The solder should flow towards the flame (G).

  Step 6—Excess solder can be removed with a bur or with a rubber wheel in a handpiece.

Complications

- Overheating the wire to cherry-red causes it to be annealed and destroys its spring temper, making it unsuitable for holding or working arch functions.

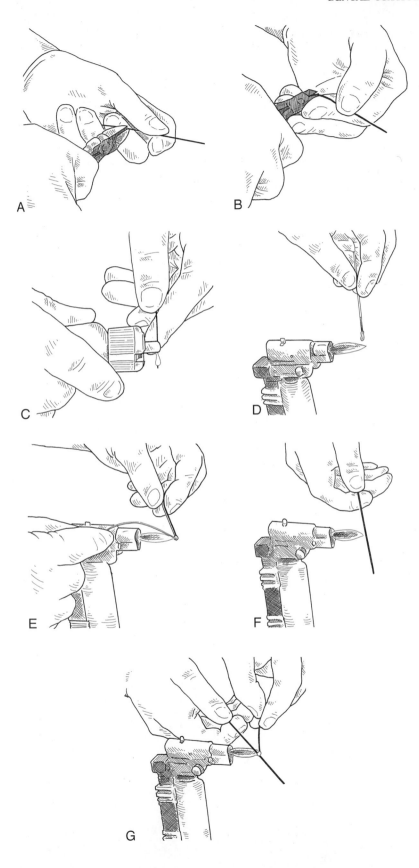

Making Acrylic Appliances

General Comment

- An acrylic appliance may be manufactured either by a dental laboratory or by the practitioner.[4, 5]

Indications

- Orthodontic tooth movement.
- Splinting of avulsed teeth.
- Splinting of oral fractures.

Contraindications

- Severely infected areas.
- Uncooperative patients that may not allow oral hygiene.

Materials

- Dental model as previously described. It is recommended that a second "working model" be manufactured, whether by taking a second impression on the patient, by pouring two models from the first impression, or by taking an impression of the first model and pouring a second model from this impression.
- Tin foil "substitute": material to inhibit bonding of acrylic to the working model.

- Rope wax.
- Sticky wax.
- Dental acrylic (denture-type material).
- Ruby laboratory burs.
- Wax-carving instrument.
- Propane or alcohol torch.

Technique (Beginning)

Step 1—The area on the model where the appliance will be built is coated with the tin foil substitute and is allowed to dry (A).

Step 2—Rope wax is placed around the area for which the appliance is to be manufactured (B).

Step 3—Any wires, such as finger springs, retaining wires, etc., are bent and placed on the model in the desired position (C).

Step 4—Sticky wax is placed by heating a wax-carving instrument and dipping it into the hardened wax so the wax melts onto the instrument (D) and flows onto the model and wire (E). When the wax cools, it will harden and hold the wire in the desired position.

Step 5—The acrylic is placed onto the model.

- Three techniques are used to place the acrylic onto the model.
- Any one or all of the techniques may be used.

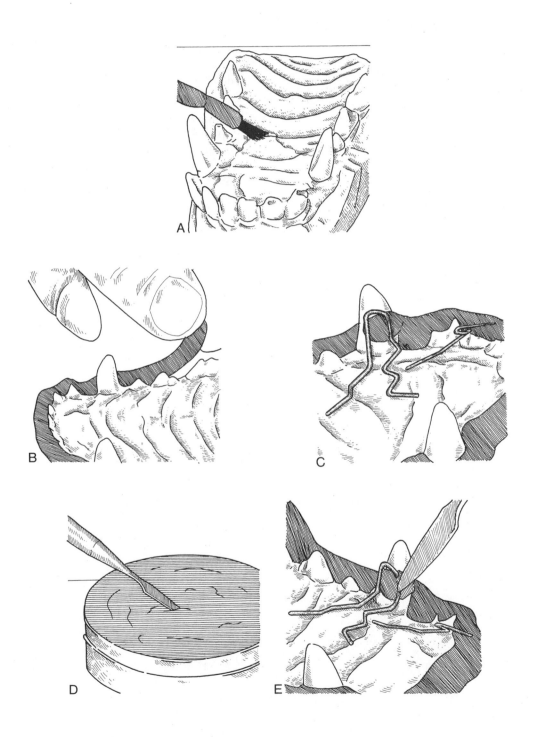

Alternative 1: "Salt and Pepper" Technique

Step 1— A light coating (1 to 2 mm) of the acrylic powder (polymer) is sprinkled from the container onto the model in the area contained by the rope wax *(A)*.

Step 2—Drops of the acrylic liquid (monomer) are dropped onto the powder *(B)*. The powder will undergo a color change as the polymer is wetted (the color depends on the brand and shade).

Step 3—Additional polymer and monomer are added to build up the appliance as desired *(C)*.

Alternative 2: Mixing Technique

Step 1—The powder is placed in a paper cup *(D)*.

- The rubber bowl used for alginate should not be used because the acrylic will destroy the bowl.
- Specially made glass or rubber bowls are made for this use.

Step 2—The liquid is added, according to the manufacturer's directions *(E)*.

Step 3—The liquid and powder are mixed with a spatula *(F)*.

Step 4—The mixture is poured onto the model *(G)*.

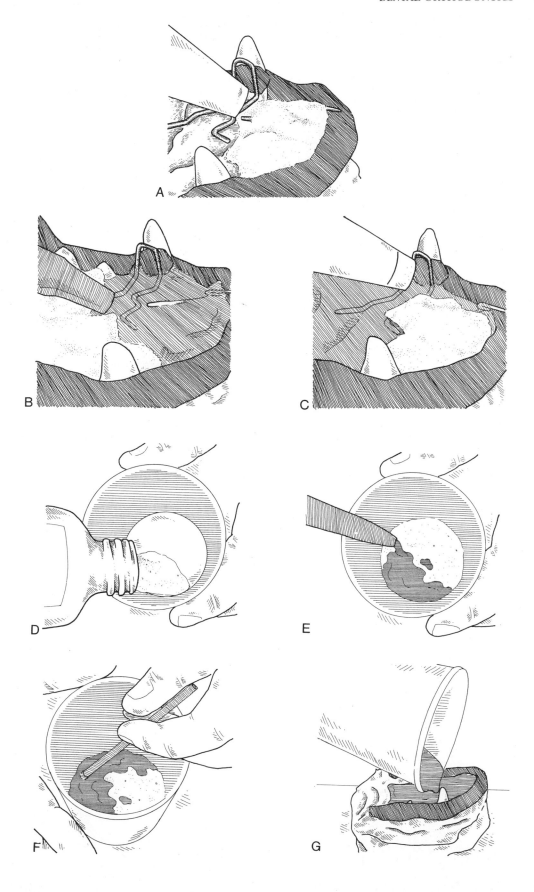

Alternative 3: Brush Technique

Step 1—The polymer and monomer are each placed in dappen dishes (A).

Step 2—A brush is dipped into the polymer (B) and then dipped into the monomer (C) to obtain a small amount of acrylic on the brush tip. The polymer absorbs the liquid monomer.

Step 3—The paste of acrylic is carried and placed on the model in the desired location (D).

• The brush technique allows a precise placement of the dental acrylic.

Technique (Conclusion)

Step 6 (optional)—The model and appliance are placed in a pressure pot, and pressure and heat are applied to eliminate air bubbles and to make a stronger appliance. Acrylic cured in this manner is more transparent.

Step 7—Once hardened, the appliance is removed from the model.

Step 8—With a laboratory bur and low-speed handpiece, the appliance is trimmed and shaped.

Step 9 (optional)—The appliance is smoothed with a polishing wheel.

Complications

Appliance Sticking to Model

• Failure to apply adequate amount of tin foil substitute or releasing agent.

Breakage of Appliance

• The appliance is too thin or needs reinforcing wires.

Breakage of Model

• Breakage of the model while manufacturing the appliance almost always occurs; therefore, a working model should be used. It is helpful to keep a duplicate model at the clinic in these cases.

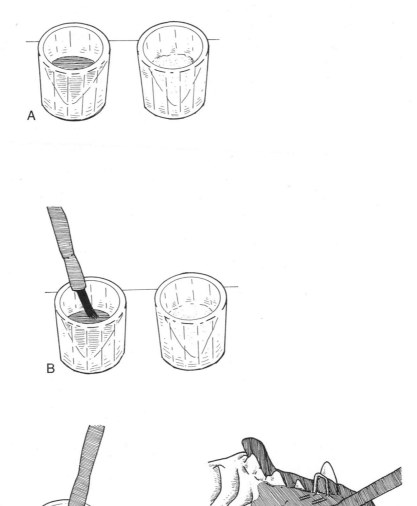

A

B

C

D

INTERCEPTIVE ORTHODONTICS

General Comments

- The "dental interlock" formed by the lower teeth occluding (locking) with the upper teeth inhibits the independent growth and development of the bony structures of the jaws.
- By interfering with this lock, the bony structures are more readily allowed to grow independently of each other and more closely reflect genetic programming.
- Interfering primary teeth are extracted to allow the mandible and faciomaxillary complex to grow independently.
- A primary tooth may be extracted to create space for an adult tooth to erupt unimpeded.

Indications

- Abnormal occlusion in a young patient before the eruption of the adult teeth. Treatment is started as early as possible to allow the longest time for correction to occur before the adult teeth erupt.
- Retained deciduous teeth; any primary tooth that is not lost by the time its homologous adult tooth has begun to erupt.[6–8]

Technique

Step 1—The bite is evaluated, and the desired movement identified. For example, in a patient with a class 2 occlusion, the mandible needs to be longer.

Step 2—Any primary tooth that is inhibiting or would inhibit the desired growth is extracted. Extract the complete tooth and root; do not damage the developing permanent tooth bud.

- In this situation it is better to extract any primary tooth that the clinician believes might be hindering growth than to err by extracting too few teeth.

Complications

- If the entire root is not extracted, eruption of the adult tooth may be hindered.
- Careless extraction techniques may damage the adult tooth.
- Choosing to "wait and watch" will reduce the available catch-up time of the short jaw before the adult teeth erupt.

ORTHODONTIC APPLIANCES

- Many types of orthodontic appliances exist; each is custom-made for the patient.

General Indication

- To correct a malocclusion that is causing or may lead to discomfort or tooth loss. Orthodontic adjustment also has a cosmetic value, which, with due considerations to ethical implications, may be desirable.

General Contraindications

- Ankylosis of teeth.
- Severe periodontal disease associated with teeth in the area of treatment.
- Untrained/unsupervised patients.
- Patients whose oral behavior cannot be controlled.
- Clients who will not comply with oral hygiene or oral hygiene examinations.
- Fraudulent intentions.

Specific Appliances

Button to Button

General Comments

- The movement of a tooth or teeth with elastics or "power chain or cords" attached to the teeth with buttons, brackets, or bands.
- Use of buttons bonded to a tooth to secure an elastic is a straightforward way to achieve simple movement of a single tooth or group of teeth, such as the lower incisors.
- Force vectors are determined by the location of the button placed on the anchor tooth and on the tooth to be moved (active tooth). These forces must be carefully evaluated while placing the buttons so as to guide the movement properly.

Objective

- To achieve tooth movement (usually bodily or tipping) using force created by elastics.

Indications

- Minor displacement of teeth.
- Rostral displacement of maxillary canines.
- Rostral tipping or displacement of mandibular canines.
- To tip mandibular incisors caudally when angled rostrally.
- To tip maxillary incisors when angled caudally.

Contraindications

- Periodontal disease in the treatment area.
- See general contraindications to orthodontic appliances.

Materials

- Orthodontic buttons.
- Preferred button: Ormesh Curved Lingual Pad with button.*
- Flour pumice.
- Prophy cups.
- Orthodontic bonding material.
- Scaler or curette.
- Bracket-holding forceps or cotton pliers.
- Orthodontic elastics of various sizes and strengths.
- Power cord* or masel chain.
- Scissors.

Technique

- Buttons are bonded to the teeth as previously described.
- One or more buttons are placed on the anchor teeth. One deciding factor involves the need for the anchor root(s) to have more total surface area than the root(s) of the active teeth. It may be necessary to unite more than one tooth by buttons and ligature wire to create an appropriate anchor.
- Another button is placed on the tooth to be moved or as support for the elastic across the lower incisors.
- Elastic (masel) chain, power cord, or orthodontic elastics of appropriate size are placed between the buttons to create the desired force on the teeth to be moved.
- The initial force on the teeth is determined by the strength of the elastic or by the number of links between the teeth when using masel chain.
- The exact force to be used depends on the type of power chain, age of patient, size of tooth, and which tooth is to be moved, etc. The best guideline is to start with a light force and increase the force in subsequent visits if the desired movement is not being obtained.

*Ormco Corporation, 1332 South Lone Hill Ave., Glendora, CA 91740

Displaced Maxillary Canines

- Occasionally (most often in Shetland sheepdogs) the maxillary canine is angled rostrally, causing interference with the mandibular canine *(A)*.
- The maxillary canine can also be displaced mesially; this pattern may be associated with a retained primary tooth. This may occur alone or in conjunction with lingually displaced mandibular canines or with one or both mandibular canines in labioversion.
- The anchor teeth are the maxillary third, fourth premolar, and first molar. Additional anchorage and force on the canine tooth can be created by bonding a button to the lingual surface of the mandibular first molar and the palatal surface of the maxillary canine tooth and attaching an elastic chain with light tension.
- The button on the canine tooth must be placed in a location to create the appropriate movement. In an angled tooth, the button may initially be placed closer to the tip of the tooth for more tipping action to move the crown into position. As the crown becomes more perpendicular, the button can be replaced to the midtooth area to achieve a bodily movement into normal position.
- When using an elastic chain between the anchor teeth and the maxillary canine tooth, the distance between the fourth premolar and the canine tooth buttons is reduced by one fourth the number of links as the starting tension. The client or clinician can adjust the tension by one link at subsequent visits until the tooth is in correct position.
- Place a ligature wire between the buttons on the fourth premolar and first molar to create a more solid anchorage and prevent displacement of the maxillary fourth premolar.

Advantages

- Direct orthodontics.
- Less expensive way to move teeth.

- Tolerated well by the patient.
- Elastic size or chain length can be adjusted easily as the tooth moves.

Disadvantages

- Buttons can be displaced by chewing on hard objects.
- Possible poor evaluation of the stability of the anchor. This can result in mesial displacement, extrusion, and possible rotation of the fourth premolar if it is used alone as the anchor tooth. The total surface area of the roots of the anchor must exceed that of the root(s) of the active tooth.

Rostrally Displaced Mandibular Canines

- Seen occasionally where one or more of the lower canines is tilted forward, often interfering with the maxillary lateral incisor and causing displacement or wear of that tooth.
- For anchorage, buttons are placed in the midtooth area of the canines and buccally or lingually on the third and fourth mandibular premolars or lingually on the lower molar.
- Orthodontic elastics, or elastic chain, is stretched between the buttons to create a light force *(B)*.
- The elastics are changed and the size adjusted as tooth movement occurs.
- Chain elastic can be adjusted by decreasing the number of links between the buttons to increase the pull or by increasing the number of links to decrease the pull. Chain elastic can be replaced as necessary.

Advantages

- Simple, less expensive movement of a displaced canine tooth.
- Tolerated well by the patient.

Disadvantages

- Dislodgment of the buttons.
- Pain and tooth damage possible by too much force placed on teeth with elastics (moving an active tooth too fast or moving the anchor teeth).
- Difficult to place buttons on small teeth in toy breeds or cats.

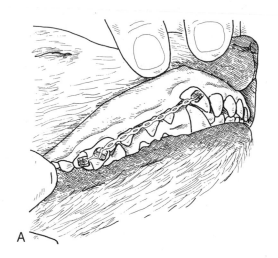

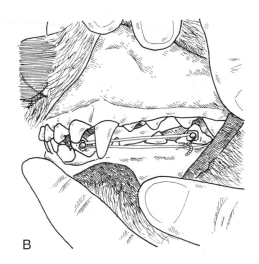

Caudal Movement of Lower Incisors

- In patients with anterior crossbite, some of the mandibular incisors can be moved caudally, either as a lone procedure or in conjunction with the simultaneous movement of the upper incisors anteriorly, to achieve a scissors occlusion.
- Buttons are placed on the buccal surface of the lower canines and on each of the second incisors.
- An appropriate-size orthodontic elastics, power cord, or masel chain is stretched across the incisors from canine to canine *(A)*.
- Another variation of this technique places small brackets on the second or third lower incisors *(B)*. An orthodontic elastic or elastic cord is placed around both canines. The two strands of elastic stretched between the canine teeth are brought in front of the incisors and are secured in the slot of the brackets. Small amounts of bonding material can be placed on the canines and central incisors to help keep the elastic from slipping.
- The buttons/brackets secure the elastics and keep them from slipping down onto or beneath the gingiva.
- Little force is needed to create the desired movement.
- These techniques should not be used until the permanent canines have a developed root as verified by radiographs (when the patient is about 7 months of age); otherwise, these teeth are not secure enough to use as anchor teeth, and they may themselves be displaced.

Advantages

- Less expensive method of moving teeth.
- Casts to design an appliance are not needed.
- Can be easily applied.

Disadvantages

- Buttons can be dislodged.
- Can create excessive crowding of teeth or may displace the canines if too much force is used.

- Does not allow for a retainer period to keep teeth in position. Elastic may be replaced with stainless steel wire placed between the buttons to maintain desired position.

Complications

- Early removal of buttons, requiring replacement with another anesthetic procedure.
- Noncompliance of clients to maintain oral hygiene with gingival irritation secondary to debris/hair wrapped around buttons.
- Sliding of elastic either caudal to the incisors or down onto or beneath gingiva. This is usually corrected by creating a ledge on central incisors with bonding material to hold the elastic in place.
- Improper application of elastic by the client; excessive force on teeth and undesirable movement/crowding are the result.
- If there is insufficient space distal to the third incisors to allow caudal movement of the incisors, crowding and loss of the curved rostral arch can occur.

Aftercare for Elastic Chains

- Home oral hygiene; taking care to keep the buttons and elastics free of hair, lint, etc.
- Recheck appointments every 7 to 14 days to monitor home hygiene and tooth movement.
- Replacement of elastics or masel chain, on a regular basis, when indicated.
- Softened food, no chew toys, and no hard treats.
- Removal of the buttons or brackets is easily accomplished using pliers. Squeeze the prongs together on brackets or use band-removing pliers for buttons or bands.
- The excess bonding material is removed with the band-removing pliers and/or an ultrasonic scaler, and the teeth are polished with a fluoride-containing pumice.
- Occasionally, the bands may have to be cut with a high-speed handpiece and cutting bur after orthodontic movement is complete. Eye protection should be worn.

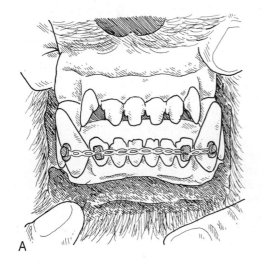

A

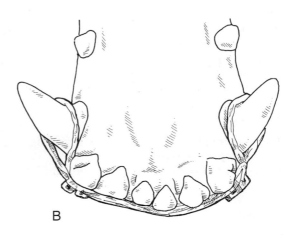

B

Arch Wires

General Comments

- Arch wires may be placed on the maxillary or mandibular teeth on either the palatal/lingual or labial surface.
- Arch wires are held in place by either bands or brackets, usually attached to the canine teeth.

Objective

- Arch wires using various activating forces, including those created by loops, arches, and finger springs, create tooth movement.

Indications

- Anterior crossbite, moving upper incisors rostrally.
- Anterior crossbite, moving lower incisors caudally.
- Movement of one or more teeth.
- Depressed mandibular central incisors.[9]

Contraindications

- Teeth so small that wire cannot be maintained in proper position.
- General orthodontic appliance contraindications.

Materials

- Patient's dental model.
- Laboratory-fabricated arch wire.
- Orthodontic wire, welder, solder, etc., if practitioner is capable of manufacturing in office.
- Brackets and bands, if not incorporated into appliance.
- Orthodontic bonding material.
- Flour pumice.
- Rubber cups.
- Scaler or curette.

Technique: General

- The technique of manufacturing the arch wire is beyond the scope of this text. This text begins with a fabricated arch wire.
- Many types of configurations can be used with the arch wire.

- The arch wire with incorporated bands is applied as described in the brackets/band bonding technique earlier in this chapter.
- Brackets are bonded to the tooth first, and the arch wire is fitted and secured with ligature wire (if an arch wire is being used by itself).

Arch Wire Elastics

- An arch wire is designed to come across the labial surface of the mandibular incisors and is welded to bands that encircle the canine teeth.
- The arch wire forms the desired position for forward movement of the teeth.
- The arch wire has small hooks approximating the location of each incisor, allowing a small elastic to be placed between the arch wire and the button on the tooth to be moved.
- Buttons or brackets are first bonded onto the teeth to be moved.
- The appliance is bonded to the canines as previously described.
- Once the bonding material is set, elastics are placed between the bracket on the tooth and arch wire *(A)*. The strength of an elastic is measured in ounces and is calibrated at approximately twice the diameter of the elastic. For example, a ⅜ inch light elastic has 3 ounces of force when stretched to a length equaling twice its diameter, which is ¾ inch.
- A combination of arch wire, bands, and elastics or power chain can be used to pull teeth into proper position *(B) (C)*.
- The elastics should be changed at appropriate intervals by the client.

Advantages

- Less expensive appliance to make than expansion devices.
- Can achieve rapid movement of teeth.
- Easy to keep clean.

Disadvantages

- Can cause irritation of upper lip.
- Client must be able and committed to change small elastics.
- Buttons or brackets can be dislodged.
- Arch wire can be bent.
- Arch wire design has to allow space for lower canines to come into normal position.

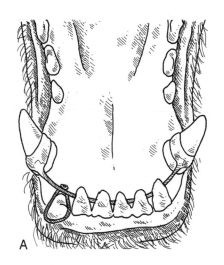

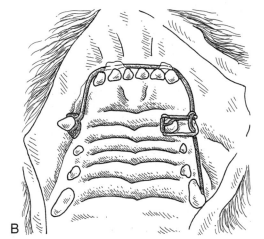

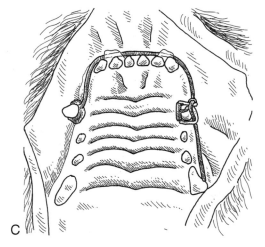

Arch Wire Finger Springs

- Bands are placed around the canine teeth, which are linked together with an arch wire that has finger springs soldered onto it, to create the desired tooth movement.
- This appliance can be designed to move a single tooth or several teeth.
- This appliance can be adapted for use in the maxilla or mandible, moving incisors forward or caudally.
- The appliance is trial-fitted, and the finger springs are adjusted with three-prong or appropriate orthodontic pliers so the spring pressure will move the teeth to their desired position *(A)*. A slight overadjustment should be anticipated; however, additional adjustments may be made later on recheck visits.
- The appliance is cemented to the canines, using the technique described on pages 412 to 415.
- The active finger spring wires are tucked behind the upper incisors, against their palatal surface *(B)*. A small ledge of composite resin or bonding material can be placed on the lingual surface of the incisors to keep the wire from slipping over the incisal edge and forward, off the teeth.

Advantages

- Simple appliance to design.
- Less expensive than expansion devices.
- Easy to keep clean.

Disadvantages

- Spring wires get caught in hair, blankets, and carpet and can become hazardous to the patient and damaging to the treatment.
- Laceration of lips/tongue from bent or broken wires.

Labial Arch Wires

- A labial arch wire uses a retention device (usually bands) connected by an arch wire that lies on the labial surface of the teeth *(C)*.
- Springs are formed by loops in the anterior diastema between the canine and lateral incisor.
- Closing these loops gradually with pliers over time creates the desired force to move the teeth.
- This type of arch wire can be used for an anterior crossbite by tipping the mandibular incisors lingually if there is a space between the incisors and canine teeth.

Advantages

- Easy appliance to design and place.
- Well tolerated by the patient.
- Can act as its own retainer when the desired tooth position is reached.
- Easy to keep clean.

Disadvantages

- Cannot be used in dogs with very small incisors.
- Wire can be bent or dislodged by oral abuse.

Complications

- Breakage of finger springs.
- Bending of finger springs.
- Hair and carpet getting caught in wires.
- Loss of appliance.

Aftercare

- Rechecks every 10 to 14 days.
- Elastics, finger springs, or loops adjusted as needed to maintain orthodontic force.
- After retainer period, the appliance is removed using band-removing pliers.
- Excess cement is removed with band-removing pliers or an ultrasonic scaler, and the teeth are polished with fluoride-containing pumice.

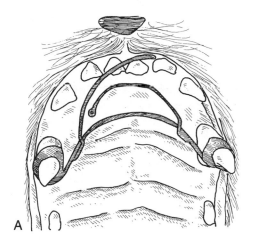

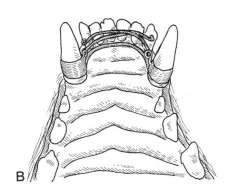

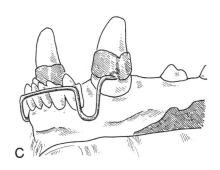

Expansion Devices

General Comments

- Expansion screws, acrylic plate, and arch wire may be used to tip teeth labially.
- Small expansion screws can be placed in acrylic appliances or attached to wires and bands to create gradual movement of the teeth by adjusting the screw that directs an orthodontic force on the teeth to be moved.
- These screws come in various sizes and with various expansion capabilities.
- Practitioners can either create their own appliance with acrylic or wires and bands or send the patient's models to a laboratory to have one fabricated.
- Either removable or fixed appliances can be designed.
- Removable appliances (usually maxillary) are designed with wire loops that lie along the palatal surface of the canines and lateral incisors. Brackets or buttons are bonded to the buccal or labial surface of these teeth near the gingival margin, and small elastics are placed over the wire on the appliance and button/bracket to hold the appliance in place.
- Removable appliances are removed for eating and allow for easier cleaning and oral hygiene.
- Fixed appliances are designed with bands around the canine teeth that are cemented in place.

Objective

- Actively create gradual tooth movement using an expansion device that places an orthodontic force on the teeth to be moved.

Indications

- Anterior crossbite, maxillary appliance.
- Lingually displaced mandibular canines.

Contraindication

- See general orthodontic appliance contraindications.

Materials

- Worm gear.
- Expansion screws; Unitek No. 440–160 Mid-Palatal Suture Expansion Screw.*

---

*Unitek Corporation, 2714 South Peck Rd., Monrovia CA 91016

- Orthodontic wire; suggested sizes: 0.016 inch, 0.020 inch, 0.022 inch, 0.028 inch, 0.032 inch, 0.036 inch, and 0.040 inch.
- Buttons/brackets.
- Orthodontic cement/bonding material.
- Flour pumice.
- Rubber cups.
- Patient's models.
- Laboratory-fabricated appliance.
- Adjusting key.

Techniques

Maxillary Acrylic or Metal Appliance for Anterior Crossbite

- An appliance is designed with the expansion screw placed front to back embedded in an acrylic shoe *(A)* or in a separated fabricated metal shoe. The shoe is cut so the front half of the screw is in a section of acrylic that will move separately against the incisors to be pushed forward.
- This can be a removable *(B)* or fixed *(A)* appliance.
- The expansion screw is adjusted using a small wire key in the hole at the center of the expansion screw that expands the screw, thus putting an increased pressure on the teeth to be moved.
- The screw is adjusted by the client, who turns the key once every 4 days. Each 90 degree turn of the key moves the active tooth 0.25 mm.
- When the teeth have moved into occlusion, the appliance is left in place for an additional 2 to 6 weeks for the retainer period.

Advantages

- A strong device that does not have loose wires that can be bent or catch on hair, etc.
- Can be designed as a removable appliance for easy cleaning *(B)*.
- Well tolerated by the patient.
- Creates a more uniform, controlled tooth movement.

Disadvantages

- Movable shoe may slip over the incisal edge of the active incisors. (Having a shoe that fits well against the cingulum of the incisors to be moved incorporated into the acrylic can help prevent this.)
- More expensive to manufacture than arch wire.
- Client must take care of home oral hygiene.
- Client must be able to make adjustments with wire key.
- An overzealous or impatient client may create pain and tooth damage in the patient.

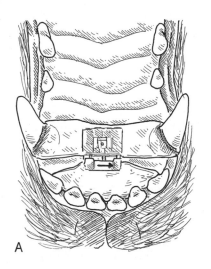

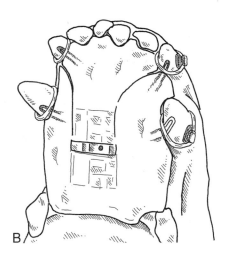

Lingually Displaced Mandibular Canines

- This common occlusion problem is usually caused by retained primary canines that do not allow the adult teeth to come into position outside the maxillary arch. It may also occur by malpositioned secondary canine tooth buds or by structurally narrow mandibles. In a condition treated similarly, the mandibular canines are oriented properly, but a class II malocclusion results in the cusps of these teeth traumatizing the palate. It is a skeletal, structural problem, but it is treated orthodontically to relieve discomfort.
- The pressure caused by the indentation of the mandibular canines on the hard palate can lead to periodontal disease of the maxillary canines, pain, necrosis of the palatal tissue, and an irritable temperament.
- The expansion screw is placed in a wire support structure with bands around the mandibular canines (A).
- This device can be used effectively when both canines need to be moved out and are located in their normal relationship mesial to distal.
- Variations on the device, such as a wire arm alongside the premolars or placed at an angle between the canines, have been used to achieve movement of a single canine without shifting position of the other.
- The device is cemented to the canines, using the technique described on pages 412 to 415.

Advantages

- Easily designed to create desired movement.
- Well tolerated by the patient.
- Easy to keep clean.
- Cannot be removed easily by the patient.

Disadvantages

- Tongue may make adjustments difficult.
- Client must be able to make the screw adjustments.
- This device will not change mesial/distal position of the canine tooth.
- The size of the patient may limit the device's use if there is not enough expansion to achieve desired tooth position.
- Appliance can be dislodged by indiscriminate oral behavior.
- In larger dogs, the splaying of the mandibular canines may be too extreme to allow installation of this appliance because the expansion screw may not be long enough. This complication can be overcome with an appliance designed as a Maryland bridge piece, with metal wings resting on the lingual surface of the canines and custom bands that can be installed and cemented to encircle the anchor tooth and its wing.

Omega or "W" Wire

- An omega/"W" wire is an orthodontic wire bent in the form of the Greek letter Ω or "W" (B). Loops designed in the bends of the "W" create an expansion action of the outer arms when activated.
- The wire is soldered to bands around the canines and can be used to move lingually displaced canine teeth.
- The appliance is trial-fitted, and the outer arms are activated with three-prong pliers to extend to the desired position of the teeth while the appliance is free from the canines.
- The wire and bands are cemented to the teeth as previously described, collapsing the expanded "W." This creates the force to move the teeth into position.

Advantages

- Easily designed appliance.
- Can be made to fit any size mouth.
- Easy to clean around appliance.

Disadvantages

- Cannot control force as easily; may move teeth too fast.
- Force created may not be sufficient to achieve desired movement.
- Can be dislodged or bent by heavy chewing on hard objects.
- Does not have a retainer function as readily as expansion-screw device.

Complications

- Noncompliance of client with home oral hygiene.
- Dislodgment or breakage of appliance.
- Alveolar bone necrosis from rapid movement of teeth.
- Premature removal of appliance, with teeth drifting back; appliance should be left in place for adequate retainer period.
- Patient discomfort if force is too great.

Aftercare

- Home oral hygiene; daily flushing around appliance.
- Expansion-screw adjustments should be

made every 3 to 4 days. (Each turn of the key expands the screw 0.25 mm; therefore, four turns equals 1 mm expansion.)

- Recheck examinations every 10 to 14 days to monitor home oral hygiene and tooth movement.
- Retaining period, provided by inactivating the wire, for 4 to 6 weeks to prevent regression.
- Appliance is removed with band-removing pliers; excess cement is removed with band-removing pliers or an ultrasonic scaler; and the teeth are polished with a fluoride-containing pumice.

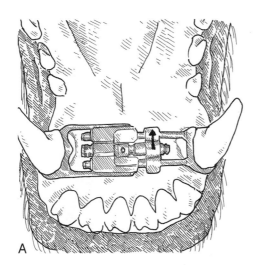

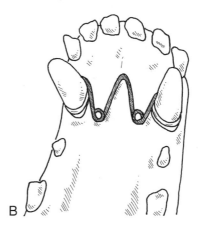

Inclined Plane

General Comments

- Inclined planes are designed of acrylic or cast metal to guide a tooth into a new movement, using normal occlusal forces. Every time the patient closes its mouth, the teeth come in contact with the inclined plane and are directed into the desired position. Orthodontically, this is an intermittent active force, the force being applied more strongly and more frequently by more orally oriented animals.
- The appliance can be used for a variety of tooth movements but is most commonly used for lingually displaced mandibular canines. It has also been successfully designed to move incisors rostrally or caudally.
- The inclined plane can be designed to allow forward or caudal canine movement along with buccal movement of the teeth.
- A telescoping inclined plane can be fabricated with a stabilizing transpalatal bar consisting of a rod from one canine anchor fitting into a sleeve from the other canine anchor. This is useful when working with young, growing patients, to allow palatal expansion during treatment.
- Desired tooth position can be readily achieved with the inclined plane design.
- The device creates an intermittent force between times of rest and mastication.

- The time necessary to create movement desired depends on distance needed to travel, amount of time arches are in occlusion, and angulation of incline.
- The more acute the angle, the faster the tipping movement and decreased tendency to create intrusion.
- Age of the patient is a factor: the younger the patient, the faster the movement.
- Another factor is the extent of oral activity of the patient.
- In mild cases of lingual displacement the palatal gingiva can be used as an inclined plane (see the subsequent section in this chapter, Gingival Wedge).
- An incline should be created on both sides of the appliance even if only one tooth orientation needs to be adjusted. This prevents shifting of the mandible and stress on the temporomandibular joint that may be created if only one canine is to be moved.

Objective

- To direct the tooth into a desired position by using normal occlusal forces.

Indications

- Lingual displacement of one or both mandibular canines (lower cuspid linguoversion.)
- Caudal displacement of maxillary incisor.

Contraindication

- See general orthodontic appliance contra-indications.

Materials

- Patient's models.
- Laboratory-designed inclined plane device.
- Orthodontic cementing materials.
- Flour pumice.
- Rubber cups.

Techniques

Acrylic

Indirect Palatal Acrylic Appliance

- An inclined plane can be designed, using the dental models in the office or at a dental laboratory, out of dental acrylic to fit against the hard palate.
- The appliance can be removable or fixed.
- The removable appliance is attached with elastics placed over buttons bonded to the buccal surface of the canines and lateral incisors, and wires are incorporated into the acrylic that lie along the palatal surface of those teeth.
- The fixed appliance is designed with bands around the maxillary canines and is cemented in place as previously described.
- The inclined plane can be reshaped, as necessary, in the mouth with an acrylic bur in a low-speed handpiece.
- Periodic adjustments are not needed with this device, because the design of the inclined plane is to create the intermittent patient-activated force necessary to move the tooth into position during natural occlusal activity.

Advantages

- Acrylic material allows for office adjustments, if necessary, during the course of treatment without removing the appliance.
- Less expensive than cast-metal appliance.
- Can be designed as a removable appliance for easy cleaning.
- No concern with heat production during curing of acrylic.
- Can create a smoother finish on appliance.

Disadvantages

- Client must maintain good home oral hygiene.
- Appliance must be designed to allow expansion between the maxillary canines for placement of the device and growth in the young patient.
- Requires an additional visit and anesthetic period to take impressions for models.
- Acrylic may be fractured by active chewing on hard objects (this occurs more often in large dogs).
- Palatal mucosal irritation with nonremovable appliances.

Direct Acrylic Full Palatal Appliance

General Comments

- Designing the acrylic inclined plane in the patient's mouth eliminates the need for a dental laboratory. It eliminates an additional anesthetic session to obtain impressions. It provides, therefore, a more rapid initiation of treatment and decreased cost and risk for the client.[10]
- The appliance can be remodeled as desired and made with minimal expense.

Advantages

- Requires only one anesthetic session to place appliance and one to remove it.
- Less expensive than cast-metal or laboratory-fabricated appliance.
- Acrylic can be adjusted in the office if necessary.

Disadvantages

- Covers the palate, with potential for mucosal irritation and necrosis.
- Does not allow for maxillary growth.
- Can be damaged or dislodged by the patient's oral abuse.
- Unless a nonexothermic acrylic, such as Merdon 7 or Tokuso Rebase (Tokuyama), or an acrylic composite combination such as Protemp Garant (ESPE America) is used, significant heat is produced during the curing period that may damage the soft tissues or the pulp tissue.

Materials

- Acrylic material (see comment above).
- Rubber prophy cups.
- Utility wax strips.
- Low-speed and high-speed drills.
- Acrylic finishing burs.
- Nonfluoride paste/pumice.
- Etching gel.
- Assorted "Dura white" low-speed polishing stones (flame and pointed cone).

Technique

Step 1—The patient is anesthetized, intubated, and placed in dorsal recumbency; the back of the pharynx is packed with gauze.

Step 2—The anterior maxillary teeth are scaled and polished with the nonfluoride pumice.

Step 3—All surfaces of the teeth are etched with a 37% phosphoric acid etching gel for 30 seconds and then rinsed and dried with oil and moisture-free air.

Step 4—A wax strip dam (3/16 inch or greater in diameter) is formed around the anterior teeth at the gingival level.

Step 5—The powder is placed to a depth of 1/4 inch within the wax dam, and the liquid is placed dropwise directly on the powder.

Step 6—Additional acrylic can be applied by repeating the process.

Step 7—Before the acrylic sets, the patient is extubated, and the jaws are occluded to create indentations that will serve as starting points for the inclined plane. The patient is reintubated.

Step 8—Using a bullet-shaped acrylic bur in a high-speed handpiece, an inclined groove is cut into the acrylic from the starting indentations to a point that will be the end point of the movement desired.

Step 9—The fine adjustments of angulation and direction can be achieved on the inclined plane with a white stone in a low-speed handpiece.

Step 10—The acrylic shavings are rinsed periodically, and the gauze is exchanged at the back of the mouth.

Step 11—The wax strip is removed, and all the surfaces of the appliance are meticulously smoothed and polished with a low-speed white stone.

Bilateral Direct Acrylic Inclined Plane

- This technique uses acrylic that is molded around the maxillary incisors and canine teeth on either side of the mouth to form an inclined plane to redirect the displaced mandibular canines.
- The two sides are separate to allow for continued maxillary development and easier oral hygiene.

Materials

- Flour pumice.
- Rubber prophy cups.
- Low-speed handpiece.
- Acrylic cutting burs.
- Finishing burs.
- Finishing stones.
- Etching gel.
- Light-cure acrylic sheets (Triad VLC, Caulk) or self-curing Bis-Acryl-Composite material.*
- Light-cure gun.

Technique

Step 1—The patient is anesthetized, intubated, and placed in dorsal recumbency.

Step 2—The maxillary lateral and intermediate incisors and canine teeth are scaled and polished with flour pumice and rinsed.

---

*Protemp Garant, ESPE America, 1710 Romano Dr., Norristown, PA 19404

Step 3—The incisors and canines are spot-etched for 30 seconds with the etching gel. They are rinsed with water and dried with oil and moisture-free air.

Step 4—The acrylic material is placed and shaped by hand to form an inclined plane anchored around and between the lateral and intermediate incisors and canine teeth on each side of the maxilla (A). The acrylic material should not be in contact with the soft tissues.

Step 5—The patient is extubated to check the occlusion of the mandibular incisors on the inclined surface (B). The mandibular canines should meet the incline at a 20 degree angle from parallel.[11] The angle is adjusted as

necessary, and the patient is reintubated. The slope of the incline can be directed mediolateral, or rostrocaudal and mediolateral, as necessary to direct the lower canines into proper alignment.

Step 6—If using the light-cured acrylic (C), the acrylic is light-cured in overlapping sections for 60 seconds each. If a self-curing acrylic is used, it is allowed to harden.

Step 7—The patient is extubated, and the occlusion is reevaluated and adjusted with acrylic burs if necessary, and the patient reintubated.

Step 8—The acrylic is trimmed and smoothed with finishing burs and stones in a low-speed handpiece with irrigation (D).

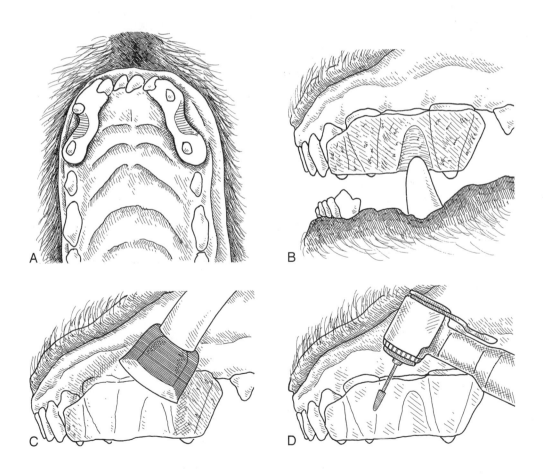

Cast Metal

- A cast-metal inclined plane is designed in an appliance with a telescoping bar across the hard palate and bands around the maxillary canines *(A)* (p. 451).
- The metal telescoping inclined plane can be designed to direct the teeth in a number of directions (rostral and buccal, or caudal and buccal) *(B)* (p. 451).
- The appliance is trial-fitted and cemented in place as previously described.

Advantages

- The telescoping bar allows for easy placement and continued maxillary growth of the patient.
- The appliance is not in direct contact with the hard palate and is easier to keep clean.
- The appliance is well tolerated by the patient.
- Because it has greater appliance strength, it is less likely to be damaged by larger patients.
- Some adjustments can be made by adding composite to the lingual surface of the lower canines to allow further lateral movement.

Disadvantages

- Adjustments in design requiring removing and remaking the appliance.
- Discoloration of inside of mandibular canines from contact with some types of metal or cement.
- Wear on the tips of mandibular canines if appliance is poorly designed or in place for a long time.
- Teeth must be fully erupted before taking the impression to manufacture the appliance.

Complications (All Techniques)

- Premature removal of appliance—prevented by using appropriate cementing material and technique.
- Inadequate appliance design creating incorrect movement or undesired move-

ment—have accurate models and bite impressions for laboratory to work with.

- Inadequate home care by client, leading to gingival irritation.
- Orally inappropriate behavior by patient, resulting in foreign objects being wedged between appliance and mouth.
- Palatal mucosal irritation. (If present, resolves quickly after appliance is removed, but has been known to result in mucosal necrosis.)
- Restriction of maxillary growth in younger patients if left in place for extended time (full palate appliance).
- Fracture/loss of appliance.
- Premature limitation of movement. If the acrylic plate is too thick over a prominent incisive papilla, canine movement will be stopped when the lower incisors come in contact with the plate.
- Acrylic material harboring bacteria and serving as a reservoir for infection.
- Staining of the teeth from etching and microleakage under the appliance.

Aftercare (All Inclined Planes)

- An Elizabethan collar may be necessary for the first few days the appliance is in place to prevent self-trauma from the patient trying to remove it.
- A curved-tip syringe with dilute chlorhexidine solution should be used 2 to 3 times daily to flush all gingival/appliance margins.
- Provide softened food, no chew toys, or hard treats while appliance is in place.
- Recheck examinations every week to monitor oral hygiene and tooth movement. Length of treatment depends on the age of the patient and the degree of movement necessary. Teeth may be moved with a well-designed appliance in as few as 7 to 10 days.
- When teeth are in desired position, the appliance is removed using band-removing pliers. Excess cement is removed from the teeth with band-removing pliers or an ultrasonic scaler, and the teeth are polished with a fluoride-containing pumice.

Gingival Wedge (Gingivoplasty of the Anterior Diastema)

- A wedge can be created in the gingival tissue anterior to the maxillary canine, using electrosurgery or a scalpel blade to remove a traumatically caused superficial pocket of palatal tissue, to direct minimally displaced mandibular canines laterally[12] (C).
- This technique can be used in patients whose teeth are still erupting to allow the teeth to come into normal position by the time eruption is complete.

Advantages

- Not necessary to take impressions and make models to correct the malocclusion.
- Easily performed by a general practitioner without additional dental equipment.
- Use in a young patient allows early correction of teeth.
- "One-stop shopping" for the client.

Disadvantages

- Only effective if mandibular canines are minimally displaced.
- Excessive use of electrosurgery may damage gingiva and create additional sloughing.
- Overaggressive surgery may create permanent change in gingival contour.

Maryland Bridge

- A cast-metal appliance that uses a variety of forces (expansion screw, elastics) to achieve the desired movement.[13]
- The Maryland bridge uses broad coverage of the lingual or palatal surface of the canines (metal "wings"), along with cast-metal partial crown covers, to attach the appliance, creating more surface area for cementation and therefore greater retention of the appliance in the mouth.
- Additional circumferential bands over the wings provides additional retention.

- The wings, cast crown covers, and band areas cemented in place using a Maryland bridge adhesive or similar luting cement (Comspan,* Panavia†).
- These appliances are very durable in the mouth and are not easily broken or dislodged.

Objective

- To improve retention of an orthodontic appliance to achieve movement of teeth through the use of increased surface contact for cementation.

Indications

- Patients with chewing habits that require a sturdy appliance.
- Patients who have broken or removed their other appliances.
- Additional cementation security.

Contraindications

- Poor client compliance with follow-up care and rechecks.
- Inability of client to adjust expansion screws or replace elastics as necessary.
- Periodontal disease of the affected teeth, weak supportive bone.

Materials

- Patient's models.
- Laboratory-fabricated appliance.
- Maryland bridge adhesive or luting cement.
- Flour pumice.
- Rubber prophy cups.
- Howe pliers.
- Scaler or curette.

---

*L. D. Caulk/Dentsply, Lakeview and Clark Avenues, P.O. Box 359, Milford, DE 19963
†J. Morita, 14712 Bentley Circle, Tustin, CA 92680

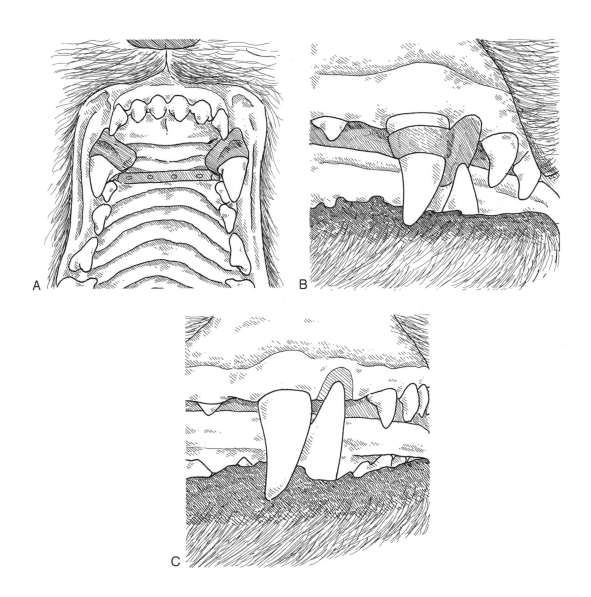

Technique

Maxillary Appliance for Anterior Crossbite

- The appliance is cemented to the maxillary canines and incisors, following the directions of the cementing product.
- An expansion screw is designed into the appliance to create gradual forward movement of the incisors.

Advantages

- A stronger appliance is beneficial in large dogs that are more likely to break an acrylic appliance.
- There are no wires, buttons, or brackets to be dislodged or caught in hair, chew toys, etc.
- The open design of the cast-metal appliance allows for easy cleaning of the hard palate area and less chance of irritation from deficiencies in home oral hygiene.

Disadvantages

- Increased expense of appliance.
- Must use special luting cements for proper retention.
- Lack of availability; not all laboratories make this style appliance.

Mandibular Appliance for Anterior Crossbite

- This appliance is cemented to the mandibular canines using the appropriate luting cement and following the instructions included with that particular cement.
- This appliance is designed to use orthodontic elastics across the front of the lower incisors to tip them caudally.
- The elastics are anchored on small hooks incorporated into the canine wings and through a notch in the incisor crown covers (*figure*).
- The elastics are changed daily, and the strength of elastic is adjusted as the teeth move into position.

Advantages

- Secure appliance to achieve caudal tipping of the lower incisors.
- Improved attachment and elastic holding to keep the appliance in place and to prevent gingival damage from slippage.
- Mandibular appliance may be used in conjunction with the maxillary appliance to achieve the desired occlusion in patients with severe anterior crossbite.

Disadvantages

- Increased expense of appliance.
- Must use special luting cements for proper retention.
- Lack of availability; not all laboratories make this style appliance.

Complications

- Noncompliance of the client to return for rechecks.
- Discoloration of teeth under wings if cement leaks, staining the tooth surfaces.
- Removal of appliance, although rarely, by patient.
- Must have enough distal room between incisors and lower canines to allow uniform movement of incisal arch without crowding.

Aftercare

- Adjusting elastics or expansion screw as necessary and recheck examination every 2 weeks to monitor tooth movement.
- Removing appliance after proper retainer period. It may be necessary to cut the bands with a diamond bur to facilitate removal. Using an ultrasonic scaler over the wings may help to fracture the cement for removal with band-removing pliers.
- Remaining cement is removed with band-removing pliers or an ultrasonic scaler.

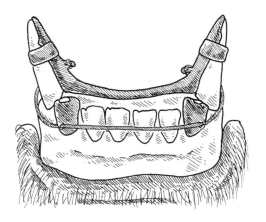

LABORATORY PRESCRIPTION (ORTHODONTIC)

- If a dental laboratory is used, a prescription should accompany the models.
- The prescription should order the type of appliance, the material to be used, and the color or shade of material, as appropriate.
- By drawing on the dental chart, the practitioner can indicate the anchorage and type of force to be applied.

REFERENCES

1. Eisner ER. Bites, Breath and Benevolent Breeding. Denver: Published by author, 1997.
2. Ross DL. Orthodontics for the dog: bite evaluation, basic concepts, and equipment. Philadelphia: W.B. Saunders Co., 1986:955–966.
3. Proffit WR. Contemporary Orthodontics. St. Louis: C.V. Mosby Co., 1986:579.
4. Wiggs RB. Orthodontics. American Veterinary Dental Society Annual Meeting. St. Louis, 1989.
5. Goldstein GS. The Removable Orthodontic Appliance. American Veterinary Dental Society Annual Meeting. Washington, D.C., 1988.
6. Weigel JP, Dorn AS. Disease of the jaws and abnormal occlusion. In: Harvey CE, ed. Veterinary Dentistry. Philadelphia: W.B. Saunders Co., 1985:106–122.
7. Ross D. Veterinary Dentistry. In: Ettinger SJ, ed. Veterinary Internal Medicine. Philadelphia: W.B. Saunders Co., 1975:1053–1054.
8. Eisenmenger E, Zetner K. Veterinary Dentistry. Philadelphia: Lea & Febiger, 1985:165.
9. Ross DL. Common Veterinary Orthodontic Indications: Identification and Classifications of Needs. New Orleans: Nabisco, 1988.
10. Luskin I. Veterinary Dentistry 1994 Proceedings. Philadelphia, 1994.
11. Hale FA. Orthodontic corrections of lingually displaced canine teeth in a young dog using light-cured acrylic resin. J Vet Dentistry 1996; 13:69–73.
12. Goldstein GS. Bite Plates: Removable and Fixed. New Orleans: Nabisco, 1988.
13. Beard GB. Interceptive Orthodontics for Prevention: Maryland Bridges for Correction. New Orleans: Nabisco, 1988.

Dental Lab Prescription

Veterinarian _____ Clinic/Hospital _____

Street Address _____ City _____ State ____ Zip _____ Telephone _____

Patient name/Identification _____ Breed _____ Age ____ Sex ____

History:

_____

_____

Diagnosis:

_____

_____

Appliance prescribed:

May we substitute, if a better appliance is available?

☐ Yes, without consultation

☐ Yes, but consult first

☐ No, design as prescribed

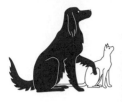

Chapter 10

DENTAL ORTHOPEDICS

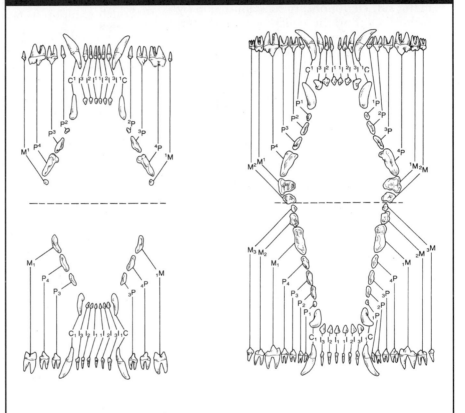

- Dental techniques may be used to stabilize or assist in the stabilization of the maxillofacial complex, of mandibular fractures, and of luxated teeth.

TAPE MUZZLE NONSURGICAL FRACTURE STABILIZATION

Indications

- Occasionally, if there is very little displacement, sufficient nonsurgical stabilization by means of fitting the patient with a leather, nylon, plastic, or in-clinic fabricated adhesive tape muzzle may effectively provide adequate stabilization for healing.[1-8]
- Appropriate cases are those with minimal displacement in which the original patient occlusion has not been altered by the trauma.
- Additionally, fractures of the vertical ramus of the mandible are partially stabilized, often well enough, for adequate healing by this conservative treatment.[3]
- Tape muzzles can also be very useful in providing enough stability in cases of periodontally caused traumatic pathologic mandibular fractures so that a functional, if not rigid, fibrous union is achieved.

Contraindications

- Malocclusion.
- Respiratory distress due to epistaxis or hematoma.
- Risk of inhalation pneumonia if patient vomits.

Materials

- 1 inch semiporous tape.
- 2 inch semiporous tape.

Technique

- To fit an adhesive muzzle to a dog or cat, two to four pieces of tape are employed (A) (p. 461).
- For the first fitting, tape wide enough to encompass most of the patient's muzzle is used: generally up to 2 inches wide. It is placed sticky side out and is oriented so that it encircles the face and jaw. It is applied loosely enough so that the patient can lap water and semiliquid food but snugly enough for the dental interlock to be maintained.

- A second layer of tape is applied, sticky side down, directly on top of the encircling tape. This second fitting is the retaining loop, a long piece the middle of which is placed behind the occiput to serve as a halter, keeping the encircling tape around the muzzle. Each side is brought forward, ventral to the ear base, drawn beneath the first encircling tape, then back over that tape and returned caudally with the sticky side down until its ends overlap each other behind the head.
- A third tape fitting can be applied to cats and short-faced dogs to add stability to the tape device. It is applied in a fashion similar to that of the retaining piece. The middle of this third tape is at the dorsal portion of the encircling tape. One piece passes above, and one piece passes below the encircling tape, and they are brought caudally, between the eyes, and fastened together behind the occiput to the retaining piece.
- A fourth (or possibly used as the third) piece can be applied, as necessary, as a throat latch and attached by being threaded around the cheek portion of the retaining piece of tape and passed ventrally beneath the throat.

- Tape muzzles are useful as a temporary first-aid treatment of maxillary and mandibular fractures, when providing stabilizing medical management before surgical intervention.

Complications

- Heat prostration.
- Dyspnea in brachycephalic patients is possible while the mouth is being maintained in a nearly closed position.
- The tape should be monitored by the owner so that tape-induced dermatitis can be treated, if necessary. Occasionally, taping the front feet is useful for preventing scratching with the front feet to dislodge the muzzle.[1]

Aftercare

- The muzzle should be maintained for 6 to 7 weeks while callous or fibrous union is being formed.
- At the conclusion of treatment, an adjustment period is often required, during which the patient regains full use of the muscles of mastication.

PARAPULPAR COMPOSITE BRIDGE

General Comments

- Another nonsurgical technique that may be used to maintain proper occlusal alignment and stabilize anterior mandibular fractures is the parapulpar pin technique.[5, 9–12]
- Parapulpar pins are inserted, either rostrally or caudally and perpendicular to the pulp chamber of all four upper and lower canine teeth.
- A composite bridge is placed, stabilizing and joining the pins of each maxillary canine to its ipsilateral mandibular counterpart (B).
- The bridges are left in place for 6 to 7 weeks, during callus formation.
- The technique for insertion of the parapulpar pins and composites employs the same principles as for handling those materials as described in Chapter 8, Restorative Dentistry.

Indications

- This technique is particularly useful in cats and small dogs, which are the most difficult patients on which to maintain a tape muzzle.
- The parapulpar technique is also useful in animals that are hypersensitive to tape.
- This technique has also worked very well in mandibular fracture cases that have additionally had reduced temporomandibular luxation.[11]

Contraindications

- The same precautions and contraindications apply as for tape muzzles, as described above.

Materials

- Small minim-pins* are used in domestic cats and small dogs.
- TMS pins* or thicker titanium pins are used in larger dogs.

---

*Whaledent, 236 5th Ave., New York, NY 10001

Technique

- The pin sites are chosen on the maxillary and mandibular canines such that a composite bridge can easily be fabricated between them and apically far enough on the crown to reduce the chance of exposing the pulp during placement.
- The occlusion should be stabilized in a partially open manner, similar to the preceding tape muzzle technique, so that the patient can lap water and semisolid food.
- The acid-etch technique of composite placement is recommended, and the applied light-cured or chemically cured composite should be finished smoothly with finishing burs or abrasive discs so as not to irritate the patient.

Complication

- If the pulp chamber is perforated, a sterile pin, coated with calcium hydroxide, should be placed in that specific hole later.

Aftercare

- If the patient, most commonly a small patient, has difficulty feeding itself, liquids can be introduced into the cheek pouch or by gastrostomy or pharyngostomy tube.
- At the end of treatment the patient is again anesthetized, the composite is removed, and the pins are either cut off at the level of the enamel and the remaining ends are polished, or the pins are twisted counterclockwise and removed and the resultant holes are filled with composite.

SPLINT BONDING

General Comments

- Bonding with wire splints between teeth is an effective method for achieving stabilization and occlusal alignment of oral structures.[7, 8]
- The strength of the bond limits this method to stabilization of minor components (such as an avulsed tooth or block of teeth with the remainder of the maxillofacial complex or mandible intact, or in fractures with other means of stabilization used).

Indications

- Repair maxillary fractures, along with other stabilization.
- Repair mandibular fractures, along with other stabilization.
- Stabilize luxated teeth.[13]
- Surgically correct misaligned teeth after other fracture repair has been performed.

Contraindication

- Severe fractures and unstable fractures without additional treatment methods.

Objective

- To create stability and proper tooth alignment that leads to fracture healing.

Materials

- 5 × 90 mm periodontal splinting material (wire mesh).*

---

*Masel Inc., 2701 Partram Rd., Bristol, PA 19007

- Composite reinforced woven mesh (Ribbond*).
- Stainless steel mesh splinting ribbon (splint mesh ribbon†).
- Nylon mesh splinting ribbon (splint grid splinting ribbon†).
- Stainless steel periodontal splinting bars (splint bars†).
- Self-curing Bis-Acrylic–composite temporary crown and bridge material (Protemp Garant‡).
- Orthodontic wire; suggested sizes: 0.016, 0.020, 0.022, 0.028, 0.032, 0.036, and 0.040 inch.
- Soft stainless steel orthopedic wire: 18, 20, 24, and 26 gauge.
- Flour pumice (not prophy paste).
- Prophy angle and rubber prophy cups.
- Dental handpiece.
- Orthodontic or light-cured enamel bonding materials.
- Acid-etch materials.

---

*Ribbond, Inc., 1326 5th Ave., Seattle, WA 98101

†Ellman International, Inc., 1135 Railroad Ave., Hewlett, NY 11557

‡ESPE America, 1710 Romano Dr., P.O. Box 111, Norristown, PA 19404

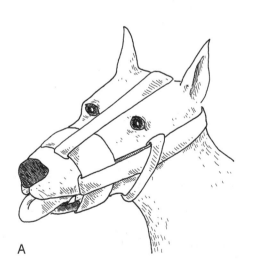

A

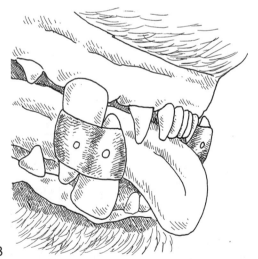

B

Technique: Avulsed Tooth Fracture, Wire or Nylon Mesh

Step 1—Radiographs are taken.

Step 2—The fracture is realigned *(A)*. (In avulsed or fractured teeth, root canal therapy or other treatment may be necessary.)

Step 3—The teeth to be splinted are scaled and polished with a slurry of flour pumice (not prophy paste).

Step 4—A phosphoric acid-etch solution or gel is applied to the enamel surface and after 15 to 30 seconds is rinsed with water for at least 30 to 60 seconds.

Step 5—The surface is air-dried.

Step 6—The wire, mesh, or splint is bent to lie over the surface to be bonded, is removed, and is set aside *(B)*.

Step 7—A light coat of a liquid, unfilled resin from the orthodontic or composite bonding kit is applied to the teeth to be bonded and to the wire or mesh *(C)*.

Step 8—The filled resin is mixed (if not light-cured) and applied to the prepared tooth surface and wire or mesh *(D)*.

Step 9—The filled resin is cured with time or light activation.

Step 10—The bonding is checked for stability by tactile pressure.

Step 11—The bonding material is smoothed with composite finishing burs *(E)*.

Technique: Avulsed Tooth Fracture, Cloth Fiber

• This technique utilizes a gas-plasma–treated, woven ultrahigh molecular weight polyethylene fabric (Ribbond bondable reinforcement ribbon).* It is 10 times stronger than steel and 35% stronger than Kevlar, but because of its multidirectional weave, it is easily adapted to the contours of the oral cavity.[14]

Step 1—Radiographs are taken.

Step 2—The fracture is realigned. (In avulsed or fractured teeth, root canal therapy or other treatment may be necessary.)

Step 3—The teeth to be splinted are scaled and polished with a slurry of flour pumice (not prophy paste).

Step 4—A phosphoric acid-etch solution or gel is applied to the enamel surface and after

---

*Ribbond, Inc., 1326 5th Ave., Seattle, WA 98101

15 to 30 seconds is rinsed with water for at least 30 to 60 seconds.

Step 5—The surface is air-dried.

Step 6—The cotton fiber is placed over the surface to be bonded and is then measured, cut, and set aside.

• Special gloves should be used while handling Ribbond, and the special scissors, supplied with each kit, should be used to cut the material.

Step 7—A light coat of a liquid, unfilled resin from the orthodontic or composite bonding kit is applied to the teeth to be bonded and to the cloth fiber.

Step 8—The filled resin is mixed (if not light-cured) and applied to the prepared tooth surface. The cloth fiber is placed on the filled resin and shaped to the teeth. Additional filled resin is placed over the cloth fiber. This procedure is very technique-sensitive, and the cloth fiber and composite resin must be handled carefully to avoid contamination.

Step 9—The filled resin is cured with time or light.

Step 10—The bonding is checked for stability by tactile pressure.

Step 11—The bonding material is smoothed with composite finishing burs.

Alternate Technique: Bis-Acrylic Composite Material[1]

• This material is very strong and can be used alone or with metal, cloth fiber, or nylon mesh as additional support in larger dogs. The material can be placed with the mixing gun or mixed separately and placed with a hand instrument.

• There is no exothermic reaction upon curing.

Step 1—Radiographs are taken.

Step 2—The fracture is reduced or tooth replaced if avulsed, and soft tissues are sutured if necessary. The opposite dental arch is covered with petroleum jelly, because after the splint material is applied, but before it has set, the mouth is closed so that the teeth can indent the material to provide for future function of the mouth without interference by the splint. The petroleum jelly on the opposite arch prevents adherence of the splint material to those teeth.

Step 3—The teeth to be splinted are scaled and polished with a slurry of nonfluoride pumice and rinsed with water.

Step 4—The enamel is spot-etched with phosphoric acid gel for 30 seconds in several places on the teeth to be splinted, rinsed with water, and air-dried. This may help with retention.

Step 5—The Bis-Acrylic composite material is injected over the tooth crowns to be incorporated into the splint; while the material is setting, the mouth is placed into occlusion to ensure proper alignment, eliminating interference with the opposing teeth.

Step 6—The material is allowed to harden, for 4 to 6 minutes, and the edges are smoothed with finishing burs.

Complications

- Failure to obtain stability (add more wire, or rebond).
- Failure to obtain proper occlusion.
- Creation of malocclusion.
- Bonded material preventing mouth from closing.
- Premature removal of appliance by patient.

Aftercare

A water pick or curved-tip syringe is used to irrigate debris from between the splint and the teeth.

- Radiographs are taken at appropriate intervals.
- When healing has occurred, as determined radiographically and clinically, the appliance is removed with band-removing instruments or a high-speed drill.

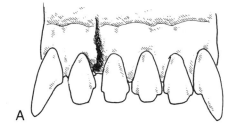

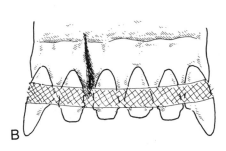

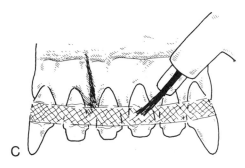

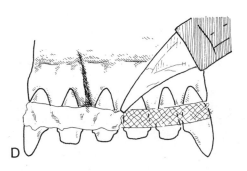

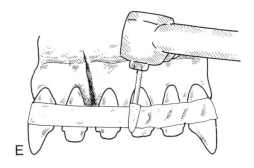

FORMING APPLIANCE IN MOUTH

General Comment

• Dental acrylics may be cast directly in the oral cavity to create an intraoral splint.[7, 8, 15–17, 19]

Indications

• Fractured maxillofacial complex.
• Fractured mandible anterior to the first molar.
• Luxated or subluxated teeth.[18]
• To increase stability of other fixation techniques.

Contraindications

• Numerous missing teeth preventing stabilization with the splint.
• Severely comminuted fractures without other techniques.

Objective

• Obtain stability so that healing may occur.

Materials

• Flour pumice (not prophy paste).
• Prophy angle and rubber prophy cups.
• Cold-cure acrylics.
• Petroleum jelly.
• Low-speed handpiece with acrylic cutting laboratory burs 75–080, 78–060.*
• Soft stainless steel (surgical or orthodontic) wire; the gauge ranges from 14 to 26, depending on patient and tooth size.

Technique: Mandibular Fracture[5, 15, 19, 20]

Step 1—Appropriate radiographs are taken, misalignments are corrected, and other therapy is performed as indicated (A). The tooth surfaces should be clean.

*Brassler USA, Inc., 800 King George Blvd., Savannah, GA 31419

Step 2—The coronal surface of the teeth (usually the canines and larger premolars) may be used for retention of the splint along with wiring techniques. The bonding sites are identified, scaled, and polished with a slurry of flour pumice (B). The oral cavity is rinsed well.

Step 3—The bonding sites are acid-etched (see Chapter 9, Dental Orthodontics, p. 412).

Step 4—Wire is bent from tooth to tooth to act as a support for the acrylic (C).

Step 5—A light coat of petroleum jelly is applied to exposed soft tissue surfaces (avoid the previously placed wire).

Step 6—A thin layer of the acrylic powder is applied (D).

Step 7—The liquid monomer is dripped onto the powder (E).

Step 8—Additional powder and liquid are alternatively applied until the appliance has been built up for sufficient strength (F).

Step 9—The appliance is trimmed and smoothed.

Step 10—The oral cavity and appliance are inspected for stability and occlusion.

Complications

• Exothermic reaction can burn the oral cavity. This is avoided by using fewer exothermic acrylics. Once curing is started, the appliance may be cooled with water spray. This may cause discoloration of the material.
• The tendency of acrylic material to flow during the setting process into portions of the soft/hard tissue may be missed in fracture cases and may inhibit healing of oral structures.
• Sharp edges may be formed at the margins.
• Stomatitis may occur secondary to food being trapped between the appliance and gingiva. This generally will resolve, without treatment, a few days after the appliance is removed.

Aftercare

• Good oral hygiene must be maintained; clients should be encouraged to flush area twice daily with 0.2% chlorhexidine.
• Radiographs are taken at appropriate intervals.
• When healing has occurred, as determined radiographically and clinically, the appliance is removed with band-removing pliers or a high-speed drill.

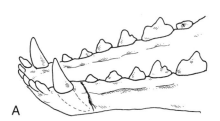

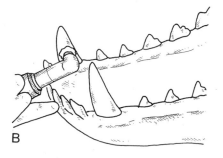

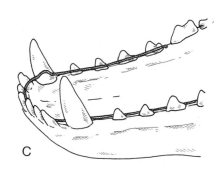

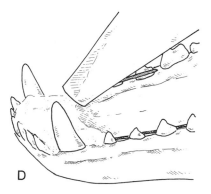

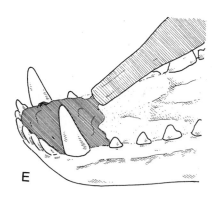

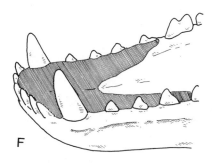

APPLIANCE FORMED ON AN ORAL CAST

General Comment

- This method adds the additional steps of creating a working model (cast) to form the splint.[20]

Indications

- Fractured maxillofacial complex.
- Fractured mandible anterior to the first molar.
- Luxated or subluxated teeth.
- To increase stability of other fixation techniques.

Contraindications

- Numerous missing teeth preventing stabilization of the splint.
- Severely comminuted fractures without other techniques.

Objective

- To obtain stability so that healing may occur.

Materials

- Flour pumice (not prophy paste).
- Prophy angle and rubber prophy cups.
- Impression trays.
- Alginate impression material.
- Rubber bowl.
- Spatula.
- Die stone.
- Rope wax.
- Dental acrylics.
- Low-speed handpiece with laboratory burs.
- Soft stainless steel orthopedic wire.
- Orthodontic wire; suggested sizes: 0.016, 0.020, 0.022, 0.028, 0.032, 0.036, and 0.040 inch.

Technique

Step 1—Appropriate radiographs are taken, misalignments are corrected, and other therapy is performed as indicated.

Step 2—The proper impression tray is selected, alginate is mixed, and an impression is taken (see Chapter 9, Dental Orthodontics).

Step 3—A stone model is poured (see Chapter 9).

Step 4—An outline of the splint is created on the model with rope wax (see Chapter 9).

Step 5—Bonding sites for wiring the appliance in place are identified.

Step 6—Wire is bent from tooth to tooth to act as a support for the acrylic.

Step 7—A thin layer of the acrylic powder is applied.

Step 8—The liquid monomer is dripped onto the powder from a dropper bottle.

Step 9—Additional powder and liquid are alternately applied until the appliance has been built up for sufficient strength.

Step 10—The appliance is trimmed and smoothed.

Step 11—The appliance is trial-fitted and inspected for fit.

Step 12—The previously identified bonding sites are cleaned, flour-pumiced, and acid-etched for 15 to 30 seconds with phosphoric acid gel or solution; then they are rinsed with water for 30 seconds and air-dried.

Step 13—The appliance is refitted.

Step 14—Orthodontic bonding material or light-cure restorative material is applied to the appliance and etched teeth to cement the appliance in place.

Complications

- The indirect formation of the cast is a longer procedure and is best suited to a team approach in cases with multiple trauma sites.
- Bone movement at the fracture site before, during, and after the impression is taken may complicate the installation of the splint.
- Open wounds should be protected from being contaminated with pumice slurry by the use of a water-soluble sterile lubricant jelly.
- Additional length of time for anesthesia is required to create the cast.

Aftercare

- Client must be instructed in the techniques of maintaining good oral hygiene. A water pick or other appliance may be used to aid in cleaning the oral cavity.
- Radiographs are taken at appropriate intervals.
- When healing has occurred, as determined radiographically and clinically, the appliance is removed with band-removing pliers or a high-speed drill.

SYMPHYSIAL FRACTURE REPAIR: ANTERIOR CERCLAGE TECHNIQUE

General Comment

• Symphysial fractures are common in cats.

Indications

• Fractures of the mandibular symphysis; rostrocaudal fractures of other portions of the anterior mandibular bone supporting the incisors.

Contraindications

• Osteomyelitis.
• Severe periodontal disease.
• Comminuted fractures.

Objective

• A wire is passed between the skin and bone around both sides of the mandible behind the canine teeth to stabilize and compress the fracture/separation.[2-4]

Materials

• Howe pliers.
• 22 gauge soft stainless steel wire.
• Large hypodermic needle (14 to 18 gauge).

Technique

Step 1—The wire is passed into the bore of the needle at the hub to make sure the wire fits through the needle (A).

Step 2—A stab incision is made, and the needle is inserted at the ventral midline, through the skin of the mandible, and passed along the surface of the bone, directed dorsally to the buccal-distal side of the canine (B).

Step 3—The needle is grasped with orthodontic pliers while the wire is pushed up, but not completely, through the needle (C). The needle is removed, leaving the wire between the bone and skin and exiting both at the access and exit sites.

Step 4—The needle is reinserted at the ventral midline into the skin of the mandible and directed dorsally to the buccal-distal side of the opposite canine, in a fashion similar to that of the first insertion (D).

Step 5—The wire is inserted into the bore at the tip of the needle (E).

Step 6—The needle is removed, along with the wire.

Step 7—While the symphysis is stabilized in proper alignment, the wire ends are clamped together at the midventral puncture site and twisted until the mandible is stable (F). A small orthopedic wire-twister is preferred, but a strong needle holder can be used, observing traditional guidelines for effective cerclage technique.

Step 8—The wire is trimmed so that approximately ¼ inch or four twists remain.

Step 9—The wire is gently bent out of the way so that the sharp edge does not protrude or irritate. A single cruciate skin stitch is placed to close the skin and cover the wire.

Complications

• Breaking the wire by overtwisting. This requires rewiring.
• Overtightening causing misalignment or necrosis of bone and subsequent malunion (misalignment prevented by evaluating the occlusion after the wire is tightened; if the occlusion is not correct, adjustments should be made, another technique used, or the patient evaluated for other fractures or temporomandibular joint problems).

Aftercare

• The wire is removed after 4 to 6 weeks, and the jaw is checked for stability.
• Failure for union to occur may not be as serious as first thought. Many patients do very well with mandibles that function independently.
• Other forms of symphysial repair.
• Transosseous cortical screw.[2, 7, 8, 21]

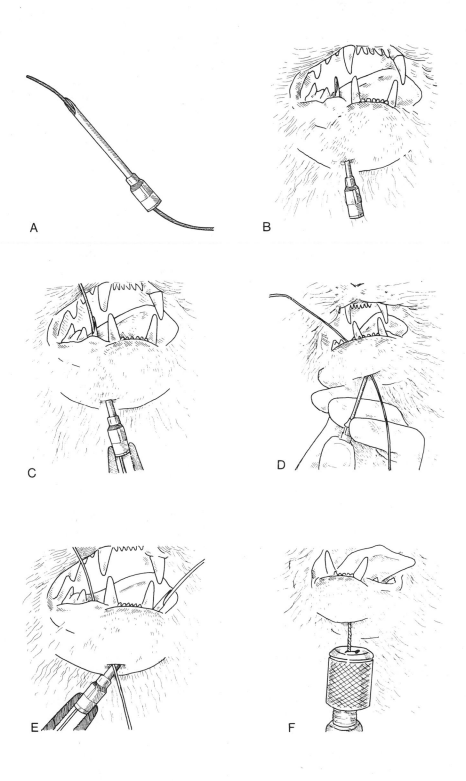

IVY LOOP WIRING TECHNIQUE

General Comment

- The Ivy loop wiring technique can be used alone or with other fracture stabilization techniques.[4, 5, 13, 17]

Indications

- Fractured maxilla.
- Fractured mandible.
- Stabilize intraoral acrylic splints.

Contraindication

- Unstable or comminuted fractures with tooth loss.

Objective

- To place a single wire interdentally, stabilizing and aligning adjacent teeth or providing anchorage for an intraoral splint.

Materials

- 24 or 26 gauge soft stainless steel wire.
- Howe pliers.
- Wire-twisting pliers.

Technique

Step 1—A length of wire is cut, and a loop is formed in the middle (A). The ends are twisted together once.

Step 2—The free ends are passed buccally to palatally/lingually in the interdental space between the two teeth to be stabilized at the gingival margin (B).

Step 3—One free end is passed rostrally and around the mesial aspect of the first tooth at the interdental space (C).

Step 4—The other free end is passed caudally and around the distal aspect of the second tooth at the interdental space (D). This wire is passed through the preformed loop rostrally and is twisted tight with the other free end (E).

Step 5—The loop can be tightened further, and the twisted ends can be bent to lie flat against the tooth surface.

Step 6—Dental acrylic or composite resin material can be placed over the wire loops for additional security of the wire and to minimize irritation of soft tissue from the loop twists (see pp. 464 to 465).

Complications

- Loosening wire with gingival irritation/recession.
- Inadequate fixation of fracture if used as a lone procedure in unstable fractures.

Aftercare

- Home oral hygiene with a water pick to keep the area clean.
- Follow-up radiographs to evaluate healing.
- Removal of wire and acrylic when healing is complete.

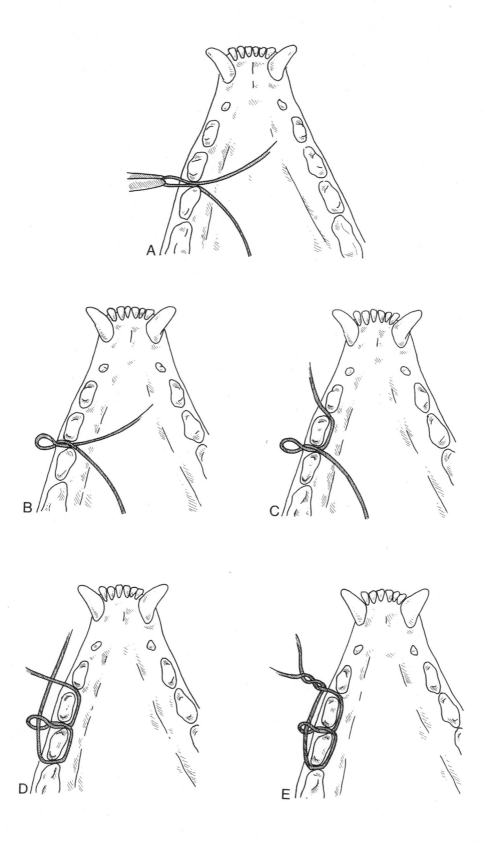

STOUT MULTIPLE LOOP WIRING TECHNIQUE

General Comments

- This technique can be used alone or with other stabilization techniques.[4, 7, 8, 13, 17, 23]
- This technique provides greater support of the dental arch than does the Ivy loop technique.

Indications

- Fractured maxilla.
- Fractured incisal bone.
- Fractured mandible.
- To stabilize intraoral acrylic splint.

Contraindication

- Unstable or comminuted fractures with missing teeth.

Objective

- To stabilize several adjacent teeth with an interdental wiring technique.

Materials

- 24 or 26 gauge soft stainless steel wire.
- Howe pliers.
- Wire-twisting pliers.

Technique

Step 1—A length of wire is cut and pre-stretched to eliminate kinks (A).

Step 2—One end of the wire is passed along the lateral surface of the teeth to be stabilized.

Step 3—The other end is passed around the distal tooth at the interdental space to the medial aspect (B).

Step 4—This end is passed back to the lateral surface at the next interdental space under the buccal wire and looped over the buccal wire and back medially through the same interdental space (C).

Step 5—The loop formed is twisted tight while the ends of the wire are held taut in place along the teeth (D).

Step 6—This process is repeated until all the teeth to be stabilized are encircled with the wire and their loops are tightened (E).

Step 7—The loop twists are bent flat against the tooth surface and can be covered with a dental acrylic or composite resin material for additional security after acid-etch preparation (F) (see Chapter 9, Dental Orthodontics, p. 412).

Complication

- Loosening of wire with gingival irritation/ recession.

Aftercare

- Home oral hygiene with a water pick to keep the area clean.
- Follow-up radiographs as necessary to evaluate healing.
- Removal of wires and acrylic when healing is complete.

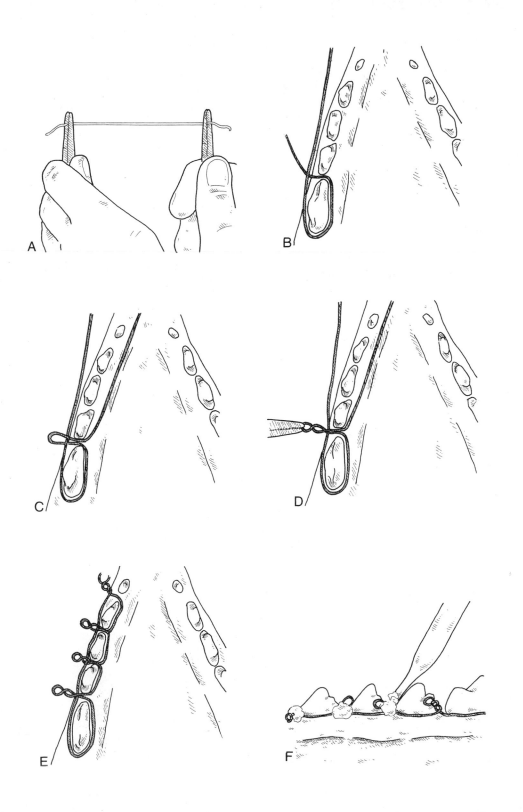

RISDON WIRING TECHNIQUE

General Comment

- The Risdon technique uses a master wire with auxiliary wires looped around the necks of the teeth and twisted around the master wire.[4, 13]

Indication

- Rostral jaw fractures.

Contraindication

- Lack of good support for teeth (periodontal disease, fractured alveolus, etc.).

Materials

- Various-gauge (18 to 26) soft stainless steel wire.
- Howe, or appropriate, orthodontic pliers.

Technique

Step 1—A length of wire is passed around the anchor tooth selected on each side of the jaw so that the midpoint is on the palatal/lingual surface and equal lengths protrude on the buccal surface (A).

Step 2—The free ends of the wires on each side of the head are twisted together for their entire length (B).

Step 3—The twisted strands from each side are brought together at the midline and are twisted together (C).

Step 4—Secondary wires are wrapped around the individual teeth in each arch and are twisted around the twisted master wire (D).

Complications

- Loosening or breaking of wires, in which case the procedure is repeated or an alternative wiring technique is chosen.
- Irritation of gingiva or soft tissue from loose ends; orthodontic wax or dental acrylic may be used to cover the sharp points of wire as prevention or treatment.

Aftercare

- Home oral hygiene with a water pick to keep the area clean.
- Follow-up radiographs as necessary to evaluate healing.
- Removal of wires and acrylic when healing is complete.

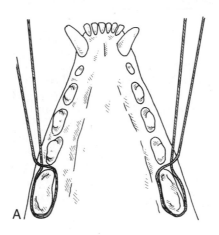

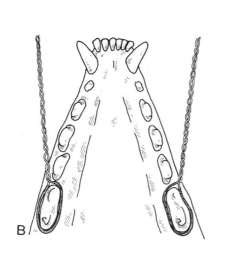

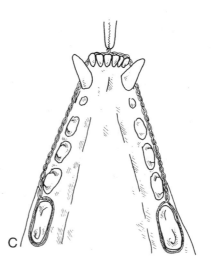

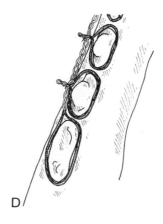

ESSIG WIRING TECHNIQUE

General Comment

- The Essig wiring technique uses a master wire looped around the teeth and twisted, with secondary wires looped around the master wires in the interproximal space and twisted tight.[4, 7, 8, 13, 17, 23]

Indication

- Alveolar fractures with loose or partially avulsed teeth.

Contraindications

- Severe periodontal disease.
- Tooth root fractures without other treatment.
- Missing teeth.

Materials

- Various-gauge (18 to 26) soft stainless steel wires.
- Howe, or appropriate, orthodontic pliers.

Technique

Step 1—The master wire is looped around the buccal and lingual surfaces of the teeth (A). If possible, four to five teeth should be used as anchors on each side of the fracture.

Step 2—The master wire is twisted at a site that is out of occlusion (B).

Step 3—The secondary wires are fed through the interproximal space, passing palatally (lingually), looped around the palatal (lingual) portion of the master wire, and passed buccally/labially through the interproximal space and around the buccal/labial portion of the master wire (C).

Step 4—The secondary wires are twisted together individually (D). Secondary wires are gradually and sequentially tightened until the palatal (lingual) master wire is tight against the teeth.

Step 5—The teeth are examined for stabilization.

Complications

- Overtightening of the wire causing unwanted orthodontic movement.
- Irritation of soft tissues.

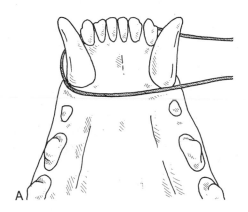

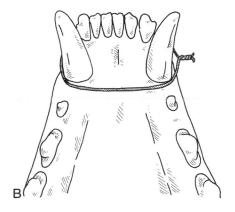

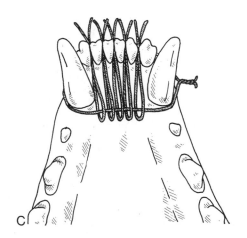

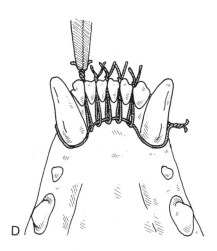

FIGURE-OF-EIGHT WIRING TECHNIQUE

General Comment

- Wire is wrapped around the canine teeth to provide stabilization in combination with dental acrylics.

Indications

- Mandibular symphysis fracture/separation.
- Avulsion (with root canal therapy) or luxation of the canine tooth.

Contraindications

- Severe periodontal disease.
- Osteomyelitis.
- Failure to perform root canal therapy in the case of avulsed teeth.

Materials

- Various-gauge (18 to 26) soft stainless steel wires.
- Howe, or appropriate, orthodontic pliers.
- Acid-etch materials.
- Orthodontic or light-cure acrylics.

Technique

Step 1—The teeth are scaled and polished with flour pumice.

Step 2—The wire is looped from the mesial aspect of one canine (A) to the distal aspect of the opposite canine (B) (A).

Step 3—The wire is looped in a buccal-mesial direction around the opposite canine (B).

Step 4—The wire is directed from canine B back toward the distal aspect of canine A (C).

Step 5—The two ends of the wire are joined together and are twisted on the distal surface (D).

Step 6—The wire and teeth are rinsed and acid-etched (see Chapter 8).

Step 7—Dental acrylic and/or composite is placed over the wire and teeth. The acrylic may be placed over the wire and mucosal tissue between the canines.

Step 8—Any rough surfaces are smoothed; then the appliance is polished.

Complications

- Breakage of wire.
- Slippage of wire from bonded teeth.
- Periodontitis from the wire.

Aftercare

- The wire is removed when healing has occurred (6 to 8 weeks).
- Depending on the case, radiographs may be necessary.
- Good oral hygiene must be maintained.

CONCLUSION

Many other more invasive forms of repair, including transosseous wiring, intramedullary pinning, plating, and Kirschner/Ehmer appliances, or combinations thereof, are described in the literature. A number of orthopedic and general surgical texts are useful for further information regarding these techniques.[2-6, 7, 8, 12, 23-28]

REFERENCES

1. Schrader SC. Dental Orthopedics. In: Small Animal Oral Medicine and Surgery. Philadelphia: Lea & Febiger, 1990:241–264.
2. Kertesz P. Oral Surgery: II. Orthopaedic Surgery of the Mandible and Maxilla. In: A Colour Atlas of Veterinary Dentistry and Oral Surgery. Aylesbury, England: Wolfe Publishers (imprint of Mosby–Year Book Europe Ltd.), 1993:165–182.
3. Manfra Marretta S, Schrader SC, Matthiesen DT. Problems Associated with the Management and Treatment of Jaw Fractures. In: Manfra Marretta S, ed. Problems in Veterinary Medicine—Dentistry. Philadelphia: J.B. Lippincott Co., 1990:220–247.
4. Wiggs RB, Lobprise HB. Oral Fracture Repair. In: Veterinary Dentistry Principles and Practice. Philadelphia: J.B. Lippincott Co., 1997:259–279.
5. Harvey CE, Emily PP. Oral Surgery. In: Small Animal Dentistry. St. Louis: Mosby, 1993:312–377.
6. Mulligan TW. Management of Mandible and Maxilla Fractures. Proceedings of the American Animal Hospital Association Dental Seminar, 1989:149–177.
7. Davidson JR. Treatment of mandibular and maxillary fractures in dogs and cats. Waltham International Focus 1993; 3:9–16.
8. Davidson JR, Bauer MS. Fractures of the mandible and the maxilla. Vet Clin North Am Small Anim Pract 1992; 22:109–119.
9. Wallace BJ, Kapatkin AS, Manfra Marretta S. Dental composite for the fixation of mandibular fractures and luxations in 11 cats and 6 dogs. Vet Surg 1994; 23:1990–1994.

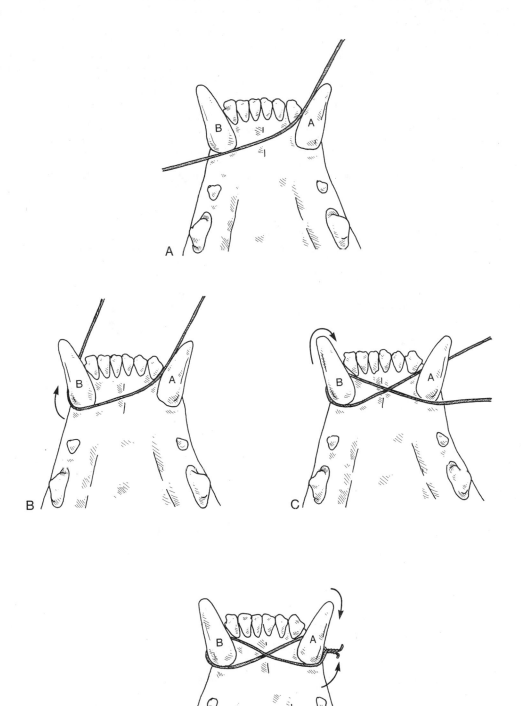

10. Zetner K. Parapulpar pin-anchored bridge for jaw fractures. Proceedings of American Veterinary Dental Society Annual Meeting. New Orleans, 1983.

11. Zetner K. Treatment of Jaw Fractures in Small Animals with Parapulpar Pin Composite Bridges. In: Harvey CE. Feline Dentistry. Vet Clin North Am Small Anim Pract 1992; November:1461–1467.

12. Shipp AD, Fahrenkrug P. Oral Surgery. In: Practitioners' Guide to Veterinary Dentistry. Beverly Hills: Dr. Shipps' Laboratories, 1992:148–167.

13. Tholen MA. Dental Orthopedics. In: Concepts in Veterinary Dentistry. Edwardsville, KS: Veterinary Medicine Publishing Co., 1983:139–143.

14. Miller TE, Margalit S, Creamer TH. Emergency direct/indirect polyethylene ribbon–reinforced composite resin, fixed partial denture: a case report. Compend Contin Educ—Dent 1996; 17:182–189.

15. Spellman G. Reduction of fractures of the mandibular symphysis using acrylic splints with circumandibular wiring. Small Anim Clin 1972; November:1213–1215.

16. Lantz GC. Maxillary splint rod for the repair of selected facial fractures. J Am Anim Hosp Assoc 1984; 20:905–910.

17. Merkley DF, Brinker WO. Facial reconstruction following massive bilateral maxillary fracture in dogs. Vet Digest 1978; March/April:22–24.

18. Henry RJ, Jerrell RG. Rationale and treatment of an avulsed permanent tooth. Compend Contin Educ—Dent 1990; 11:6:346–353.

19. Emily P. Simple mandibular fracture repair in dogs with acrylics. Vet Forum 1994; March:74.

20. Emily P. Noninvasive Mandibular Fracture Repair. Proceedings of the Tenth Annual Dental Forum. Houston, 1996.

21. McOwen, JS. Intraoral dental acrylic splint for mandibular fractures. Comp Anim Pract 1987; 1:17–18.

22. Wolff EF. Use of a cortical screw in repair of fractured mandibular symphysis in the cat. Vet Med Small Anim Clinician 1974; July:859–862.

23. Shulak FB. Complicated fracture of the mandible repaired with a simple wiring technique. Vet Med Small Anim Clinician 1977; Feb:174–177.

24. Chaffee VW. A technique for fixation of bilateral mandibular fractures caudal to the canine teeth in the dog. Vet Med Small Anim Clinician 1978; July:907–909.

25. Renegar WR, Leeds EB, Olds RB. The use of the Kirschner-Ehmer splint in clinical orthopedics: I. Long bone and mandibular fractures. Compend CE 1982; 4:381–392.

26. Biner WO, Piermattei DL, Flo GS. Fractures and dislocations of the upper and lower jaw. In: Handbook of Small Animal Orthopedics and Fracture Treatment. Philadelphia: W.B. Saunders Co., 1990:230–243.

27. Egger EL. Skull and mandibular fractures. In: Slatter DJ. Textbook of Small Animal Surgery, 2nd ed. Philadelphia: W.B. Saunders Co., 1993:1910–1921.

28. Taylor RA. Mandibular fractures. In: Bojrab MJ, ed. Current Techniques in Small Animal Surgery, 3rd ed. Philadelphia: Lea & Febiger, 1990:890–894.

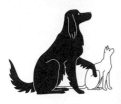

Chapter 11

ANESTHESIA AND PAIN MANAGEMENT IN DENTAL AND ORAL PROCEDURES

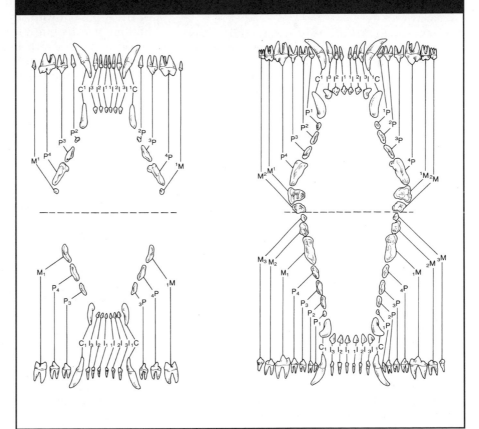

There is a vast amount of information about anesthesia that is beyond the scope of this book in terms of the nuances, idiosyncrasies, and precautions that should be more thoroughly investigated by the reader. This chapter is intended to serve as a user-friendly guide to some convenient anesthesia practices, routes of administration, and management suggestions before, during, and after operative dentistry on the small-animal patient.

GENERAL ANESTHESIA

General Comments

- General anesthesia is a necessary part of most dental procedures to provide immobility and safe and total access to the oral cavity.
- Dental patients are usually categorized, according to the American Society of Anesthesiologists (ASA) classification, as class I or II (normal patient or patient with mild systemic disease; see the following chart). In clinical practice, a notable exception to this is the geriatric patient or the patient that is immunologically or metabolically compromised.
- Safe anesthetic protocols are available even for young puppies and kittens so they can be placed under general anesthesia for various dental procedures such as interceptive orthodontic extractions.
- General anesthesia is often a major concern of the client, particularly when multiple anesthesia sessions are required.
- A significant portion of the cost of any dental procedure is generated by anesthesia, supportive measures during anesthesia, and preoperative laboratory tests before anesthesia.
- Attention and adjustment to correct the physiologic changes that occur during anesthesia, such as reduced body temperature, decreased blood pressure, and reduced circulation, will ensure a safer anesthesia session.
- With proper attention to their physiologic needs, healthy geriatric patients or patients with mild systemic diseases can be safely anesthetized. These patients can be treated for their dental disease and will benefit from improved oral health.
- Anesthesia records should include administration time, route, and duration of anesthetic drugs; dosages used; fluids administered; catheter type, size, and location; endotracheal tube size; and monitoring parameters.
- Charting heart rate and respiratory rate is beneficial. Adverse reactions or delayed recovery should be noted so that future anesthetic protocols can be adjusted.
- To prevent aspiration during dentistry, food is withheld for 12 hours before induction of anesthesia, except for young patients and diabetics to prevent hypoglycemia. Water should not be withheld until the morning of the procedure.

Chart: ASA Classifications[1]

ASA I: A normal patient with no organic disease.
ASA II: A patient with mild systemic disease.
ASA III: A patient with severe systemic disease limiting activity but not incapacitating.
ASA IV: A patient with incapacitating disease that is a constant threat to life.
ASA V: A moribund patient not expected to live 24 hours with or without surgery.

- Patient evaluation prior to anesthesia includes (1) signalment (species, breed, age, sex), (2) a complete physical examination, (3) the chief complaint, and (4) the prior medical history.

Preprocedure Work-Up

- Patients are generally classified into one of two age groups for preanesthesia laboratory work-ups. It is recommended that generally healthy patients younger than 6 years of age be screened with the following tests: hematocrit level, total protein, liver and kidney function tests, and a urine specific gravity. Patients older than 6 years of age generally should have a complete blood count and chemistry profile performed as a minimum database. Additionally, tests of thyroid function, feline leukemia and feline immunodeficiency virus (for cats), urinalysis, electrocardiogram, and thoracic radiography should be scheduled, depending on the patient's condition and the client's permission.
- Other considerations for determining the anesthetic protocol include weight, temperament, procedure to be performed, length of anticipated procedure, concurrent diseases (e.g., epilepsy, heart disease, kidney disease, liver disease, endocrine disease,

gastrointestinal disease, or bleeding disorders), medications administered previously or concurrently, previous anesthesia experiences, and dietary history.[2]

Preanesthetic Medications

Comments

- Preanesthetic medications are used to reduce the anxiety level of the patient and to reduce secretions and may also be used to provide analgesia.
- These drugs are usually given subcutaneously or intramuscularly 10 to 40 minutes before induction of general anesthesia.
- In some instances they can be administered intravenously immediately before the induction agent.
- Intravenous administration in compromised patients may cause a more profound effect than desired; it is preferable to administer these drugs intramuscularly or subcutaneously.
- Dosages provided here are for young, healthy patients; older or debilitated patients may require reduced dose amounts.

Anticholinergics

Comments

- To maintain heart rate and cardiac output so as to counteract strong vagal tone caused by the parasympathetic nervous system.
- To help dry the respiratory passages and to reduce salivary secretions.
- Two commonly used drugs are atropine and glycopyrrolate.

Atropine

- Dose: cat/dog—0.02 to 0.04 mg/kg intramuscularly or subcutaneously.[3, 4]

Advantages

- Short time of onset.
- Can be given intraoperatively to increase heart rate if sinus bradycardia develops.

Disadvantages

- Duration of 60 to 90 minutes.
- Can cause sinus tachycardia.

Glycopyrrolate

- Dose: cat/dog—0.01 mg/kg intramuscularly or subcutaneously.[3, 4]

Advantages

- Less effect on heart rate than atropine.
- Lasts longer than atropine (2 to 3 hours).

Disadvantages

- Takes 30 to 45 minutes to reach peak effect.
- More expensive than atropine.
- Indicated, instead of atropine, for use in patients with tachycardia.

Tranquilizers/Sedatives

Comment

- Reduce nervousness; reduce the amount of induction agent required to allow intubation; smooth the transition to gas anesthetic; and reduce the amount of inhalant anesthetic required to maintain anesthesia.

Acepromazine

- Dose: cat/dog—0.01 to 0.06 mg/kg intramuscularly or subcutaneously (maximum dose 3 mg).[4]

Advantages

- Produces a significant calming effect on most patients.
- Inexpensive.
- Can be protective of heart arrhythmias related to catecholamine release.

Disadvantages

- Not for use in compromised patients.
- Can cause peripheral vasodilation, potentiating hypotension and hypothermia.
- Requires biotransformation in the liver; can have a prolonged effect in some patients, and they may remain sedated at the time of hospital release.
- No analgesic effect.
- Potentiates seizures.

Diazepam

- Dose: cat/dog—0.2 to 0.5 mg/kg intravenously or intramuscularly.[3, 4]

Advantages

- Minimal central nervous system or cardio-vascular depression.
- Produces muscle relaxation.
- Protects from seizures.
- When used with ketamine, can provide short-term anesthesia or be used as a combination induction agent.
- When used with a narcotic, provides good sedation and tranquilization.

Disadvantages

- When administered intramuscularly it can provide unpredictable absorption.
- Rapid intravenous injection can lead to hypotension and bradycardia.
- More expensive than acepromazine.

Narcotics

Comments

- The use of narcotics as a preanesthetic medication can provide analgesia as well as sedation.
- Butorphanol is effective for cases with mild to moderate pain potential.
- Morphine and oxymorphone produce greater pain relief but also greater respiratory depression.
- Administering narcotics as preanesthetic medications can dramatically reduce the amount of anesthetic agent required to maintain anesthesia.
- Meperidine HCl is approximately one eighth as potent as morphine but produces a similar level of respiratory depression as morphine at equal levels of anesthesia. It does not suppress the cough at doses lower than the anesthetic dose. It is the only used opioid that causes vagolytic and negative inotropic effects at clinically used doses.[5] It should be used cautiously in greatly debilitated patients as well as in those with hypothyroidism, severe renal insufficiency, and adrenocortical insufficiency. The same precautions and contraindications should be observed as with other opiates. Other central nervous system depressants, phenothiazines, antihistamines, tranquilizers, or alcohol used in combination with meperidine may cause increased central nervous system or respiratory depression.[5]

Dosages

- Butorphanol: cat/dog—0.2 to 0.4 mg/kg intramuscularly or subcutaneously and 0.1 mg/kg intraveneously.[3, 4]
- Morphine: dog—0.5 to 1.0 mg/kg subcutaneously or intramuscularly.[3, 4]
- Meperidine: cat/dog—2.0 to 5.0 mg/kg intramuscularly or subcutaneously[4]; dog—2.5 to 6.5 mg/kg or cat—2.2 to 4.4 mg/kg may be used as a preanesthetic.
- Oxymorphone: cat/dog—0.04 to 0.06 mg/kg intramuscularly or subcutaneously.[4]

Advantages

- Provide analgesia.
- Produce a calming effect.
- Can be given with phenothiazine for additional sedation in aggressive patients.
- Reduce anesthetic requirements.
- Do not depress myocardial contractility.
- Narcotic effect can be reversed with a narcotic antagonist such as naloxone.

Disadvantages

- Can cause sinus bradycardia; risk reduced by administration in conjunction with anticholinergic.
- Can cause respiratory depression.
- Can cause behavioral changes in some patients (vocalization).
- May cause panting.
- Can create startle response with loud noises.

α_2-Adrenoreceptor Agonist

Fentanyl Citrate

Advantages
- Very potent opiate, with the same indications and cautions as other narcotics.
- Compatible with dextrose 5% in water (D$_5$W), dextrose 5% in lactated Ringer's solution (D$_5$LRS), physiologic saline solution (PSS), potassium chloride (KCl), glycopyrrolate, heparin sodium, hydrocortisone, sodium succinate, KCl, and sodium bicarbonate (NaHCO$_3$).[5]
- Causes tranquilization and sedation, although may be less than that provided by phenothiazine tranquilizers.
- May be used alone for minor procedures or in combination with more potent general anesthetics for major surgical procedures.

- Duration of effect is 30 to 40 minutes; sedation remains for several hours.
- Naloxone is an antagonist and can be used to reverse fentanyl citrate's effects.

Disadvantages

- May cause defecation, flatulence, respiratory depression, panting, and nystagmus; if the patient is not pretreated with atropine or glycopyrrolate, may also cause bradycardia and salivation.
- Overdosing may cause marked central nervous system or respiratory depression. In severe cases, cardiovascular collapse, tremors, neck rigidity, and seizures have been reported.[6]
- Naloxone may have to be repeated in cases of severe overdosage.

Preanesthetic Use in Dogs

- As an ingredient in a preanesthetic recipe.[7]

Technique

- A sterile vial of diluted acepromazine is prepared by adding 9.0 ml physiologic saline to 1.0 ml acepromazine. The diluted solution is stored at room temperature.
- The dose of fentanyl is 1.0 ml/5 kg subcutaneously (maximum of 8.0 ml). In the same syringe as the fentanyl, add the diluted acepromazine, using 0.1 ml acepromazine per calculated 1.0 ml fentanyl.

Comments

- Glycopyrrolate, at a dose of 1.0 ml/22 kg, can be added to the same syringe or administered subcutaneously from a separate syringe.
- Fentanyl reaches peak levels 40 minutes after subcutaneous administration.
- Anesthetic induction is administered to effect when sedation is clinically apparent (approximately 20 minutes).
- An appropriately reduced dose of induction medications, such as equal parts of ketamine hydrochloride and diazepam, should be used as it would be with any narcotic preanesthetic.

Xylazine

- Dose: dog—0.2 mg/kg intramuscularly; cat—0.5 to 1 mg/kg intramuscularly.[3]

Advantages

- Produces muscle relaxation and a sleep state.
- Produces a sedative effect that can last 1 to 2 hours.

- Can be given in combination with narcotic or ketamine for more profound sedation.
- Can be reversed with yohimbine HCl.

Disadvantages

- Can produce bradycardia, second-degree heart block, and increased peripheral resistance.
- Can lead to hypotension.
- May cause respiratory depression, emesis, and bloating in large dogs.
- Requires hepatic metabolism.
- Not an analgesic.

Neuroleptanalgesia

Comments

- Combines a narcotic agent with a tranquilizer as a preanesthetic medication.
- Combination dosages:

    Cat/dog—acepromazine 0.02 to 0.05 mg/kg + meperidine HCl 4.0 to 5.0 mg/kg subcutaneously or intramuscularly.[4]
    Cat/dog—acepromazine 0.02 to 0.05 mg/kg + oxymorphone 0.04 mg/kg subcutaneously or intramuscularly.[4]
    Cat/dog—acepromazine 0.02 mg/kg + butorphanol 0.1 mg/kg subcutaneously or intramuscularly.[4]

Advantages

- Provides analgesia.
- Provides sedation.
- Reduces amount of induction agent required.
- Good for aggressive patients.
- Provides adequate sedation for quiet mask induction.
- Narcotic portion can be reversed.

Disadvantages

- Can create excessive sedation.
- Can create respiratory depression.
- Can create bradycardia.
- Can create dysphoria.

Induction Drugs

Comments

- Induction drugs are used to induce unconsciousness in a smooth, struggle-free manner.

- These drugs are generally administered fairly rapidly intravenously before intubation.
- Adverse effects of these drugs are dose-dependent; therefore, it is beneficial to give them in small, rapid increments to minimize adverse reactions.

Barbiturates

Thiopental Sodium
- Dose: dogs and cats—10 mg/kg.[4]
- A 2.5% solution is used for dogs.[4]
- A 1.25% solution is used for cats.[4]

Advantages
- Inexpensive.
- Rapid, smooth induction.
- Good relaxation for intubation.
- Relatively short acting.

Disadvantages
- Requires redistribution to fat and muscle for termination of effect. Contraindicated in sight hounds and obese patients.
- Requires hepatic transformation.
- Can cause severe reactions if given extravenously (in greater than 2% solutions).
- Can cause hypotension, arrhythmias, heart block, and apnea.

Dissociative Agents

Ketamine
- Dose: cat—5.0 to 10.0 mg/kg intramuscularly.[4]
- Can be given intravenously with diazepam as an induction agent.

Advantages
- Relatively inexpensive.
- Minimal effect on cardiac output, blood pressure, and respiration.
- Causes immobility and dissociation from the environment.
- No tissue reaction if accidentally given extravenously (but is painful, especially in cats).
- Alone as a single agent or in combination with another agent is good for short period of restraint.

Disadvantages
- Causes increased salivation. Anticholinergics must be given before use.
- Can cause central nervous system excitement; possibly seizures.
- Causes renal excretion in cats, biotransformation by the liver in dogs.
- Poor analgesic.

Propofol

Comments
- A safe, short-acting anesthetic agent that is milky white for intravenous injection.
- Dose: cats/dogs—4.0 mg/kg intravenously with sedation; 6.0 mg/kg without sedation.[3, 4]

Advantages
- Short duration of anesthesia; can be given as repeated injections or continuous infusion.
- Rapid recovery (approximately 15 to 30 minutes until patient is standing unaided) without hangover effect.

Disadvantages
- Can cause significant respiratory depression if given too rapidly.
- Expensive.
- Vial of anesthetic does not contain preservatives; not suitable for multiple procedures from one vial without risk of contamination.
- Required doses vary slightly between genders and between dogs and cats; drug should be administered slowly, intravenously, and to effect.[8-15]
- Most prevalent adverse effect is apnea and is seen most often after rapid administration.[14]
- One dog has been reported to have prolonged excitement and seizure-like activity on recovery from propofol (dog had been previously diagnosed with idiopathic epilepsy).[13]

Induction Agent/Drug Combinations

Ketamine/Diazepam

- Dose: cat/dog—diazepam (5.0 mg/ml) with ketamine (100 mg/ml) given as a 50/50 mixture 1 ml/9 kg body weight[3] intravenously; alternatively, 0.5 mg/kg diazepam + 5.0 mg/kg ketamine intravenously.[4]
- Mix in same syringe just before induction, after premedication with anticholinergic and tranquilizer of preference.

Advantages
- Safe induction agent.
- Minimal cardiovascular effects.
- Same as individual drugs.

Disadvantages
- Patient may be semiconscious for intubation and may resist procedure.

- Can produce apnea.
- Patient may have rough, hyperactive recovery from ketamine.

Thiopental Sodium/Diazepam

- Dose: cat/dog—thiopental sodium 10.0 mg/kg + diazepam 0.2 to 0.5 mg/kg intravenously.[4]
- Give each drug separately intravenously; start with one-half dose thiopental sodium, then flush with saline, follow with one-half dose diazepam, and flush. Repeat the sequence with one-quarter dosages until patient is relaxed enough to permit intubation.

Advantages
- Smooth induction.
- Lower dose of thiopental sodium given for decreased undesirable cardiovascular effects.
- Patient relaxed for intubation.
- Smooth recovery.

Disadvantages
- Slower induction when administering drugs alternatively and waiting for effect.
- Requires intravenous catheter.

Propofol/Diazepam

- Dose: cat/dog—4.0 mg/kg propofol and 0.2 to 0.5 mg/kg diazepam intravenously.[4]
- Administered similarly to above combination, with similar advantages and disadvantages. One effective protocol, with or without a preanesthetic, is to use 4.0 mg/kg propofol and 0.3 mg/kg diazepam intravenously and slowly in separate syringes in the following format: install an intravenous catheter, inject 25% of the propofol dose, flush with PSS, inject 50% of the diazepam dose, and flush with PSS; then if necessary, inject 25% of the propofol dose, flush with PSS, follow as necessary with 50% of the diazepam dose, flush with PSS, and intubate.[8]

Inhalant Anesthetics

Methoxyflurane

Advantage
- Inexpensive.

Disadvantages
- Prolonged recovery.
- Does not use precision vaporizer.

- Greater hepatic metabolization than other inhalant anesthetics (up to 50%).[3]

Halothane

Advantages
- Inexpensive.
- Rapid induction and recovery.
- Can be used for mask or chamber induction.
- Precision vaporization for control of level of anesthetic administered.

Disadvantages
- Can cause heart arrhythmia.
- Taken up by body fat.
- Produces dose-dependent respiratory and cardiovascular depression.
- Requires some hepatic metabolization (25%).[3]
- Needs longer time to be removed from system than does isoflurane.

Isoflurane

Advantages
- Slightly more rapid induction than halothane.
- Can be used for mask or chamber induction.
- Because it is less soluble in blood and tissue than halothane, isoflurane provides a quicker recovery than halothane.
- Almost no hepatic metabolization (less than 1%).[3]
- Causes less cardiovascular depression and fewer arrhythmias than halothane.

Disadvantages
- May cause hypotension at high levels.
- Causes dose-dependent cardiovascular and respiratory depression.

Mask or Chamber Induction

Comments

- The use of gas anesthetics such as halothane or isoflurane can be used after preanesthetic medication by application of a mask or chamber box to induce anesthesia.
- The patient is given a period of straight oxygen before the anesthetic is introduced in small increments up to a maximum of 3 to 5%.
- As the patient becomes relaxed in the chamber, the patient can be removed, and additional anesthetic can be administered via mask until the patient is ready to intu-

bate (do not use these techniques in patients that are vomiting).

Advantages

- Chamber induction can be used on smaller patients that are too fractious to restrain safely for intravenous induction.
- Can induce anesthesia without additional drugs to be metabolized.
- Allows for more rapid recovery from anesthetic when no other induction drugs are used.

Disadvantages

- Difficult to use on larger patients that are harder to restrain during induction phase.
- Uses more anesthetic agent and is therefore more costly.
- Short time to intubate.
- Patients will be in a lighter plane of anesthesia without additional induction drugs.
- May initially require a higher percentage of anesthetic.
- Higher degree of environmental contamination with anesthetic vapors released into the operatory environment.

Monitoring

General Comments

- Monitoring the patient during the anesthesia period is becoming the standard of practice and is necessary in order to provide safe anesthesia.
- No one method is completely adequate or accurate; therefore, it is best to monitor more than one body system during anesthesia.[16]
- Physical responses can be observed. Heart rate, respiratory rate, eye position, palpebral reflex, blood pressure rate and character, mucous membrane color, and capillary refill can be easily monitored by an assistant and should be measured and charted at regular, frequent intervals.
- Adjustments in the flow of anesthetic should be made to keep the patient at a stable level of anesthesia.
- In private practice, physical monitoring is often inadequate due to a limited number of personnel. Electronic monitoring devices are therefore advantageous for detecting changes in the patient's anesthetic condition before a crisis occurs.

Pulse Oximeter

Comments

- This is believed to be the most sensitive indicator of the patient's condition, because it measures the percentage of oxygen saturation of hemoglobin in the arterial vascular supply.
- This parameter is the first to drop before other changes in heart rate or respiratory rate are noticed.
- The oximeter can be used on the tongue, ear flap, vulva, rectum prepuce tissue, or toe web *(A) (B)*.
- A reading between 96 and 100 SpO_2 is considered normal.[17]

Advantages

- Can be placed in areas away from the mouth.
- Various models available, some able to monitor additional parameters.
- Noninvasive method for monitoring arterial oxygenation.

Disadvantages

- Expensive.
- Oximeter may become dislodged when patient is moved.
- Some oximeters do not measure oxygen saturation well other than on the tongue.
- Skin pigmentation, icterus can cause abnormal readings.

Blood Pressure Monitor

Comments

- Arterial blood pressure is created by heart rate, stroke volume, and peripheral resistance.
- Many preanesthetic agents and most general anesthetic agents affect these parameters and may cause hypotension.
- In addition, blood loss may decrease venous return and thus stroke volume, causing a decrease in stroke volume and blood pressure. Blood pressure may be measured directly or indirectly.
- Direct measurement requires placement of a catheter and the measurement of a column of fluid suspended above the patient or the use of an aneroid manometer.
- Indirect blood pressure monitoring uses external equipment to obtain the measurement.
- Blood pressure may be indirectly monitored by manual indirect sphygmomanometry, Doppler monitor, and oscillometrics.

Manual Indirect Sphygmomanometry

- A cuff is attached to a pressure gauge and a pump, and the pulse is ascertained with a stethoscope.
- Air is pumped into the cuff, occluding the artery; the pulse is no longer heard.
- As the pressure is released, blood again begins to flow.
- A pulse is heard, and the needle on the gauge is seen to oscillate.
- The beginning of the oscillation is the systolic pressure.
- The point at which the needle no longer oscillates is considered the diastolic pressure.

Doppler Blood Pressure Measurement

- Doppler blood pressure measurement uses a small piezoelectric crystal over an artery.
- This crystal emits an ultrasonic pulse that is reflected back from moving tissues at a slightly different frequency.

- This shift in tone is converted to an audible tone that can be heard and/or measured.
- A mean systemic blood pressure above 50 to 60 mm Hg in an anesthetized patient is necessary for adequate cardiovascular function and tissue perfusion.[6, 18] Pressure readings should be taken frequently so that trends can be followed.

Oscillometric Instruments

- The method that oscillometric instruments use to measure blood pressure is similar to that of manual measurement.
- A cuff is placed around an extremity, and a probe is placed over the digital artery on the palmar aspect of the foot, proximal to the central pad (C). The appropriate cuff is used, the width being approximately 40% of the circumference of the extremity. It is placed proximal to the probe.
- Systolic, mean, and diastolic blood pressure and heart rate are computed and displayed. Many of these instruments can be set to measure blood pressure at preset intervals.

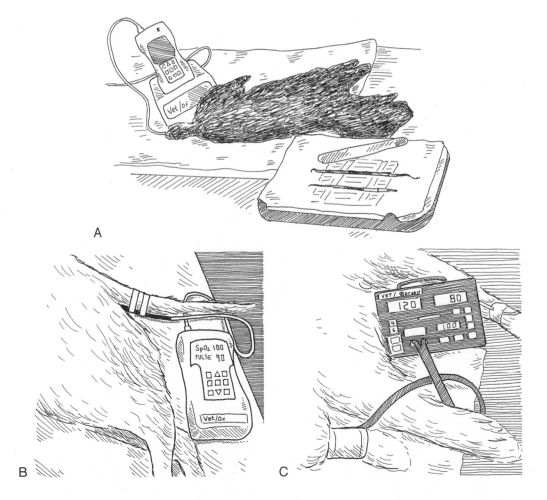

Advantages

- Give early monitoring of physiologic status of blood pressure before crisis occurs.
- Out of the way of the oral cavity.
- Provide reading of pulse rate and rhythm.
- Can monitor response to anesthetic adjustments and increased fluid flow.

Disadvantages

- Expensive.
- Inaccurate readings in very small patients, due to sizes of cuffs available.
- Difficult to get reading on some patients.
- Probe can be dislodged when patient is repositioned.
- Battery-operated units may lose charge during procedure.

Respiratory Monitor

Comments

- Adequate respiratory function is essential to maintain adequate tissue oxygenation and carbon dioxide elimination; therefore, monitoring respiration is important.
- These monitors have an attachment to the endotracheal tube that measures each respiration.
- The monitors can be preset to sound an alarm if apnea is present. They also provide an audible beep with each respiration. The respiratory rate should be a minimum of 8 to 10 breaths per minute.[17]

Advantages

- Inexpensive.
- Can be used easily on a patient of any size.
- Provides early recognition of changes in respiratory rate.
- Monitor is not in the way.

Disadvantages

- Does not measure depth of respiration.
- Less sensitive monitoring than Doppler monitor or pulse oximeter.

Combined Respiratory and Heart Monitor (The Beeper*)

Comments

- Attaches to the endotracheal tube and has a two-lead attachment to front legs to monitor heart rate.

---

*Spencer Instrumentation, Inc. 17286 Citron, Irvine, CA 92612

- Provides two separate readings and beeps for heart rate and respiratory rate.
- Alarm can be set for either function.

Advantages

- Gives two continuous parameters of patient status.
- Only moderately expensive.
- Attachments are not in the mouth.

Disadvantages

- Less sensitive than pulse oximeter, Doppler monitor, or electrocardiogram monitor.

Electrocardiogram Monitor

Comments

- Clamps or needles are attached to the skin near the elbows and flanks and attached to leads to provide continuous electrocardiogram and cardiac rhythm readings.

Advantages

- Monitors heart rate and rhythm.
- Can get accurate measurement of cardiac response to anesthesia.
- Can get information on oxygen saturation (depressed ST segment), electrolyte disturbances, abnormal beats and type of arrhythmias that may not be detected by other monitoring techniques.

Disadvantages

- Expensive.
- Can have interference from other electrical systems (electrocautery).
- Must be monitored closely for subtle changes or periodic abnormal complexes.
- Can have a normal electrocardiogram and still have a serious condition or change in anesthetic status occurring.
- Best to use in conjunction with other monitoring.
- Clamps or needles may be dislodged when the patient is repositioned.

Esophageal Heart Monitor

Comments

- A probe is inserted orally into the esophagus to a level near the heart, and it records the heartbeat on an audible amplifier.
- Normal heart rates for dogs during anes-

thesia should range between 60 and 140 beats per minute; for cats, between 80 and 160 beats per minute.[17]

- Bradycardia during anesthesia can be caused by increased vagal tone, too deep an anesthetic plane, hypothermia, hypoxia, hypertension, and hyperkalemia.
- Tachycardia during anesthesia can be caused by the patient's being too light and responding to painful stimuli, hypotension, hypoxia, hypercarbia, or hyperthermia.

Advantages

- Inexpensive.
- Monitors heart rate to measure patient's response to anesthesia.
- May also hear breathing sounds.

Disadvantages

- Places an additional tube in the patient's mouth during a dental procedure.
- Secondary noise can be distracting when patient is moved or tube is moved.
- Is not an early detection of the patient's changes in physiologic response to anesthesia.

Temperature Monitor

Comments

- Body temperature changes of the patient can affect its response to anesthesia. This can be a problem with prolonged procedures.
- Prevention of hypothermia can be easily accomplished by using a circulating water heating pad. Further conservation of body heat can be achieved by covering the patient's body with a towel or blanket. This conservation can be further enhanced if the towel is just removed from a clothes drier.
- Wrapping small dogs and cats in bubble wrap or a plastic bag will also help retain body heat.
- Administering warm oral flushing solutions, keeping the patient as dry as possible during dental procedures, and maintaining the ambient temperature at a comfortable level is helpful.
- Hypothermia is the most common temperature change that occurs during anesthesia.
- Hypothermia most frequently occurs in small, short-coated pets, but it can also occur in large, heavy-coated dogs.
- Malignant hyperthermia is a rare pathologic complication that occurs during anes-

thesia. The body temperature can rise fatally. Body temperature can be monitored with a standard rectal mercury thermometer or by using rectal or esophageal probes that record body temperature.

- These thermometers should be able to read a decrease as well as an increase in body temperature, unlike a fever thermometer.

Body Changes with Hypothermia

- Body temperature below 100 degrees F.
- Prolonged recovery from anesthesia.
- Bradycardia.
- Less anesthetic required.
- Hypotension.
- Shivering creating an increased oxygen demand.

Body Changes with Hyperthermia

- Body temperature above 104 degrees F.
- Tachycardia.
- Increased respiratory rate.

Changes in Anesthesia Status During Procedure

Problem

Anesthetic plane too light.

- Changes noticed in patient's status.
- Increased respiratory and heart rate.
- Movement of eyes, jaw, or limbs.
- Increased blood pressure reading.

Correction

- Check anesthetic level in vaporizer.
- Check vaporizer setting.
- Check equipment circuit.
- Check freshness of carbon dioxide granules.
- Check placement of endotracheal tube and connection to anesthetic hose.
- Check oxygen flow.
- Check vaporizer calibration.

Problem

Anesthetic plane too deep.

- Changes noted in patient's status.
- Decreased heart and respiratory rate.
- Lowered blood pressure reading.

Correction

- Check vaporizer setting.
- Check patient positioning.
- Check oxygen setting.
- Ventilate patient as necessary.

Additional Considerations for General Anesthesia

- A proper-sized endotracheal tube with an inflated cuff is used in dental and oral surgery patients to keep water, blood, and calculus debris from being aspirated.
- The endotracheal tube should be stabilized to prevent accidental extubation and/or leakage around the tube. Gauze ties, rubber bands, or used intravenous tubing can be used to secure the tube.
- It may be desirable for patients undergoing major oral surgery, such as fracture repair, where intraoperative evaluation of occlusion is necessary, to have the endotracheal tube exit through a pharyngotomy incision in order to keep the oral cavity clear. (Continuous infusion of propofol or other intravenous anesthetic agent is an alternative protocol during fracture repair.)
- It is appropriate during prolonged procedures for intravenous fluids to be administered. Older, more brittle patients can maintain a better fluid balance if fluid therapy is started before the procedure and continued after the procedure until they are alert, stable, and their swallow reflex has returned.
- Less stable patients will often benefit by receiving intravenous fluids on the day before and after the procedure.

Regional/Local Anesthesia

General Comments

- Local dental nerve blocks can be administered in conjunction with general anesthetic for greater pain relief and reduced general anesthetic levels during oral surgery procedures. Local anesthesia will also provide increased postoperative analgesia.
- Longer acting anesthetics, such as 0.5% bupivacaine, can provide analgesia for 6 to 10 hours; 2% lidocaine without epinephrine gives a shorter duration (less than 2 hours); 2% mepivacaine provides a moderate duration (4 hours).[1]
- Regional blocks are introduced at the nerve foramen and create anesthesia of the regional teeth and associated soft tissues.
- Local blocks are accomplished by injecting anesthetic into the periodontal space and/or gingiva surrounding the tooth. Local blocks provide anesthesia only for the limited area directly perfused by local infiltration.

- Total maximum dose of bupivacaine for cats and dogs is 2 mg/kg.[4]
- A 1.5-in 27 gauge needle on a dental anesthetic syringe is designed to be used with the anesthetic Carpule and works most effectively. Alternatively, a 1 ml^3 syringe with a 27 gauge hypodermic needle can be used to withdraw the anesthetic from the Carpule and infiltrate it into the site.
- Use of regional anesthetic can significantly reduce the level of general anesthetic required.
- With practice, nerve blocks can be performed accurately and can be very efficacious.

Technique[19, 20]

Infraorbital Nerve Block

Caudal

- The injection site is located where the infraorbital nerve enters the maxillary foramen.
- The injection site in the dog is dorsal to the last maxillary molar at the ventral-most junction of the zygomatic bone on the maxilla.
- Advance the needle tip to the pterygopalatine fossa, and inject anesthetic adjacent to the nerve.
- This provides anesthesia to all the maxillary teeth and soft tissues on that side.

Cranial

- The injection site is located at the rostral end of the infraorbital canal.
- The infraorbital canal foramen can be palpated dorsal to the distal root of the third premolar.
- Advance the needle into the canal approximately 0.5 to 1.0 cm, and inject anesthetic adjacent to the nerve.
- The infraorbital nerve block desensitizes the maxillary incisors, canine, first two premolars, and the soft tissues on that side.

Mandibular Alveolar Nerve Block

- The mandibular foramen is on the lingual aspect of the mandible at the base of the coronoid process.
- It is palpated, and the needle is inserted perpendicular to the ventral border of the mandible.
- The needle is advanced 1 to 2 cm, and anesthetic is injected adjacent to the nerve.
- The mandibular nerve block desensitizes all the mandibular teeth on that side.

Mental Nerve Block

- Use the middle mental foramen; it is the largest of the three foramina.
- It is palpated ventral to the mesial root of the second premolar.
- The needle is inserted 0.5 to 1.0 cm, and the anesthetic is injected adjacent to the nerve.
- The mental nerve block desensitizes the mandibular incisors, canine tooth, first two premolars, and associated soft tissues on that side.

Advantages
- Provides pain relief during the procedure and postoperatively.
- Reduces anesthetic requirements.

Disadvantages
- Can add additional time to procedure.
- Potential nerve injury.

Pain Management

General Comments

- Pain recognition and its management is becoming an important part of dental treatment.
- Animals have an evolutionary stoicism; in the wild, if an animal appears sick or injured, it may be eliminated by the group or attacked by predators[21]; therefore, patients can be adept at hiding behaviors that indicate pain. This seems to be the case with dental disease; it is often quite advanced, and many patients exhibit minimal signs of discomfort.
- There are individual, species, and breed variations in the response to painful stimuli.
- Signs of pain can be expressed by a change in behavior, vocalization, aggression, shivering, restlessness, reluctance to move or eat, guarding or avoidance of touch, and increased salivation.
- Dilated pupils, tachycardia, hypertension, possible increase in respiratory rate, heart arrhythmias, and hyperglycemia can also be noted in pained patients.[22]
- Control of pain is important physiologically. (1) As pain increases, there is an increased sympathetic nervous system stimulation with a catecholamine release; this can lead to vasoconstriction and tachycardia, which can increase the cardiac workload. (2) Pain results in decreased gastrointestinal motility. (3) Pain stimulates the release of antidiuretic hormone, which can lead to changes in body fluid balance. (4) Pain increases the level of patient stress, with potential negative effects on healing and the immune system. These can be related to decreased water and food consumption.[1]
- Preventing and managing pain associated with dental procedures is humane.
- The goal of pain management is to reduce the ongoing pain stimuli and thereby reduce the patient response.
- It is more beneficial to the patient to administer pain treatment before onset of pain.[23] This leads to an increased usage of narcotics as a preanesthetic medication, which can reduce the amount of general anesthetic needed. Administration of an injectable analgesic before the patient reaches consciousness (when inhalant anesthetic is discontinued) is the preferred time of injection for control of postoperative pain and allows for a smaller dose to be given.
- When major oral manipulation is anticipated, regional blocks are beneficial in managing pain during anesthesia and immediately postoperatively.
- Regional blocks can eliminate the need for initial postoperative narcotic analgesics, which may interfere with postanesthesia management.
- There are four times for pain management: preoperative, intraoperative, immediate postoperative, and later owner-administered. Preoperative medications that include narcotics can reduce pain before and during dental procedures. More complete pain relief can be obtained with regional or local analgesia that will continue into the postoperative period, depending on duration of drug used.

Postoperative and Owner-Administered Pain Management

Comments

- There has been a hesitation in using postoperative narcotics because of the lack of approved narcotics for use in cats and dogs for pain control; other reasons are short duration or inconsistency of duration of some drugs, expense, and the potential for abuse of class II narcotics.[6, 21]
- Providing dispensed or prescribed pain medication after involved dental proce-

dures allows clients to participate in their pet's recovery and satisfies their need to reduce perceived pain.

Drugs

Aspirin
- Dose: dog—10–25 mg/kg orally two to three times per day.[5]

Comments
- Aspirin is a common nonsteroidal anti-inflammatory drug (NSAID) that reduces pain, inflammation, and fever.
- Aspirin also decreases platelet aggregation.
- A buffered, encapsulated, or enteric-coated form is preferred to minimize gastrointestinal ulceration.
- Providing aspirin with food is preferred; therefore, aspirin is best reserved for postoperative care when the patient is eating.
- Not recommended for patients with liver, renal, or respiratory disease; gastrointestinal ulceration; hypoalbuminemia; bleeding disorders; or for patients taking corticosteroids or other NSAIDs.[24]

Advantages
- Inexpensive.
- Can be given orally with food.
- Decreases fever and inflammation.
- Convenient over-the-counter medication.

Disadvantages
- Good only for mild pain relief.
- With doses in excess of 50 mg/kg twice daily, patient may get gastrointestinal ulceration, followed by hepatic necrosis, renal damage, and bone marrow alteration.[24]
- Not acceptable for patients with renal or kidney disease.

Carprofen (Rimadyl: Pfizer)
- A non-narcotic NSAID.
- Dose for dogs is 2 mg/kg by mouth every 12 hours.
- Supplied in 25, 75, and 100 mg scored caplets, in bottles of 100 or 250 caplets. Dosage should be calculated in half-caplet increments.

Advantages
- Relieves pain and inflammation in dogs.

Disadvantages
- This drug is not for use in cats.
- Hepatopathies have been noted. It is advisable to pre-evaluate liver function before use of this product.
- NSAIDs have been reported in association with renal and gastrointestinal toxicity.

- Patients at greatest risk for complications are those on concomitant diuretic therapy and those with renal, cardiac, or hepatic dysfunction.
- This drug should be used with caution in conjunction with other anti-inflammatory drugs, such as corticosteroids and NSAIDs.

Opioid Medications
- Opioids (narcotic medications) interact with specific receptors to inhibit pain signal transmission from the dorsal root zone of the spinal cord, inhibiting the pain impulse transmission in the neurologic pathways.
- A number of oral and injectable drugs are available for use in cats and dogs.

Butorphanol

Comments
- The use of large-animal Torbugesic (10 mg/ml)* makes administration more cost-effective.[12] (Torbugesic SA (0.5 mg/ml)* for small animals is available for cats and small dogs.)
- Duration of relief varies from 1 to 4 hours.
- Dose: cat/dog—0.2 to 0.4 mg/kg subcutaneously or intramuscularly.[11, 12]

Advantages
- Unscheduled narcotic.
- Also supplied in an oral form.
- Good for mild to moderate pain relief.
- Economical cost of injectable form.
- Little respiratory depression.
- Torbutrol is also supplied as oral tablets in 1 mg and 5 mg sizes.

Disadvantages
- Oral form can become expensive for larger dogs.
- Short duration of pain relief, often only 1 to 2 hours.
- Stings when given parenterally.

Oral Formulation of Torbugesic Injectable with Corn Syrup[25]
Small: 4 to 9 lb

1.5 ml of the large-animal strength (10 mg/ml) Torbugesic may be mixed with 2 oz corn syrup and administered orally at a dose of 1 ml/5 lb. This gives a concentration of 0.25 mg/ml butorphanol.

---

*Fort Dodge Laboratories, 800 Fifth St. NW, Fort Dodge, IA 50501

Medium: 10 to 19 lb

3 ml of the large-animal strength (10 mg/ml) may be mixed with 2 oz (60 ml) of corn syrup and administered at a dose of 1 ml/10 lb. This gives a concentration of 0.5 mg/ml.

Large: 20+ lb

6 ml of the large-animal strength (10 mg/ml) may be mixed with 2 oz (60 ml) of corn syrup and administered at a dose of 1 ml/20 lb. This gives a concentration of 0.5 mg/ml.

Buprenorphine

- Comes in vials; one vial treats a 30 lb dog.
- Dose: cats—0.005 to 0.01 mg/kg; dogs—0.01 to 0.02 mg/kg subcutaneously or intramuscularly.[6, 23]

Advantages

- Good for mild to moderate pain relief.
- Duration is longest of any of the opioids.
- Parenteral administration.
- Reasonable cost.

Disadvantages

- Comes in single-use vial.
- No oral form.
- Class V narcotic.

Codeine

- Dose: dog—0.5–1 mg/kg orally every 6 to 8 hours.[5]
- Can be special-ordered by itself or used in a preparation with acetaminophen or aspirin in dogs.

Advantages

- Most cost-effective oral narcotic for dogs.
- Good for mild to moderate pain relief.

Disadvantages

- Class III narcotic.
- May cause vomiting.

Meperidine HCl

- Dose: cat/dog—2 to 10 mg/kg subcutaneously or intramuscularly.[6, 22]

Advantages

- Parenteral or oral administration.
- Good for moderate pain.
- Moderate cost.

Disadvantages

- Short duration of 1 to 2 hours.
- Class II narcotic.

Morphine

- Dose: cat—0.05–0.1 mg/kg; dog—0.5–1 mg/kg subcutaneously or intramuscularly.[5]
- Available in oral forms.

Advantages

- Least expensive narcotic.
- Strongest analgesic.
- Moderate duration of 4 hours.

Disadvantages

- May cause vomiting.
- May cause excessive sedation.
- Class II narcotic.

Oxymorphone

- Dose: dog—0.1 to 0.2 mg/kg; cat—0.05 to 0.2 mg/kg subcutaneously or intramuscularly.[6, 22]

Advantages

- Effective for severe pain.
- Can be used with tranquilizer for neuroleptanalgesia.

Disadvantages

- More expensive than morphine.
- Class II narcotic.
- Variable duration of 1 to 3 hours.
- No oral form.
- May be difficult to obtain.
- Can cause respiratory depression.

Fentanyl Transdermal Patches (Duragesic*)

- These are small patches that adhere to the skin on a clipped hair area at the shoulder blades or metatarsal area under a bandage.
- Duragesic 25 has 2.5 mg fentanyl good for cats and dogs up to 40 lb.
- Duragesic 50 has 5 mg fentanyl and is good for dogs greater than 40 lb.
- Drug acts by increasing patient's tolerance for pain and decreasing perception of suffering.

Advantages

- Easy to apply.
- Moderate cost.
- Provides continuous pain relief for 72 hours.

Disadvantages

- Need to clip hair to place patch (metatarsal area makes patch less noticeable).
- For best effect, patch needs to be placed 24 hours before pain stimulus.
- Patch could be displaced or ingested.
- Class II narcotic.
- With the options that are available in veterinary medicine for pain, this treatment modality should be included as part of dental case management.

---

*Jansen Pharmaceuticals, 1125 Trenton-Harbourton Rd., PO Box 200, Titusville, NJ 08560[24]

REFERENCES

1. Paddleford RR. Manual of Small Animal Anesthesia. New York: Churchill Livingstone, 1988.
2. Muir W, Hubbell J. Handbook of Veterinary Anesthesia. St. Louis: C.V. Mosby Co., 1989.
3. Hellyer PW. General anesthesia for dogs and cats. Vet Med 1996; April:314–325.
4. Pasco PJ, Ilkiw J. Veterinary Medical Teaching Hospital. University of California, Davis, California Small Animal Anesthesia Protocol Sheet, 1995.
5. Plumb DC. Veterinary Drug Handbook, pocket ed. White Bear Lake, MN: Pharma Vet Publishing, 1991.
6. McCoy D. Practical use of narcotic analgesics in small animals. Trends Magazine 1995; February/March:39–41.
7. Dunlap B. Personal communication in 1994 at Colorado State University Anesthesia Service.
8. Yin S. Anesthesia. In: Small Animal Veterinary Handbook. Davis, CA: Cattledog Publishing Co., 1994:1.0–1.9.
9. Thurman IC, Tranquilli WI, Benson GI. Lumb and Jones Veterinary Anesthesia, 3rd ed. Philadelphia: Lea & Febiger/Williams & Wilkins, 1996:232–34, 773–793.
10. Morgan DWT, Legge K. Clinical evaluation of propofol as an intravenous anaesthetic agent in cats and dogs. Vet Rec 1989; 124:31–33.
11. Weaver BMQ, Raptopoulos D. Induction of anaesthesia in dogs and cats with propofol. Vet Rec 1990; 126:617–620.
12. Ko JCH et al. Propofol: a new intravenous anesthetic. Vet Tech 1995; 16:734–737.
13. Smedile LE, Duke T, Taylor SM. Excitatory movements in a dog following propofol anesthesia. J Am Vet Med Assoc 1996; 32:365–368.
14. Smith JA et al. Adverse effects of administration of propofol with various preanesthetic regimens in dogs. J Am Vet Med Assoc 1993; 202:1111–1115.
15. Hansen BD. Therapeutics in practice: analgesic therapy. Compend Contin Educ 1994; 16:868–875.
16. McCurnin D. Surgical Patient Monitoring: Is It Part of Practice Management? Veterinary Product News 1996; May/June:16.
17. Jones JL. Noninvasive monitoring techniques in anesthetized animals. Vet Med 1996; April:326–336.
18. Paddleford RJ. The Case for Routine Intraoperative Blood Pressure Monitoring. In: Haskins SC, Kilde AM, eds. Vet Clin North Am. Philadelphia: W.B. Saunders Co., 1992; 22:444–445.
19. Anthony J. Proceedings Veterinary Dentistry 1995. Veterinary Dental Forum, Vancouver, British Columbia.
20. Tholen M. Concepts in Veterinary Dentistry. Philadelphia: Lea & Febiger, 1984.
21. Hustead D. Pain, Analgesia: The Relief of Pain and Suffering: A DVM's Responsibility in Controlling Patient Suffering. Fort Dodge Animal Health, February 1993.
22. Raffe M. How to Effectively Manage Pain in Seriously Ill Patients. Vet Forum 1995; March:26–40.
23. Carroll GL. How to manage perioperative pain. Vet Med 1996; April:353–357.
24. Lewis L, Small D. A Review of Pain With Potential Therapy. Vet Forum 1995; December:28–31.
25. Mooney J. Henry Schein handout.

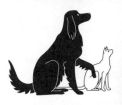

Chapter 12

ERGONOMICS AND GENERAL HEALTH SAFETY IN THE DENTAL WORKPLACE

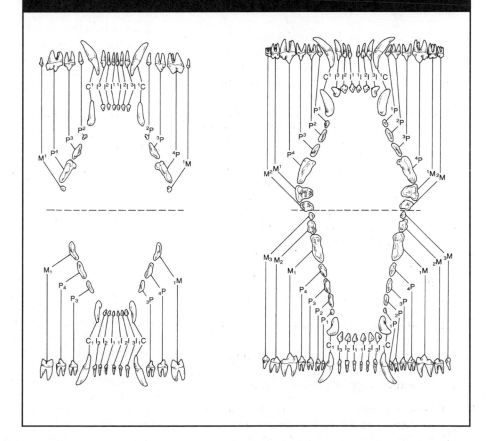

ERGONOMICS IN VETERINARY DENTAL PRACTICE

General Comments

- Veterinary dentistry in small animal clinical practice is a service that is needed on a regular periodic basis by all dogs and cats active in that practice.
- Routine professional prophylactic care exposes the staff to repetitive stress syndrome (RSS).
- Reducing the stress and maintaining a clinic's productive level benefits the practice.
- Occupational hazards can be classified as ergonomic, psychosocial, biologic, chemical, and physical.[1]

Cumulative Trauma Disorder

- The most common occupational hazards for the dental worker are ergonomic and are described as cumulative trauma disorder (CTD). CTD problems arise as a direct result of tasks being repeated on a regular basis to a point of fatigue and muscular exhaustion. The most common disease in this group of musculoskeletal problems is carpal tunnel syndrome (CTS).
- The purposes of this chapter are to make veterinarians and veterinary technicians aware of these hazards and to offer suggestions that can be incorporated into the workplace so as to enhance staff health and services in daily practice.
- The incidence of CTD can be reduced by:

  High-quality equipment.
  Maintenance of instruments on a regular schedule.
  Staff education in proper use of instruments.
  Ergonomic design of the dental operatory, instruments, and equipment.
  Education of staff in proper posture.

- CTDs of the hand, arm, and neck in dental practice share many of the same symptoms, all of which deserve prompt attention.
- The dental worker can reduce the severity and incidence of debilitating problems with proper habits and exercises. Table 12–1 lists common CTDs, areas affected, and symptoms.[1]

PERSONNEL HEALTH AND SAFETY

General Comments

- Neck, arm, and hand pain can be caused by poor posture, incorrect work habits, or a poorly designed workstation.
- A quality veterinary dental prophylactic procedure takes a minimum of 20 minutes for a cat and often in excess of 1 hour for large dogs. The incidence of periodontal disease in a general small animal practice is high enough that, if the dental department is providing appropriate service to adequately care for its patients, that service will keep two veterinary technicians occupied full time providing prophylactic dental care and assisting the clinicians in subsequent dental procedures generated as a result of the dental examination and charting during prophylactic care.
- The veterinary technician should be seated on an adjustable stool or chair and maintain good posture: head centered over the upper body when possible, an inward curve in the lower back, hips level with the knees, and feet resting flat on the floor or on a footrest (figure).
- The technician should take opportunities to change work posture frequently. The wrists should be kept in a fixed neutral position.[2]
- Additional health safeguards, including anesthetic scavenging equipment, should be present and in compliance with Occupational Safety and Health Administration (OSHA) policies. Because of the aerosolization of fomites, the technician should wear protective equipment, such as eye protection, a cap to protect the scalp and hairline, and a mask to protect the respiratory system from nosocomial infection. A clinic jacket or smock, used only for dental prophylaxis, will protect other patients from cross contamination, and gloves will protect the technician's fingernail beds from bacterial assault.
- Radiation protection training should be updated periodically, and monitoring devices should be worn by all personnel in areas where radiographic equipment is used. Equipment should also be inspected periodically and maintained in compliance with state laws.
- Technicians need to be trained in proper use of hand instruments to prevent tendini-

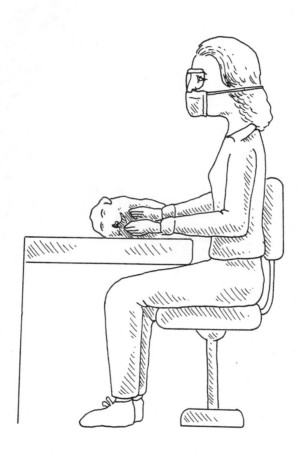

Table 12–1 • COMMON CTDS, AREAS AFFECTED, AND SYMPTOMS

Illness	Area Affected	Symptoms
Carpal tunnel syndrome	Median nerve in wrist and hand	Tingling, pain, or numb thumb, pointing finger, middle finger, and half finger. Symptoms may oc back of the hand and in t and may be more severe du sleep. Temperature sensitivity loss of strength may also resul
Ulnar nerve compression at the elbow (cupital tunnel syndrome)	Ulnar nerve at elbow, forearm, and hands	Tingling, pain, or numbness in th little finger, half the ring finger, and the ulnar side of the hand and forearm. Weakness of the hand.
Ulnar nerve entrapment at the wrist (Guyon's canal syndrome)	Ulnar nerve in the wrist and hand	Decreased hand strength.
Thoracic outlet syndrome	Neurovascular compression affecting shoulder, arm, and hands	Tingling or numbness in the fingers and hands. Atrophy of the hand muscles. Weakness of the hands. Pale or bluish hands. Chronic pain or tired arm sensation.
Reynaud syndrome	Vascular compression in the hands and fingers	Tingling or numbness in the hands and fingers, which can lead to loss of control. Sensitivity to cold. Pale or bluish hands, especially after exposure to cold.
Tenosynovitis	Connective tissue or sheath of any tendon overused or injured	Pain, especially when the hand or arm is used. Inflammation or swelling may occur.
de Quervains disease	Connective tissue at base and side of thumb	Aching and weakness in thumb. Muscle atrophy.
Tendinitis	Connective tissue in the shoulder, elbow, or forearm	Pain or irritation, especially when the hand or arm is used.
Rotator cuff tendinitis	Connective tissue in the shoulder	Pain, often intense, or tenderness in the shoulder.
Lateral epicondylitis (tennis elbow)	Connective tissue at the outside of the elbow	Pain and tenderness at the outside of the elbow, radiating along the back of the forearm.

tis and CTS, which is an occupational hazard for dental hygienists. RSS and injury cases are frequently seen in workers' compensation claims. Following is a list of considerations for the ergonomic dental station.[3]

Posture and Movement

- The patient should be kept as close as possible to the technician.
- As much as possible, the technician should avoid hunching the back and bending or twisting the neck.
- As much as possible, the technician should vary finger movements to avoid muscular exhaustion.

Clinician's/Technician's Chair

- The seat should be able to swivel to avoid making the operator twist the back.
- The chair should have five castors to provide greater stability and mobility.
- Height adjustments should be available; ideally (although sometimes not practical for veterinary conditions) an adjustable backrest should preserve the natural forward curve of the lower back.

Work Surface

- The patient's mouth should be at elbow height so that the operator's hands can be level with the elbow.

- If the operator's feet are not in touch with the floor, a smooth or sloping footrest, rather than a bar rest, should be available.

Equipment Positioning

- Equipment and controls should be positioned to avoid excessive reach forwards or sideways.
- A radius of 20 inches or less from the patient and all controls is ideal.
- Equipment and controls should be positioned directly in front of the operator whenever possible.
- More frequently used instruments and equipment should be closest to the operator.

Leg Room

- Knee-hole or cantilevered tables at the area of the patient's head should provide 16 inches from the bottom of the work surface to the level of the chair to allow for comfortable leg room.
- Foot room should allow 24 inches forward for periodic stretching.

Arm and Wrist Factors

- Hands and elbows should be well below shoulder level to maintain a relaxed shoulder position and to avoid neck and shoulder complaints.
- Type of grasp, pinch force, and instrument weight should be evaluated and addressed to avoid serious accumulative musculoskeletal traumatic disorders of inflammation and entrapment.
- Other instrument features that help reduce RSS are:

  Optimum working angles and curved tips to help prevent bending at the wrist.
  Sharp instruments to lessen operator effort.
  Hollow handles to make instruments weigh less but not so light that they increase grasp pressure and pinch force.
  Size 4 or larger handles to open the grasp and to reduce the pinch force, minimizing nerve inflammation and entrapment.

- Employers and employees can help reduce the incidence of RSS injuries by arranging workstation redesign, more appropriate instrument selection, adjustable fixtures, job rotation, and breaks.

Carpal Tunnel Syndrome

General Comments

- The most common of the nerve compression injuries for dental workers as well as for the general population is CTS.[4]
- The carpal tunnel is on the palmar side of the hand. The structures affected are the median nerve, blood vessels, and the nine extrinsic flexor tendons of the fingers. These structures pass through a tunnel bordered by the eight carpal bones and the transverse carpal ligament, which is attached beneath the ulnar nerve to the carpal bones deep to the muscles at the base of the thumb and muscles to the little finger.[2]
- CTS is a painful condition produced by compression of the nerves, vessels, and tendons passing through that tunnel.

Prevention of Carpal Tunnel Syndrome

- Table 12–2 is a veterinary modification of a checklist that is used specifically for preventing CTS in clinical dental hygiene.[1, 5, 6]

Treatment for Carpal Tunnel Syndrome

- Treatments for CTS are either surgical or nonsurgical. Surgery is the most definitive and common therapy, although more conservative treatments may be prescribed initially that may prove to be the definitive therapy.[2]
- The most common surgical treatment involves a complete release of the transverse carpal ligament. The surgery has a high degree of success and is performed as an outpatient procedure incorporating a local anesthetic.[7, 8]
- Nonsurgical treatments include the use of splints, localized injections of steroids, oral anti-inflammatory drugs, pyridoxine (vitamin B_6) if a deficiency exists, diuretics (if premenstrual association is suspected), ultrasound treatments, and appropriate adjustments to the work environment and lifestyle.[2, 6]

Table 12–2 • CARPAL TUNNEL SYNDROME: DENTAL HYGIENE OCCUPATIONAL RISK FACTORS

Risk Checklist	Preventive Strategies
Repetitiveness • Are you scheduling more than two consecutive root-planing appointments? • Are you scheduling more than two consecutive large-breed patients? • Within an appointment, are you repeating same hand motion or posture for prolonged periods (e.g., scaling for 30–45 minutes, then doing other procedures)? • Do you use ultrasonic or sonic scalers infrequently or not at all?	*Repetitiveness* • Allow sufficient time to treat the needs of the patient. • Regulate the total number and scheduling of patients requiring hand-intensive motions. • Alternate débridement and root planing within the same procedure. • Vary hand-intensive activities by interspersing procedures such as radiographs, selective polishing with débridement, and root planing. • Use very sharp instruments. • Shorten the patient's recall interval. • Maximize use of ultrasonic scalers.
Posture • Operator posture —Are your shoulders elevated? Is one higher than the other? —Are your wrists flexed or extended during scaling? • Operator/patient position —Are your elbows elevated more than 30 degrees? —Is your back bent, and is your head unsupported by your spine?	*Posture* • Relax your shoulders: keep them even and parallel to the floor. • Resist elevating elbows above 30 degrees. • Avoid prolonged ulnar deviation. • Reduce wrist flexion and extension: keep wrist in a neutral position with the hand/arm straight (patient height will help control this). • Use full-arm strokes rather than wrist or finger action.
Force • Are you using a constant, pinching grasp during both exploring and working strokes? • Are your instrument handles smooth?	*Force* • Use minimum pressure in instrument grasp. • Increase pressure with grasp only when deposits are engaged or in the early stages of root planing. • Use instruments of adequate weight. • Select instrument handles that are serrated or textured.
Mechanical Stresses • What is the diameter of your instruments? • Are your instrument handles hexagonal? • Are the cords on your handpieces short or curly? • Are your handpieces unbalanced? • Are your gloves ill-fitting?	*Mechanical Stresses* • Choose larger-diameter, round instrument handles. • Use contra-angled instruments in various treatment areas if they help maintain neutral wrist position. • Avoid heavy and unbalanced handpieces. • Select contra-angled rather than right-angled prophy angles. • Avoid short and curled cords or retractable cords that pull on the wrist. • Wear properly fitted gloves.
Temperature • Is your operatory cold, or is there a cold air vent directed toward you? • Are your instruments cold when you use them? • Do you wash your hands with cold water?	*Temperature* • Avoid cold drafts and air exhaust, especially on cold hands. • Work in warm rooms or wear warm clothing. • Use warm water to wash hands; maintain 77 degree finger temperature. • Exercise hand for muscle warm-up and to relax muscles between patients.

Modified from Gerwatowski LJ, McFall DB, Stach DJ. Carpal tunnel syndrome: Risk factors and prevention strategies for the dental hygienist. J Dent Hygiene 1992; 65:90.

Reducing Operator Fatigue

General Comments

• The dental worker can reduce fatigue and injury by incorporating a number of strategies: alternating tasks, intermittent scheduling of prolonged procedures, careful designing or modifying of the workstation, selecting and maintaining instruments properly, and exercising.

• Table 12–3 is a list of exercises suggested by a physical therapist that will reduce operator fatigue and increase strength.[1]

Table 12–3 • EXERCISE TO REDUCE OPERATOR FATIGUE AND INCREASE STRENGTH

Area of Body	Purpose	Directions
Back	Stretch and strengthen lower back muscles	1. Lie on the floor, pull knees up to chest, and wrap arms around knees. 2. Hold for a count of 3, release arms, resist arching back, and slowly straighten legs. 3. Perform 5 repetitions.
	Stretch out trunk muscles	1. Stand with arms straight down along body. 2. Laterally flex back on one side and then the other. 3. Perform 5 repetitions.
	Increase natural flexibility of lower spine	Extension: 1. Extend back by bending backward with arms held over head for balance. 2. Hold in position for a count of 2 and straighten. 3. Perform 5 repetitions. Flexion: 1. Sit on a chair or stool, lean forward and arch back, with arms hanging toward the floor. 2. Hold in position for a count of 2 and straighten. 3. Perform 5 repetitions.
Upper back and shoulders	Stretch pectoral muscles	1. Stand facing a corner of a room, approximately 2 feet from the corner. 2. Place palms of both hands on side walls in front of shoulders at shoulder height. 3. Lean toward corner, supporting your weight with your hands. 4. Hold for a count of 3, return to original position. 5. Perform 3 repetitions.
	Stretch upper back and pectorals	1. Clasp hands behind head (not neck). 2. Pull elbows back to squeeze shoulder blades together. 3. Hold for a count of 3, then relax. 4. Perform 3 repetitions.
	Encourage stability of upper back and shoulder muscles	1. Lift shoulder blades, squeeze shoulder blades together, lower shoulders, and then relax. 2. Perform 3 repetitions.
	Relax shoulder muscles	1. Roll shoulders backward, or in a clockwise direction, in circles for 5 circles.
Neck	Stretch scalenes	These stretches should be completed on one side and then reversed to stretch the muscles on the other side of the neck. 1. Sit on a chair or stool, with the lower back supported. 2. Grasp the edge of the chair with the right hand. 3. Place head toward the left shoulder, then slightly rotate head to the right. 4. Pull head toward the left shoulder, then slightly rotate head to the right. 5. Hold for a count of 6, and repeat 3 times.

Acknowledgments to the late Larynne Hashimoto, P.T.

Table continued on following page

Table 12–3 • **EXERCISE TO REDUCE OPERATOR FATIGUE AND INCREASE STRENGTH** *Continued*

Area of Body	Purpose	Directions
Neck *(Continued)*	Stretch upper trapezius	1. Sit on a chair or stool, with the lower back supported. 2. Grasp the edge of the chair with the right hand. 3. Facing forward, turn head halfway to the left. 4. With the left hand on the back of head, pull head forward and down in a diagonal direction. 5. Hold for a count of 6, and repeat 3 times.
	Stretch levator scapulae (maintains erect head/neck posture)	1. Sit on a chair or stool, with the lower back supported. 2. Place right hand on left knee. 3. Drop chin to chest. 4. Drop left ear to left shoulder, rotate head slightly to the left. 5. Hold for a count of 6, and repeat 3 times.
Wrist	Encourage gliding of radial, median, and ulnar nerves.	Stretches should be completed with one arm and then repeated with the opposite arm. 1. Extend right arm, elbow straight, palm up, out in front of the body. 2. Flex wrist so the palm of the hand is facing the head. 3. Extend the wrist by dropping fingers toward the floor. 4. Bend and drop the elbow to the side of the body. 5. Perform 3 repetitions. —— 1. Extend the arm, elbow straight, palm up, out to the side of the body. 2. Rotate the arm backward. 3. Stretch the neck by leaning the left ear to the left shoulder. 4. Perform 3 repetitions. —— 1. Flex wrist, bend elbow, and raise hand so that fingers are against the forehead. 2. Extend wrist so that wrist is against the forehead, and slowly straighten elbow until the arm is extended in front of the body. 3. Perform 3 repetitions. —— 1. Raise arm to the side, flex wrist, and raise hand to form a 90 degree angle at the elbow. 2. Rotate arm backward. 3. Stretch the neck by leaning the left ear to the left shoulder. 4. Perform 3 repetitions.

SAFETY IN THE VETERINARY DENTAL OPERATORY

General Comments

- Workers and patients in the dental operatory should be protected from harm. Potential injury may be inflicted from contact with human blood, sharp instruments, or equipment, as well as from contact with chemicals in use or the patient itself.
- Workers in the dental operatory should be provided with protective wear, and patients should be protected from the instruments, chemicals, water spray, and lights used by the workers.

Personal Protective Equipment for the Worker

- Dental personnel should have equipment to protect clothes, skin, eyes, and mouth.[9]
- Although veterinary personnel are exposed primarily to animal and equipment hazards, they are also susceptible to human communicable disease via open sores, wounds, and respiratory disease from colleagues and clients.
- Personnel who are at a reasonable risk of exposure should be trained to assume that all human blood is infectious and periodically instructed in taking the necessary protective measures to be in compliance with OSHA standards.[9]
- Following is a list of personal protective equipment particularly important for the veterinary dental worker:

  Safety glasses with wing shields, or a face shield, to protect the eyes from fomites and possible broken burs or flying bits of teeth.
  Examination or surgical-grade gloves to protect against open sores or fomite infection of the nail bed.
  Clinic jacket or smock to be used only in the dental operatory to reduce chance of fomite transfer to other patients.
  Cap and mask to protect the respiratory passage and the hairline from bacterial aerosol.
  Appropriate radiographic shielding and monitoring devices to comply with radiologic safety standards for the equipment in use.

  Convenient color-coded, puncture-resistant, and leak-proof sharps container for disposal of used endodontic files, burs, scalpel blades, and suture needles.
  An easily accessible handwashing station as well as an eyewash station for decontamination after working with each patient.

Protective Equipment and Protocol for the Patient

- General anesthesia so that competent subgingival care can be administered safely.
- Inhalant anesthesia so that anesthesia levels can be adjusted more quickly.
- Intubation equipment:

  To safeguard against aspiration of dislodged calculus or small pieces of broken equipment (e.g., files, burs).
  To safeguard against drowning during ultrasonic scaling or other procedures using water spray.
  To regulate gas anesthesia quickly and safely.

- Anesthetic monitoring for early detection of metabolic abnormalities.
- A gauze sponge or other device placed in the oral pharynx to protect against swallowing of undesirable objects.
- An ophthalmic preparation to protect the cornea from abrasion or injury from the operating light.
- A cloth covering to protect the face from soiling and the eyes from foreign objects and debris.

BLOODBORNE PATHOGEN STANDARDS

- The Centers for Disease Control and Prevention (CDC)[10, 11] and OSHA[12] work together to provide standards to safeguard dental health-care professionals and veterinary personnel to reduce the risk of disease transmission in the dental environment.
- It is advisable for veterinary dental personnel to review current requirements of occupational health safety as pertains to the country in which they work. A set of such requirements is included in the references at the end of this chapter.[10] The original standards[11, 12] are also suggested as im-

portant material to have in the veterinary dental department files.

CONCLUSION

- The production of the dental department depends on many factors; the health and well-being of its staff are only one factor.
- Careful evaluation of ergonomic factors and implementation of preventive strategies can greatly affect the efficiency of the dental department.
- No one strategy, however, will provide a complete safety net for the department; psychosocial factors, such as stress and burn-out as well as career and job satisfaction, also greatly affect the efficiency of the department as do biologic factors such as microbial aerosols, contaminated wastes, and infectious disease, which must be controlled to prevent employee illness.
- Chemical factors, such as mercury vapor, sterilizing products and disinfectants, latex allergy, and chemicals used in manufacturing latex gloves, must also be considered.
- Physical hazards such as radiation; high frequency noise; and eye injury, strain, and damage must all be included in continuing personnel safety refresher courses in order to make the dental operatory as safe as possible for dental workers.

REFERENCES

1. McFall DB. Taking Care of the Body and Hands That Feed You: Occupational Hazards for the Dental Hygienist. Illinois Dental Hygienists' Association Mid-Winter 1996.
2. McFall DB, Stach DJ, Gerwatowski LJ. Carpal tunnel syndrome: Treatment and rehabilitation therapy for the dental hygienist. J Dent Hygiene 1993; 67:126–132.
3. Pollack R. Dento-ergonomics: The key to energy-saving performance. Cal Dent Assoc J 1996; April:63–68.
4. Stewart JD, Aguayo AJ. Compression and entrapment neuropathies. In: Dyck PJ, et al, eds. Peripheral Neuropathy, vol. 2. Philadelphia: W.B. Saunders Co., 1984.
5. Armstrong TJ, Lifshitz Y. Evaluation and design of jobs for control of cumulative trauma disorders. In: Ergonomic Interventions to Prevent Musculoskeletal Injuries in Industry. Chelsea: Lewis Publishers, Inc., 1987.
6. Gerwatowski LJ, McFall DB, Stach DJ. Carpal tunnel syndrome: Risk factors and preventive strategies for the dental hygienist. J Dent Hygiene 1992; 66:89–94.
7. Phalen GS. The carpal tunnel syndrome. J Bone Joint Surg Am 1966; 48A:211–228.
8. Dawson DM, Hallett M, Millender LH (eds.). Carpal tunnel sydrome. In: Entrapment Neuropathies, 2nd ed. Boston: Little, Brown & Co., 1990:25–92.
9. Mack and Parker, Inc. and the Atlantic Mutual Companies. Safety Bulletin: Bloodborne Pathogens. AVMA Professional Liability Insurance Trust, Chicago, 1995; 3:1.
10. Menage BK. CDC Guidelines versus The OSHA Bloodborne Pathogen Standard. J Pract Hygiene 1994; January/February 3:1.
11. Centers for Disease Control and Prevention. Recommended infection-control practices for dentistry. MMWR CDC Surveill Summ 1993; RR8:42.
12. OSHA Standard for Occupational Exposure to Bloodborne Pathogens. Title CFR 1910.1030. Federal Register 56 (235):64004–64182, December 6, 1991.

MANUFACTURERS AND SOURCES OF DENTAL MATERIALS

3M Dental Products Division
Bldg. 260-28-09
3M Center
St. Paul, MN 55144
(800) 634-2249; (612) 733-1110
FAX: (612) 733-9973
Products: Many dental products

3M Unitek Corp.
2724 S. Peck Rd.
Monrovia, CA 91016
(800) 423-4588; (800) 634-6300
FAX: (818) 574-4826
Products: Orthodontic supplies

Addison Biological Laboratory, Inc.
507 N. Cleveland Ave.
Fayette, MO 65248
(800) 331-2530; (816) 248-2215
FAX: (816) 248-2554
Products: Home dental care products;
MaxiGuard Gel

Allerderm, Inc.
P.O. Box 162059
Ft. Worth, TX 76161
(800) 338-3659
FAX: (817) 831-8327
Products: Professional prophylactic and home
dental care products

Almore International, Inc.
10950 SW 5th, Ste. 270
Beaverton, OR 97005
(800) 547-1511; (503) 543-6633
FAX: (503) 643-9748
Products: Dental products, clip-on loupes,
fracture finders

Amadent/American Medical & Dental
1236 Brace Rd., Bldg. B
Cherry Hill, NJ 08034
(609) 429-8297; (800) 289-6367
FAX: (609) 429-2953
Products: Ultrasonic scaler, apex locator

Analytic Technology Corp.
15233 NE 90th St.
Redmond, WA 98052
(800) 428-2808; (206) 883-2445
FAX: (206) 882-3128
Products: Touch 'n Heat, apex locator, other
dental products

Arista Surgical Supply, Inc.
67 Lexington Ave.
New York, NY 10010
(800) 223-1984; (212) 679-3694
FAX: (212) 696-9046
Products: Dental and surgical instruments

Aseptico, Inc.
19501 144th Ave. NE
Suite B-400
Woodinville, WA 98072
(800) 425-5913; (206) 487-2808
FAX: (206) 487-2808
Products: Dental supplies and equipment

Astra Pharmaceutical Products, Inc.
50 Otis St.
Westborough, MA 01581
(800) 225-6333; (508) 366-1100
FAX: (508) 366-7406
Products: Surgical face masks

**ASVDT (American Society of Veterinary
Dental Technicians)**
316 Shore Rd.
Venice, FL 34285
(800) 613-3647; (941) 488-7802
FAX: (941) 484-1439
Product: Society membership

AVLS
P.O. Box 67127
Lincoln, NE 68506
(800) 444-3634
FAX: (402) 466-3501
Products: Client education aids

Bioplant Inc.
20 N. Main St.
South Norwalk, CT 68541
(800) 432-4487
FAX: (203) 899-0278
Products: Bioplant HTR implant materials

Brasseler USA, Inc.
800 King George Blvd.
Savannah, GA 31419
(800) 841-4222; (912) 925-8525
FAX: (912) 927-8671
Products: Burs, files, diamonds, instruments

Buffalo Dental Manufacturing Co.
99 Lafayette Dr.
Syosset, NY 11791
(800) 828-0203
FAX: (516) 496-7751
Products: Orthodontic bowls, knives, spatulas,
vibrators, bench engines, vacuum formers,
burs, handpieces

Burns Veterinary Supply
Nationwide Office
1900 Diplomat Dr.
Farmers Branch, TX 75234
(800) 922-8767; (972) 620-9941
FAX: (972) 620-1071
Products: Veterinary distributor; dental products and equipment

Butler Co.
5000 Bradeton Ave.
Dublin, OH 43017
(800) 848-5983; (614) 761-9095
FAX: (614) 761-9096
Products: Complete veterinary supply distributor; dental products and equipment

Calcitek, Inc.
2320 Faraday Ave.
Carlsbad, CA 92008
(800) 854-7019; (619) 431-9515
FAX: (619) 431-9753
Products: Dental implants

Cameron-Miller, Inc.
3949 S. Racine Ave.
Chicago, IL 60609
(800) 621-0142; (312) 523-6360
FAX: (312) 523-9495
Products: Electrosurgery equipment

CBI
3625 N. Andrews Ave.
Fort Lauderdale, FL 33309
(954) 561-8597
FAX: (954) 563-1124
Products: Dental equipment

C.D.M.V. Inc.
C.P. 608.2999 Choquette
St. Hyancinthe
Quebec, CANADA J25 7C2
(514) 773-6073
FAX: (514) 773-4370
Products: Complete veterinary supply distributor; dental products and equipment

Centrix, Inc.
770 River Rd.
Shelton, CT 06484
(800) 235-5862; (203) 929-5582
FAX: (203) 929-6804
Products: Centrix syringe, bonding agents

Charles Brungart, Inc.
2625 N. Andrews Ave.
Oakland Park, FL 33309
(800) 654-5705; (954) 561-8597
FAX: (954) 563-1124
Products: Electric motor-driven handpieces, nitrogen air-driven dental equipment, air scalers, ultrasonic scalers

Cislak Manufacturing, Inc.
1866 Johns Dr.
Glenview, IL 60025
(800) 239-2904; (847) 239-2904
FAX: (847) 729-2994
Products: Hand instruments, feline elevator kit, sharpening aids, full-service dental supplier

Colgate Oral Pharmaceuticals
One Colgate Way
Canton, MA 02021
(800) 225-3756; (617) 821-2880
FAX: (617) 828-7330
Products: Viadent mouthwash and gingival flush

Coltene/Whaledent
750 Corporate Dr.
Mahwah, NJ 07430
(800) 221-3046; (201) 512-8000
FAX: (201) 529-2103
Products: Parapulpar pins and endodontic posts, hand instruments

Confi-Dental Products Co.
416 S. Taylor Ave.
Louisville, CO 80027
(800) 383-5158; (303) 665-7535
FAX: (303) 666-4320
Products: Glass ionomers and composite restorative materials

Cosmedent, Inc.
5419 N. Sheridan Rd.
Chicago, IL 60640
(800) 621-6729; (312) 989-6844
FAX: (312) 989-1826
Products: Cements, composites, hybrids, instruments, polishing discs, polishing strips, cups, points, polishing pastes

Cottrell, Ltd.
7399 S. Tucson Way
Englewood, CO 80112
(800) 843-3343; (303) 799-9401
FAX: (303) 799-9408
Products: Dental disinfectants and sterile packs

Crescent Dental Manufacturing Co.
7750 W. 47th St.
Lyons, IL 60534
(800) 323-6952; (708) 447-8050
FAX: (708) 447-8190
Products: Germicidal trays, cleaning brushes

Danville Engineering
1901 San Ramon Valley Rd.
San Ramon, CA 94583
(800) 827-7940; (510) 838-7940
FAX: (510) 838-0944
Products: Etcher and dust box

Den Mat Corp.
2727 Skyway Dr.
Santa Maria, CA 93456
(800) 433-6628; (805) 922-8491
FAX: (805) 922-6933
Products: Restorative products, bonding
agents, composites, glass ionomers

Dentalaire
17165 Newhope St., Suite J
Fountain Valley, CA 92708
(800) 866-6881; (714) 540-9969
FAX: (714) 540-9947
Products: Air compressors, complete dental
supplies; handpiece repair

Dental Enterprises
1976 S. Bannock St.
Denver, CO 80223
(800) 466-1466; (303) 777-6717
FAX: (303) 777-6726
Products: Complete line of new and used
dental equipment; equipment and handpiece
repair

Denticator International, Inc.
11330 Sunrise Park Dr., Ste. A
Rancho Cordova, CA 95742
(800) 227-3321; (916) 638-9303
FAX: (916) 638-0319
Products: Prophy cups and angles

Dentsply Implant
15821 Ventura Blvd, Ste. 420
Encino, CA 91436
(800) 877-9994; (818) 783-1517
FAX: (818) 789-3928
Products: Prosthodontics

Dentsply International
570 W. College Ave.
P.O. Box 872
York, PA 17405
(800) 877-0020; (717) 845-7511
FAX: (717) 849-4376
Products: Scalers, infection control paste

Dentsply/Gendex Division
4379 S. Howell Ave., Ste. 2
Milwaukee, WI 53207
(800) 769-2909; (414) 769-2888
FAX: (414) 769-2868
Products: Dental radiograph machines and
processors

Dentsply/Rinn Division
1212 Abbott Dr.
Elgin, IL 60123
FAX: (800) 544-0787
Products: Radiographic supplies

Dr. Shipp's Dental Laboratory
351 N. Foothill Rd.
Beverly Hills, CA 90210
(310) 550-0107
FAX: (310) 550-1664
Products: Dental models, full-service dental
supplies

Eastman Kodak Co.
HSD/ Dental Products
343 State St.
Rochester, NY 14650
(800) 933-8031; (716) 724-5631
FAX: (716) 724-5797
Products: Intraoral and panoramic
radiographic film and supplies

Easy Tray, Inc.
2209 N. 56th
Seattle, WA 98103
(800) 726-1628; (206) 545-7971
FAX: (206) 545-8011
Products: Custom trays

Ellman International, Inc.
1135 Railroad Ave.
Hewlett, NY 11557
(516) 569-1482
FAX: (516) 569-0054
Products: Radiosurgical instruments, nylon
and metal splint materials

Espe America
1710 Romano Dr.
P.O. Box 111
Norristown, PA 19404
(800) 344-8235; (800) 548-3987;
(610) 277-3800
FAX: (610) 239-2301
Products: Restorative materials

Fort Dodge Laboratories
800 Fifth St. NW
Fort Dodge, IA 50501
(800) 383-6343; (515) 955-4600
FAX: (800) 846-8626
Products: Nolvadent antimicrobial dentifrice,
Torbugesic SA, Torbutrol

Friskies Petcare Co.
800 N. Brand Blvd.
Glendale, CA 91203
(818) 543-7749
FAX: (818) 549-6509
Product: Chew-eez

G. C. America Inc.-Fuji Products
3737 W. 127th St.
Alsip, IL 60803
(800) 323-7063; (708) 597-0900
FAX: (708) 371-5103
Products: Dental cements, restorative materials

Gelkam International
P.O. Box 80004
Dallas, TX 75380
(800) 527-0222; (972) 233-2800
FAX: (972) 239-6859
Products: Gelkam, Xero-lube Scherer

George Taub Products
277 New York Ave.
Jersey City, N.J. 07307
(800) 828-2634; (201) 798-5353
FAX: (201) 659-7186
Products: Dental products

Gingi-Pak
4820 Calle Alto
P.O. Box 240
Camarillo, CA 93011
(800) 437-1514; (805) 484-1051
FAX: (805) 484-5076
Products: Gingival packing cord, instruments

Great Southwest Dental Laboratory
6709 E. 38th Ave.
Denver, CO 80207
(800) 332-0142; (303) 320-0324
Products: Crowns and orthodontic appliances

Harry J. Bosworth
7227 Hamlin Ave.
Skokie, IL 60076
(708) 679-3400
FAX: (708) 679-2080
Product: Super EBA

Heinz Pet Products
One Riverfront Place
Newport, KY 41071
(606) 655-5042
Products: Educational dental booklet, dental
home care products

Henry Schein Inc.
135 Duryea Rd.
Melville, NY 11747
(800) 872-4346; (516) 843-5500
FAX: (516) 843-5696
Products: Complete supply of veterinary and
dental products

Heska Corp.
1825 Sharp Point Dr.
Fort Collins, CO 80525
(800) 464-3752; (970) 493-7272
FAX: (970) 493-7333
Products: Heska Peridontal Disease
Therapeutic

Hills Pet Nutrition, Inc.
P.O. Box 148
Topeka, KS 66601
(800) 354-4557; (913) 354-8523
FAX: (800) 442-9910
Products: Dog and cat food beneficial to
dental hygiene

Hu-Friedy Manufacturing Co., Inc.
3232 N. Rockwell St.
Chicago, IL 60618
(800) 483-7433; (312) 975-6100
FAX: (312) 975-1683
Products: Scalers, probes, dental instruments

IDE-Interstate Dental, Inc.
1500 New Horizons Blvd.
Amityville, NY 11701
(800) 666-8100; (516) 957-8300
FAX: (516) 957-5781
Products: Dental materials, pharmaceuticals

IDEXX Laboratories
One IDEXX Dr.
Westbrook, ME 04092
(800) 551-0998
FAX: (207) 856-0625
Products: Laboratory equipment

iM3, Inc.
12013 NE 99th St., Ste. 1670
Vancouver, WA 98683
(360) 254-2981
FAX: (360) 254-2940
Product: Air-driven dental system

Image Imprints
P.O. Box 1029
North Hampton, MA 01061
(413) 586-4439
FAX: (413) 586-4439
Products: Imprinted toothbrushes

Innovative Technology Sales
149 John Deese Dr.
Ft. Collins, CO 80524
(970) 482-9077
FAX: (970) 484-1618
Product: Portident tabletop dental system

Interplak
P.O. Box 427
Eatontown, NJ 07724
(800) 633-6363; (732) 386-4500
FAX: (732) 389-4998
Product: Rotoplus

Interpore International
181 Technology Dr.
Irvine, CA 92718
(800) 722-4489; (714) 453-3200
FAX: (714) 453-0102
Products: Synthetic bone graft materials

Ivoclar North America, Inc.
175 Pineview Dr.
Amherst, NY 14228
(800) 533-6825; (716) 691-0010
FAX: (716) 691-2285
Products: Restorative materials

J. Morita USA, Inc.
14712 Bentley Cir.
Tustin, CA 92780
(800) 752-9729; (714) 544-2854
FAX: (714) 730-1048
Products: Composite resins, dental adhesives,
restorative materials, x-ray machines, video
imaging system

Jansen Pharmaceuticals
1125 Trenton-Harbourtin Rd.
P.O. Box 200
Titusville, NJ 08560
(800) 526-7736; (609) 730-2000
FAX: (609) 730-2461
Product: Fentanyl patch (Duragesic)

JEM Systems
14550 E. Easter Ave., Ste. 1000
Englewood, CO 80112
(800) 203-5406; (303) 766-0376
FAX: (303) 766-8584
Products: Delivery systems, compressors,
radiograph units, burs, handpieces, hand
instruments

Jeneric/Pentron Inc.
53 N. Plains Industrial Rd.
Wallingford, CT 06492
(800) 243-3969; (203) 265-7397
FAX: (203) 265-7397
Products: Dental materials

**Johnson & Johnson Dental Products
Division**
Johnson and Johnson Plaza
New Brunswick, NJ 08933
(800) 526-3967; (908) 524-0400
FAX: (908) 874-2545
Product: Surgicel

Jorgensen Laboratories, Inc.
1450 N. VanBuren Ave.
Loveland, CO 80538
(970) 669-2500
FAX: (970) 663-5042
Products: Dental instruments

Kerr Corp.
28,200 Wick Rd.
Romulus, MI 48174
(800) 537-7123; (714) 516-7633
Products: Composites, impression materials,
amalgam, laboratory products, endodontic
instruments

Kilgore International, Inc.
P.O. Box 68
Coldwater, MI 49036
(800) 892-9999; (517) 279-9000
FAX: (517) 278-2956
Products: Educational models

Lang Dental Manufacturing Co., Inc.
175 Messner Dr.
P.O. Box 969
Wheeling, IL 60090
(800) 222-5264; (708) 215-6680
FAX: (708) 215-6680
Products: Acrylics

Lares Research, Inc.
295 Lockhead Ave.
Chico, CA 96973
(800) 347-3289
FAX: (916) 345-1870
Products: Handpieces

L. D. Caulk/Dentsply
Lakeview and Clark Avenues
Milford, DE 19963
(800) 532-2855; (302) 422-4511
Products: Composite restoratives, bases, liners, cements, amalgam restoratives, impression materials

Lee Pharmaceuticals
1434 Santa Anita Ave.
P.O. Box 3836
South El Monte, CA 91733
(800) 950-5337; (818) 442-3141
FAX: (818) 443-5161
Products: Restoratives and other dental materials

Lifelearn
MacNabb House
University of Guelph
Ontario NIG 2W1
(800) 375-7994
FAX: (519) 767-1101
Products: Audiovisual dental educational materials

Lippincott-Raven Publishing
227 E. Washington Square
Philadelphia, PA 19106
(215) 238-4200
FAX: (215) 238-4227
Products: Dental texts

Macan Engineering & Manufacturing Co.
1564 N. Damen Ave.
Chicago, IL 60622
(773) 772-2000
FAX: (773) 772-2003
Products: Electrosurgery equipment

Masel Inc.
2701 Partram Rd.
Bristol, PA 19007
(800) 423-8227; (215) 785-1600
FAX: (215) 785-1680
Products: Orthodontic instruments, materials, wire-splinting products

Matrix Medical, Inc.
145 Mid County Dr.
Orchard Park, NY 14127
(800) 847-1000; (716) 662-6550
FAX: (716) 662-7130
Products: Dental compressors, anesthesia, emergency care products

Medidentia
39-23 62nd St.
P.O. Box 409
Woodside, NY 11377
(800) 221-0750; (718) 672-4670
FAX: (718) 672-4670
Products: Endodontic instruments, handpieces

Microcopy
3120 Moon Station Rd.
P.O. Box 2017
Kennesaw, GA 30144
(800) 235-1863; (404) 425-5715
FAX: (404) 423-4996
Products: X-ray developer, portable darkrooms

Midwest Dental Products Corp.
901 W. Oakton St.
Des Plaines, IL 60018
(800) 800-7202; (847) 640-4800
FAX: (847) 640-6165
Products: Electric delivery systems, handpieces, burs

Miltex Instrument Co., Inc.
6 Ohio Dr. - CB 5006
Lake Success, NY 11042
(800) 645-8000; (516) 775-7100
FAX: (516) 775-7185
Products: Hand instruments, burs, extraction forceps

Minxray
3611 Commercial Ave.
Northbrook, IL 60062
(800) 221-2245; (847) 564-0323
FAX: (847) 564-9040
Products: Portable radiographic equipment

Nephron Corp.
P.O. Box 1974
321 E. 25 St.
Tacoma, WA 98401
(800) 426-3603; (206) 383-1002
FAX: (206) 383-2751
Products: Hand instruments and dental products

Nutramax Laboratories, Inc.
5024 Campbell Blvd., Ste. B
Baltimore, MD 21236
(800) 925-5187
FAX: (800) 925-0361; (410) 931-4009
Products: Consil, a synthetic bone graft
material; Cosequin

Nylabone Products
P.O. Box 427
Neptune, NJ 07753
(800) 631-2188; (201) 988-8400
FAX: (908) 988-5466
Products: Home-care chewing aids

Obtura Corp.
1727 Larkin Williams Rd.
Fenton, MO 63026
(800) 344-1321; (314) 343-8733
FAX: (314) 343-5794
Products: Warm gutta-percha equipment

Omni Products
P.O. Box 762
Bountiful, UT 84011
(800) 777-2972; (801) 298-7663
FAX: (801) 298-2984
Products: Diamond burs

Omni Products International
P.O. Box 100
Gravette, AR 72736
(800) 284-4123; (501) 787-5232
FAX: (501) 787-5516
Products: Fluoride gels, rinses, toothbrushes,
implants

Orascoptic Research, Inc.
5225-3 Verona Rd., Building 3
P.O. Box 44451
Madison, WI 53744-4451
(608) 278-0111
FAX: (608) 278-0101
Products: BodyGuard Seating System (loupes,
lights, stools), zeon illuminator

Ormco Corp.
1332 S. Lone Hill Ave.
Glendora, CA 91740
(800) 854-1741; (909) 596-0100
FAX: (714) 516-7633
Products: Orthodontic supplies

Osada, Inc.
8242 W. Third St., Ste. 150
Los Angeles, CA 90048
(800) 426-7232; (213) 651-0711
FAX: (213) 651-4691
Products: Dental supplies and equipment

Oxyfresh USA, Inc.
East 12928 Indiana Ave.
Spokane, WA 99220
(800) 333-7374; (509) 924-4999
FAX: (509) 924-5285
Products: Home-care products

Parkell
155 Schmitt Blvd.
Farmingdale, NY 11735
(800) 243-7446; (516) 249-1134
FAX: (516) 249-1242
Products: Impression materials, bonding
materials, electrosurgical units, ultrasonic
scalers

Pascal Co., Inc.
2929 NE Northrup Way
Bellevue, WA 98004
(800) 426-8051; (206) 827-4694
FAX: (206) 827-6893
Products: Dental products

Patterson Dental Co.
1031 Mendota Heights Rd.
St. Paul, MN 55120
(800) 328-5536; (612) 686-1600
FAX: (612) 686-9331
Products: Dental supplies

Pearson Dental
13847 Delsur St.
San Fernando, CA 91340
(800) 535-4535; (818) 362-2600
Products: Vibrators, amalgamators, dental
materials, equipment, supplies

Periogiene
2625 Midpoint Dr., Ste. A
Ft. Collins, CO 80525
(800) 368-5776; (970) 493-8616
FAX: (970) 498-0543
Product: Odontoson scaler

Pets Veterinary Dental Laboratory
803 W. College Ave.
P.O. Box 867
Waukesha, WI 53187
(800) 558-7734; (414) 542-5100
FAX: (414) 542-1717
Products: Full-service dental laboratory

Pfizer Animal Health
812 Springdale Dr.
Exton, PA 19341
(800) 733-5500; (610) 363-3100
FAX: (800) 228-5176
Product: Clavamox (antibiotic)

Pharmacia & Upjohn
7000 Portage Rd.
Kalamazoo, MI 49001
(800) 253-8600 x32404 [technical services];
(616) 833-2404
FAX: (616) 833-3305
Products: Antirobe (antibiotic), client home-care education and office visual aids

Precision Ceramics Dental Laboratory
9591 Central Ave.
Montclair, CA 91763
(800) 223-6322
Products: Full-service dental laboratory

Premier Dental Products
3600 Horizon Dr.
King of Prussia, PA 19406
(800) 344-8235; (610) 239-6000
FAX: (610) 239-6171
Products: Restoratives, cements, dental supplies

Pro-Dentec
633 Lawrence St.
Batesville, AR 72503
(800) 228-5595; (501) 698-2300
FAX: (501) 793-5554
Products: World Health Organization Sensor Probe

Pro Vet/American Vet
2010 Ackerman Rd.
San Antonio, TX 78219
(210) 661-9500
FAX: (800) 441-4412
Products: Pharmaceuticals/equipment

Pulpdent Corp.
80 Oakland St.
P.O. Box 780
Watertown, MA 02272
(800) 343-4342; (617) 926-6666
FAX: (617) 926-6262
Products: Dental products

Quintessence Publishing Co., Inc.
551 N. Kimberly Dr.
Carol Stream, IL 60188
(800) 621-0387; (708) 682-3223
FAX: (708) 682-3288
Product: Human dental publication

Ribbond Inc.
1326 5th Ave., Ste. 640
Seattle, WA 98101
(800) 624-4554; (206) 340-8870
FAX: (206) 382-9354
Products: Splinting materials

Richmond Dental Co.
P.O. Box 34276
Charlotte, NC 28234
(800) 277-0377; (704) 376-0380
FAX: (704) 342-1892
Products: Cotton pellets and products

Rocky Mountain Orthodontics
P.O. Box 17085
Denver, CO 80217
(800) 525-6375; (303) 592-8200
FAX: (303) 592-8209
Products: Orthodontic supplies

Roth International Ltd.
669 W. Ohio St.
Chicago, IL 60610
(800) 445-0572; (312) 733-1478
FAX: (312) 733-7398
Products: Endodontic sealers

Rx Honing Machine Corp.
1301 E. Fifth St.
Mishawaka, IN 46544
(800) 346-6464; (219) 259-1606
FAX: (219) 9163
Products: Sharpening equipment

SS White/Burs, Inc.
1145 Towbin Ave.
Lakewood, NJ 08701
(800) 535-2877; (732) 905-1100
FAX: (732) 905-0987
Products: Burs

San Francisco Dental Supply
2201 S. Oneida
Greenbay, WI 54304
(800) 948-4048
Products: Distributor of dental products

Sensor Devices Incorporated
407 Pilot Court, Ste. 400A
Waukesha, WI 53187
(414) 524-1000
FAX: (414) 524-1009
Products: Diagnostic monitors

Shofu Dental Corp.
4025 Bohanon Dr.
Menlo Park, CA 94025
(800) 827-4638; (415) 324-0085
FAX: (415) 323-3180
Products: Glass ionomers

Shor-Line, Schoer Manufacturing Co.
2221 Campbell St.
Kansas City, MO 64108
(800) 444-1579; (816) 471-0488
FAX: (816) 471-5339
Products: Scalers, compressors, tables

Siemens/Pelton & Crane
11727 Fruehauf Dr.
Charlotte, NC 28273
(800) 659-6560; (704) 523-3212
FAX: (704) 588-5770
Products: Sterilizers

Silverman's Dental
22 Industrial Park Dr.
Port Washington, NY 11050
(800) 448-3384; (516) 484-7660
FAX: (516) 484-7645
Products: Distributes general dental supplies
and equipment through Henry Schein Inc.

Sontec Instruments
6341 S. Troy Cir.
Englewood, CO 80111
(800) 821-7496; (303) 790-9411
FAX: (303) 792-2606
Products: Hand instruments

Spartan USA, Inc.
1727 Larkin Williams Rd.
Fenton, MO 63026
(800) 325-9027; (314) 343-8300
FAX: (314) 343-5794
Products: Piezo scalers

St. Jon Laboratories
1656 W. 240th St.
Harbor City, CA 90710
(800) 969-7387; (310) 326-2720
FAX: (310) 326-8026
Products: Toothpastes, fluoride foam,
toothbrushes

Star Dental Products
1816 Colonial Village Lane
Lancaster, PA 17601
(800) 422-7827; (717) 291-1161
FAX: (717) 291-3249
Products: Titan-S scaler, handpieces, ultrasonic
equipment

Suburban Surgical Co., Inc.
275 Twelfth St.
Wheeling, IL 60090
(800) 323-7366; (708) 537-9320
Products: Compressors, handpieces, tables

Sullivan Dental Products, Inc.
10920 W. Lincoln Ave.
West Allis, WI 53227
(800) 558-5200; (414) 321-8881
FAX: (414) 321-8865
Products: Scalers, anesthetic infection control

Sultan Chemists, Inc.
85 W. Forest Ave.
Englewood, NJ 07631
(800) 637-8582; (201) 871-1232
FAX: (201) 871-0321
Products: Pharmaceuticals and endodontic
sealants

Summit Hill Laboratories
P.O. Box 535
Navesink, NJ 07752
(800) 922-0722; (201) 291-3600
Products: Scalers, electrosurgery units,
anesthetic machines

Surgitel/General Scientific Corp.
77 Enterprise Dr.
Ann Arbor, MI 48103
(313) 996-9200
FAX: (313) 662-0520
Products: Magnification loupes and light
systems

Tanaka Dental
5135 Golf Rd.
Skokie, IL 60077
(800) 325-5266; (708) 679-1610
FAX: (708) 674-5761
Products: Dental laboratory products, shading
kits

Teledyne-Getz
1550 Greenleaf Ave.
Elk Grove Village, IL 60007
(800) 323-6650; (312) 593-3334
Products: Alginate, cements, trays, light-cure
materials, surgical dressing, prophy cups

Temerex
112 Albany Ave.
P.O. Box 182
Freeport, NY 11520
(800) 645-1226; (516) 868-6221
FAX: (516) 868-5700
Products: Cements, bleaching etchants

Thermafil
5001 E. 68th St.
Tulsa, OK 74136
(800) 662-1202; (918) 493-6598
FAX: (800) 597-2779
Products: Warm gutta-percha products

THM Biomedical, Inc.
325 S. Lake Ave.
Duluth, MN 55804
(800) 327-6895; (218) 720-3628
FAX: (218) 720-3715
Product: Polylactic acid granules

Tulsa Dental Products
5001 E. 68th St., Ste. 500
Tulsa, OK 74136
(800) 662-1202; (918) 493-6598
FAX: (918) 493-6599
Products: Endodontic materials and supplies;
Thermafil, Profile 29 files

Ultradent Products, Inc.
505 W. 10200 South
South Jordan, UT 84095
(800) 555-5512; (801) 572-4200
FAX: (801) 572-0600
Products: Tissue management products,
impression trays, precomposite materials,
sealant materials, gingival packing cord,
hemostatic solution

Ultrasonic Services, Inc.
7126 Mullins Dr.
Houston, TX 77081
(800) 874-5332
Product: Ultrasonic repair

Union Broach Dental Products
Division of Moyco Industries
589 Davies Dr.
York, PA 17402
(800) 221-1344; (717) 840-9335
FAX: (717) 840-9347
Products: Dental files, mirrors

Unitek Corp.
2714 S. Peck Rd.
Monrovia, CA 91016
(800) 423-4588; (818) 445-7960
FAX: (818) 547-4500
Products: Othodontic supplies and equipment

Universal (USA) Ltd.
3095 Kerner Blvd.
San Rafael, CA 94901
(800) 835-3003; (415) 459-0367
FAX: (415) 459-0553
Products: General dental supplies

Veratex/Medarco Corp.
P.O. Box 4031
Troy, MI 48007
(800) 872-4346
Products: Complete dental supplies distributed
through Henry Schein, Inc.

Veterinary Dental Laboratory of America
7733 Main St.
Fairview, PA 16415
(814) 474-5806
Products: Fabricated orthodontic appliances
and restoratives

Veterinary Medicine Publishing Co.
9073 Lenexa Dr.
Lenexa, KS 66215
(800) 255-6864; (913) 492-4300
FAX: (913) 492-4157
Products: Veterinary dental books and journals

Veterinary Stainless, Inc.
2213 Fairlawn Dr.
Carthage, MO 64836
(800) 299-9525, (417) 358-4466
FAX: (417) 358-4716
Product: Dentistry wet tables

Vetko
4931 North Park Dr.
Colorado Springs, CO
(719) 598-8782
Products: Ultrasonic scalers, circulating hot-
water pads

Vetoquinol U.S.A., Inc., Immunovet
5910-G Breckenridge Parkway
Tampa, FL 33610
(813) 621-9447
FAX: (813) 621-0751
Products: Stomadhex, Bioadhesive Patch

Vident
3150 E. Birch St.
Brea, CA 92621
(800) 828-3839; (714) 961-6200
FAX: (714) 961-6299
Products: Inceram indirect restoratives

Vivadent
5130 Commerce Dr.
Baldwin Park, CA 91706
(800) 828 3839; (714) 960-7531
FAX: (714) 961-6299
Products: Restoratives, ceramics, abrasives,
cosmetic products

W.B. Saunders Co.
Independence Square West
Philadelphia, PA 19106
(215) 238-7832
FAX: (215) 238-8483
Products: Medical publications

W. L. Gore & Assoc., Inc.
1500 N. Fourth St.
P.O. Box 2500
Flagstaff, AZ 86003
(800) 282-2182; (520) 526-3030
FAX: (520) 526-1822
Products: Guided tissue regeneration products,
orthopedic devices

Welch Allyn Dental Systems
4619 Jordan Rd.
P.O. Box 187
Skaneateles Falls, NY 13153
(800) 867-3832; (315) 685-9514
FAX: (315) 685-7905
Products: Cameras, lights

Whaledent International
236 5th Ave.
New York, NY 10001
(800) 221-3046; (212) 696-8000
FAX: (212) 532-1644
Products: Dental supplies, endodontic
instruments, electrosurgical equipment

Whip Mix Corp.
361 Farmington Ave.
Louisville, KY 40217
(800) 626-5651; (502) 637-1451
FAX: (502) 654-4512
Product: Quick-setting dental stone

Young Dental
13705 Shoreline Court East
Earth City, MO 63045
(800) 325-1881; (314) 344-0010
FAX: (314) 344-0021
Products: Prophy paste, fluoride, instruments

INDEX

Note: Pages in *italic* indicate illustrations; those followed by t refer to tables.

ISBN 0-7216-5839-3

9 780721 658391

90038